TOVAR'S CLASSIC BEAUTY

TOVAR'S CLASSIC BEAUTY

*By Tovar
with Lydia P. Encinas*

Contemporary Books, Inc.
CHICAGO ■ NEW YORK

Library of Congress Cataloging-in-Publication Data

Tovar, Michael.
  Tovar's classic beauty.

  1. Beauty, Personal.   2. Hairdressing.
3. Cosmetics.   I. Encinas, Lydia Proenza.   II. Title.
III. Title: Classic beauty.
RA778.T65   1986   646.7'042   86-16772
ISBN 0-8092-4867-0

Photographs by Charles William Bush

Copyright © 1986 by Michael Tovar
All rights reserved
Published by Contemporary Books, Inc.
180 North Michigan Avenue, Chicago, Illinois 60601
Manufactured in the United States of America
Library of Congress Catalog Card Number: 86-16772
International Standard Book Number: 0-8092-4867-0

Published simultaneously in Canada by Beaverbooks, Ltd.
195 Allstate Parkway, Valleywood Business Park
Markham, Ontario L3R 4T8 Canada

CONTENTS

ACKNOWLEDGMENTS *vii*

INTRODUCTION—WHAT IS A CLASSIC BEAUTY? *1*

1 HOW YOU CAN BECOME A CLASSIC BEAUTY *5*

2 STYLES FOR YOUR LIFESTYLE *19*

3 MAKING THE BEST OF YOUR HAIR *33*

4 THE CUT *57*

5 COLORS AND PERMS *67*

6 STYLING—THE LOOK THAT'S RIGHT FOR YOU *83*

7 MAKEUP—DOS AND DON'TS *123*

8 CLASSIC BEAUTIES AND THEIR STYLES *143*

9 THE TOTAL LOOK *227*

INDEX *237*

ACKNOWLEDGMENTS

The authors wish to offer a very special mention and thanks to two people who became as important in the creation of this book as we were. Mickey Song performed makeup magic on most of the celebrities and models photographed for this book and shared his vast knowledge and experience with us. Charles Bush did all the photography and put in time and effort above and beyond the call of duty. Thank you both.

Tovar wishes to thank the following people for all their help and support: Michael Pollack, Jane and Jerry Weintraub, Larry Parker, Lani Higa, Paul Premo, Bill Sykes, Rosetta Akyempon, Monte Anderson, Fran Beiser, Leslie Bohr, Brian Burner, Cecilia Calderon, Rando Celli, Larry Cilento, Jeanette Cohen, Ron Crawford, Antonio DuBois, Charles Ferderber, John Gale, Adelina Gutierrez, Dalee Henderson, Bonnie Hoffman, Danielle Hollender, Karine Lasquade, Alegra Levi, Michael Macahalig, Renee Manacher, Soraya Saketchow, Laurence Roberts, Michel Schwert, Mark Sekera, Charles R. Taylor, Rima Uranga, Jillian Van Sice, Steve West, Deborah Lee Wilson, Tammy Worsham, and Zito.

Lydia Encinas wishes to thank Charles Bush's staff, Deidre Lamb, studio manager; and Chuck Belongie, assistant, for their wonderful help and assistance.

Makeup for Ellen Bry, Catherine Hickland, Debi Richter, Abby Dalton, Melody Anderson, and Jayne Kennedy Overton by Ron Mathews/Cloutier Agency. Makeup for Heather Locklear and Joan

Green by Angelica Schubert/Cloutier Agency. Makeup for Emmylou Harris by Antonio Dubois of the Tovar Salon. Priscilla Barnes's haircolor by Francois Noel of the Tovar Salon.

Information for the haircolor and perm chapter by Francois Noel, Karine Lasquade, and John Gale. Information for chemical straightening by Dalee Henderson.

TOVAR'S CLASSIC BEAUTY

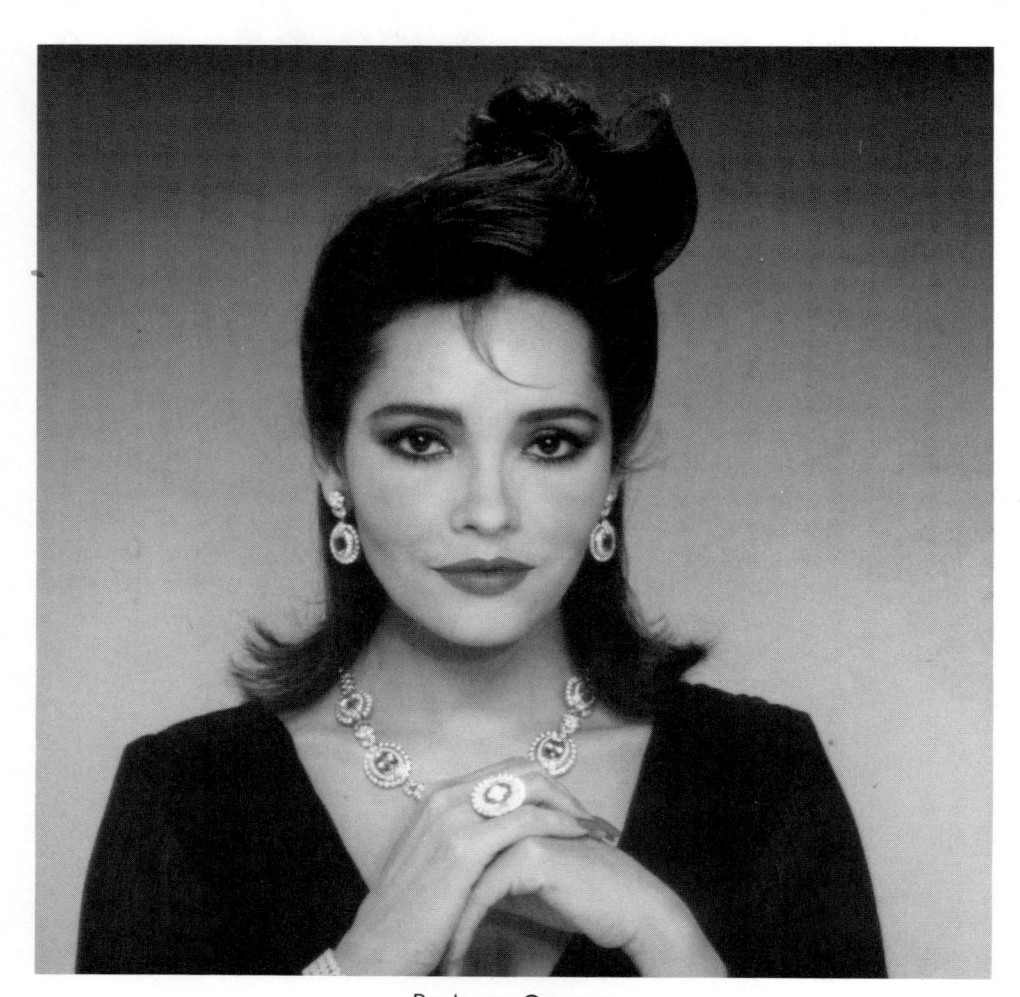

Barbara Carrera

INTRODUCTION— WHAT IS A CLASSIC BEAUTY?

A classic beauty is a woman who is an excellent model for her own kind of look—a look that is not necessarily understated or simple but is timeless, individual, and truly unique.

The stars I have chosen to represent classic beauty in my book did not start life out as classic beauties. Many of them had the basic qualities, but I believe that *every* woman is born with those qualities. With the proper guidance, every woman can achieve her full beauty potential.

At one time the term *classic beauty* was used to describe a certain type of woman. Garbo, Harlow, Monroe, Hepburn, Kelly, and Taylor—at one time or another all these famous beauties have been called classic beauties, yet they are all very different types.

In today's eclectic times, traditional styles have changed. Many different types of women can be called classic beauties. At one point during the photography of this book, a group of friends looked at the photos with me. After seeing how different all the women looked, they asked whether I still wanted to call this book *Tovar's Classic Beauty*.

I gave it some thought, but after studying the photographs many times, I realized that they confirmed and reaffirmed my belief about what makes a woman a classic beauty. Yes! All my models are classic beauties, and they reflect the freedom of choice the woman of the eighties has. Just like people, classic beauty comes in many different styles.

TOVAR'S CLASSIC BEAUTY

Barbara Carrera is a classic beauty with her cool, dark, million-dollar look. But so is Heather Locklear with her fresh-faced, all-American flawless beauty. And what about black being beautiful? Look at Jayne Kennedy Overton, a ravishing beauty; Tina Turner, an outrageous beauty; and Roxie Roker, a very stylish beauty. How about the unique and flamboyant style of Dolly Parton? Or Merete Van Kamp's stunning looks? Or Erin Gray's classic style? Pat Klous's sensational off-screen sexpot look? Abby Dalton's sassy look? Claire Yarlett's flawless beauty? I could go on and on. But you will see them soon in the following pages.

Why should classic beauty be represented by a small group of women with certain physical characteristics? Every woman has the potential and the right to develop her look into a classic.

Introduction—What Is a Classic Beauty?

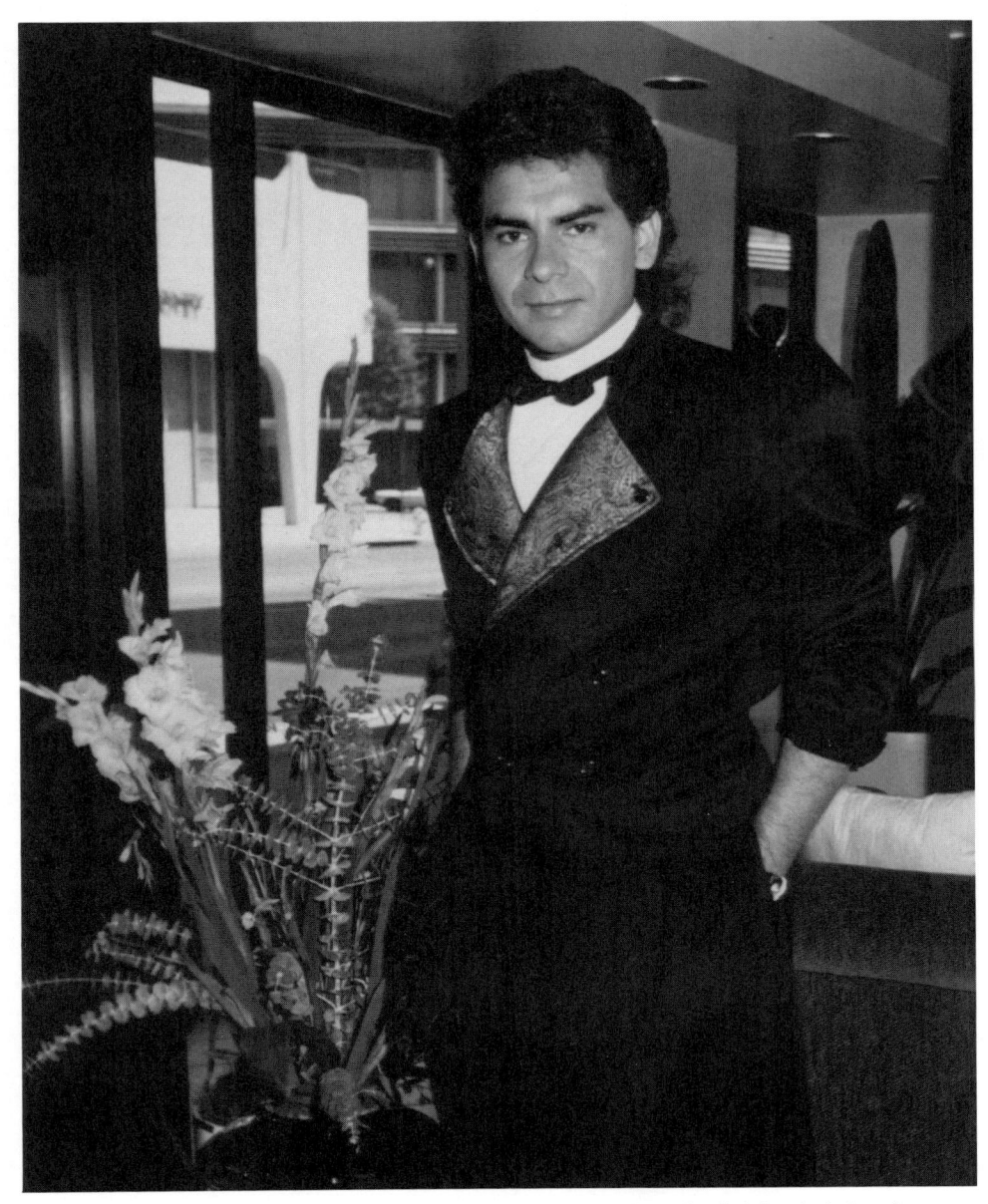

In my Beverly Hills salon I take great care in creating individual styles for each and every one of my clients.

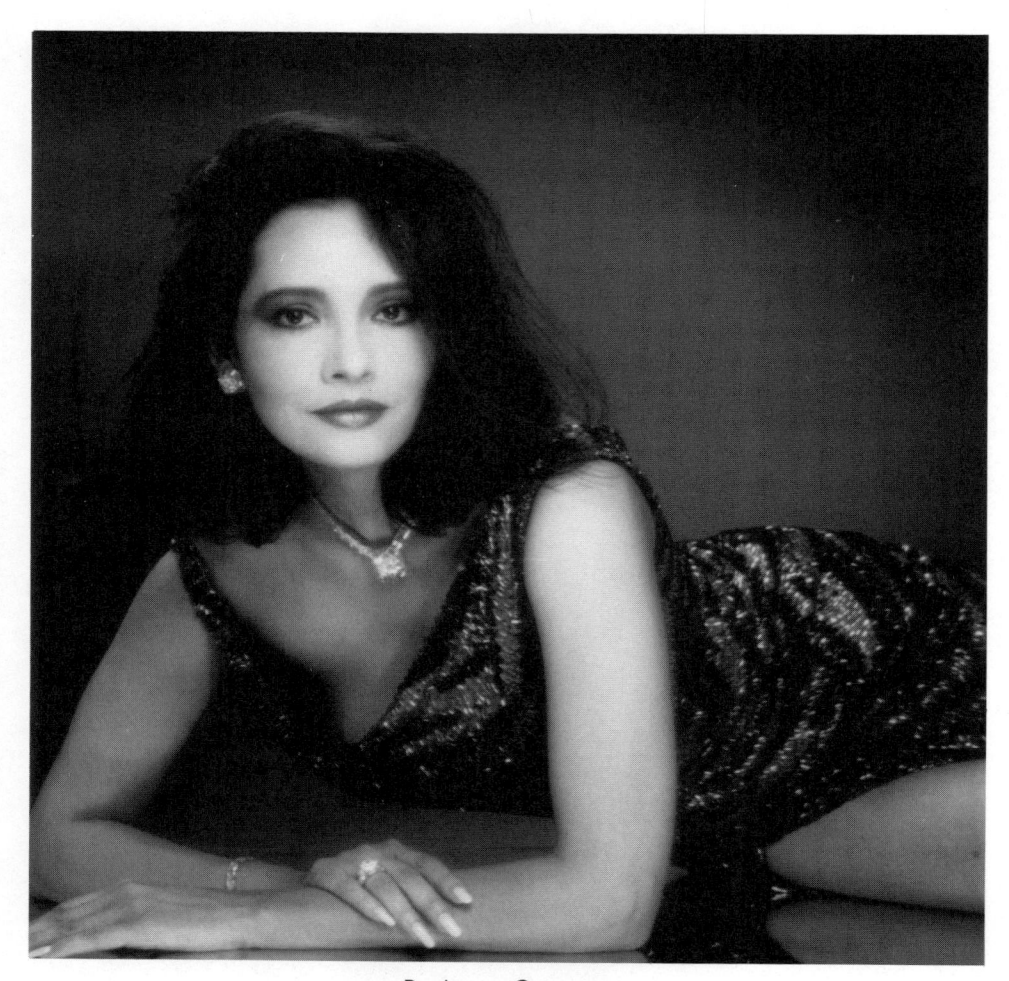

Barbara Carrera

1
HOW YOU CAN BECOME A CLASSIC BEAUTY

During a recent interview, I was asked which was the famous Tovar look—which was the hairstyle I was known for? Do I tell all my clients to wear their hair long, or do I think short hair is what every woman should wear this season?

Of course, the question did not take me by surprise. At one time or another most famous hairdressers use a specific look as their "claim to fame," such as Farrah's famous waves, Dorothy Hamill's wedge, and Toni Tenille's bob, as well as a number of other looks.

The fact is that I don't want to be known for having designed just one look or for specializing in any one type of haircut or style.

I don't create clones—and to me, the beauty of the work I do is my ability to give each client a truly individual look. Any woman who puts her looks in my hands deserves the very best—whether she is a star, a businesswoman, a society matron, or a housewife. Whoever she is, she is entitled to a look that is all hers.

The "cookie cutter" approach is not the style we use at my Beverly Hills salon. Individual and personalized styling is my trademark, as you will see with the stars and models that were photographed to illustrate this book.

Hair is the most significant part of a woman's looks, and a star's looks are her trademark and image. That is why stars will do anything to have the hairstyle that makes the most of their looks. My star clients will go to any length to have their hair look right. Some of them, like Dolly Parton and Tina Turner, pay thousands of dollars for their famous wigs. Others fly me all over the world just to do their hair.

Once a client and a hairstylist establish that one-to-one relationship, it is very difficult to replace. That is why women follow their favorite hairdresser from salon to salon and why wealthy clients are known to fly their favorite crimpers halfway around the world for the right hairstyle. That's why I have clients who come to Beverly Hills from all over the country to have me cut their hair regularly.

Why can't just any other hairdresser do it? Once a client likes your work and feels that you capture that special thing that makes her look great, she doesn't want to let you go. Especially women in the public eye, whose hairstyle is part of their image. Their looks are so important to them that, once they find the right hairstylist, they won't let anyone else touch their hair.

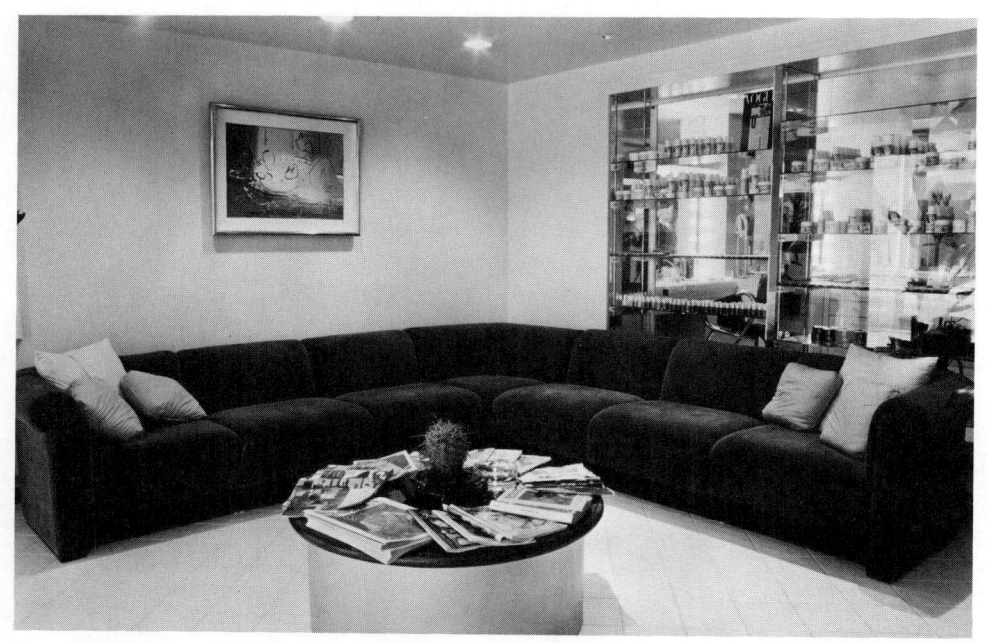

The waiting area of my salon with its sleek, plush, and comfortable sitting area and some of Peter Max's artwork on the walls.

Every woman has the potential to look her best if she knows how to make the best of her looks. Although most of the women photographed for this book were born with certain outstanding natural attributes (and almost everyone is), I and other beauty

How You Can Become a Classic Beauty

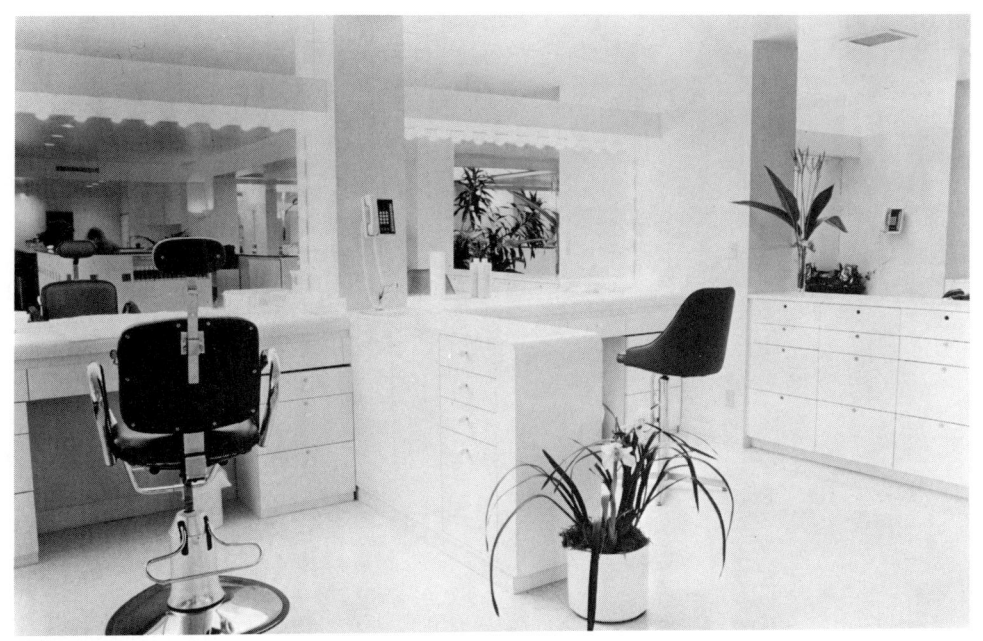

The brightly lit makeup area, pristine white with some green plants and flowers to add a colorful touch. The clean white look and brightly lit mirrors help the makeup artist concentrate on the subject.

professionals have worked with them to create their looks. You too have that potential. You can develop your own individual look by following the advice I give to my star clients and outline in this book.

My hairstyling philosophy is based on one single principle: *don't create clones*. I don't like to see women walking out of my salon all looking the same. To me, diversity is what hairstyling is all about. Also if your haircut can be worn only one way, most likely you will become bored with it. The more versatile your haircut is, the more fun you will have with your hairstyle. The photos of the stars in this book are a perfect example of that styling versatility.

Barbara Carrera (my cover girl) is to me the classiest, most chic woman in the world. She has incredible bone structure and a flawless face. Everything about her is as near perfection as a human being can be—her skin is like porcelain; her hair shines; her eyes sparkle. She likes elegant, stylish clothes and jewels; she has always been that way. Elegance has been her trademark. And one of the things that I am very proud of her for is that she is trying to bring glamour and elegance back to Hollywood.

For a while Hollywood was acting punky and funky. It was full of Madonnas and Cindy Laupers and their look-alikes—the wild hair with the multicolor streaks, the makeup and the clothes to go with it.

TOVAR'S CLASSIC BEAUTY

While that was fun for a while, it is not a look that suits everyone. Someone like Barbara Carrera will always look impeccable and elegant. That is why I selected her to represent the classic beauty look on the cover of this book.

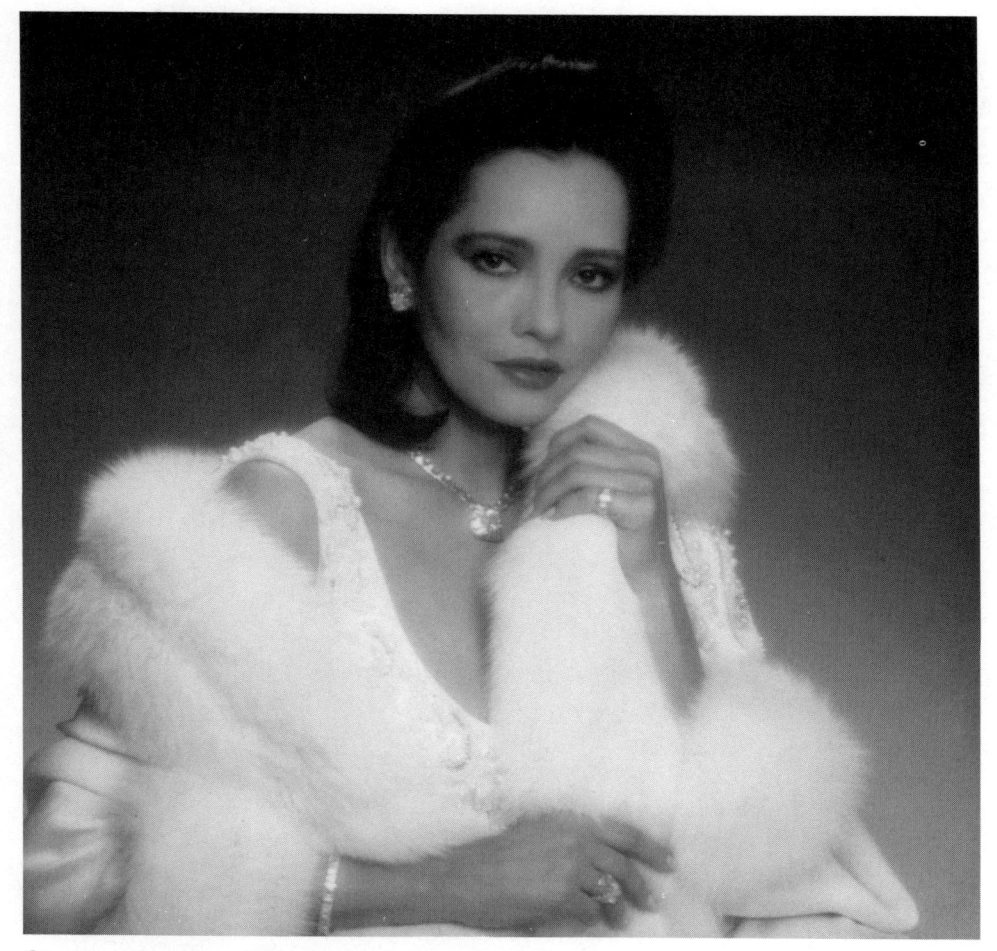

Classic elegance is Barbara Carrera's trademark.

Heather Locklear is another classic beauty, yet her looks are as different from Barbara's as the different colors of their hair. Classic beauty is not one look, one hairstyle, one face. Classic beauty is a feeling. Heather, Barbara, and the other women in this book are all different, all unique, all known for their beauty, yet they are all classics, ranging from the elegance of Barbara Carrera to the wild look of Tina Turner.

How You Can Become a Classic Beauty

My clients have a wide range of looks. Tina Turner's wicked mane for the video "We Don't Need Another Hero" from the film *Mad Max Beyond Thunderdome* is actually a $3,000 silver-blond wig. It prompted Erma Bombeck to come to me for a makeover that was filmed for "Good Morning America."

Another makeover prompted by Tina Turner's look was that of the fabulous Madame (the puppet), whom I love and adore and who sometimes makes you think she is human. Although Madame is a puppet, she has become one of my closest friends. I treat her like a person, and she comes to my salon to have her hair done once a week when she is in town. Madame used to have gray yarn hair, naturally woolly and boring. I have turned her on to synthetic wigs. She wears every color, from silver blond to brunette to redhead, and she carries them off great.

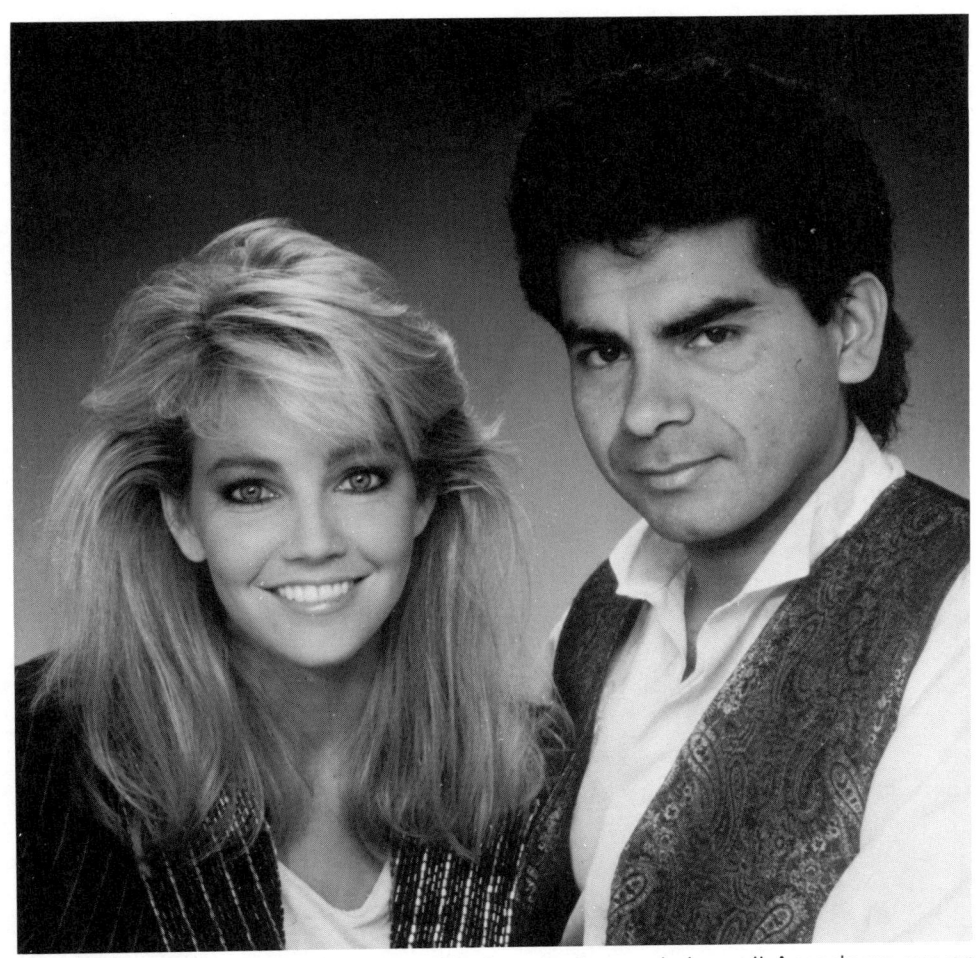

Heather Locklear's naturally styled hair complements her all-American cover girl look.

TOVAR'S CLASSIC BEAUTY

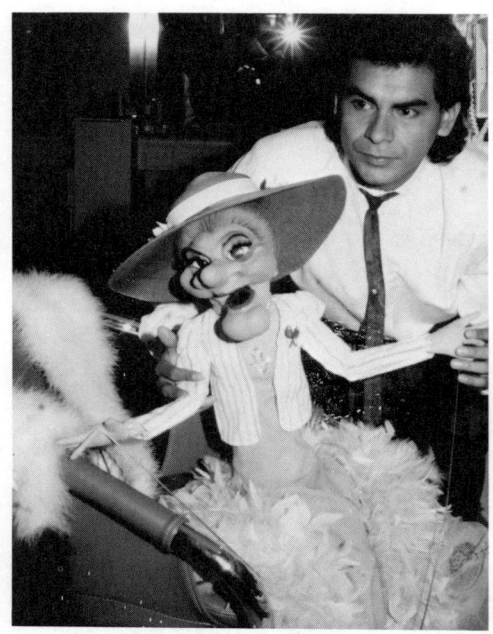

Madame, the famous puppet, became one of my clients when she saw the look I had given Tina Turner for *Mad Max Beyond Thunderdome*. She came to me to have something done about her naturally wooly gray yarn hair.

Madame insisted I introduce her to famous male model Attila (who was having his hair cut at the salon) after her makeover. Here, she selected a platinum white wig with silvery strands to meet the famous hunk.

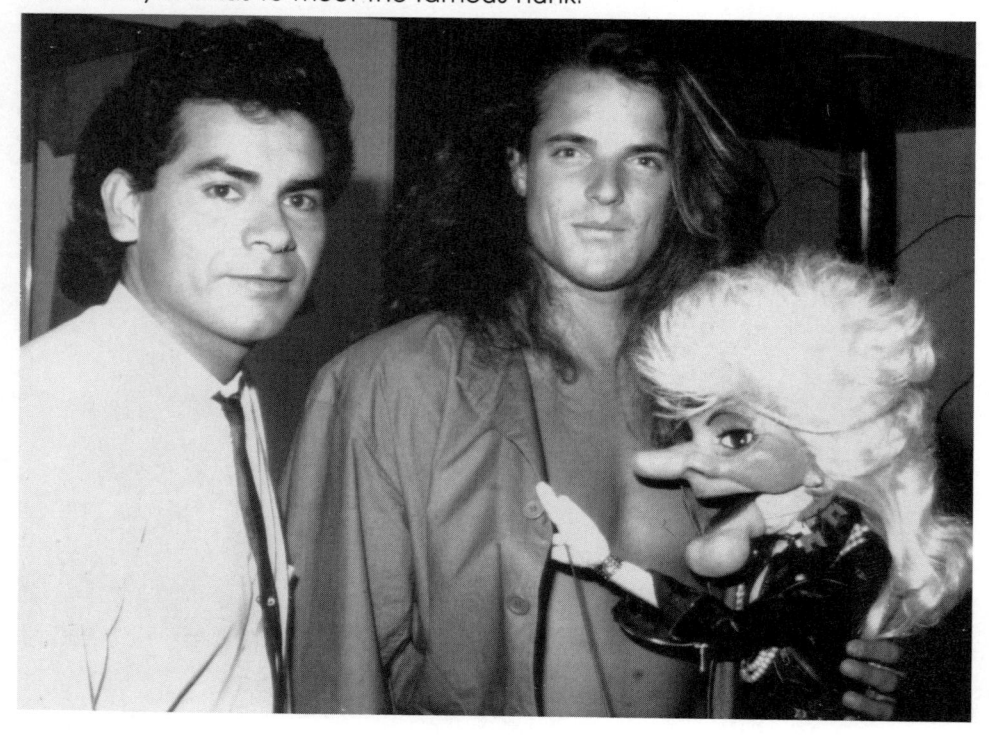

How You Can Become a Classic Beauty

Talking about my famous makeovers, Emmylou Harris has been one of my greatest. Do you remember what she used to look like? All that long, long hair, sprinkled with gray. She called me one day and said, "I am so bored with my look." And I said, "You're bored? Look at your hair—you need a drastic change. Trust me, just trust me." So Emmylou flew in from Nashville, and I gave her a totally new look. I cut and layered her hair, colored it and gave it highlights, and added a perm for body. And Emmylou has never looked better. No more long hair; now it is soft and fluffy, and she just looks great!

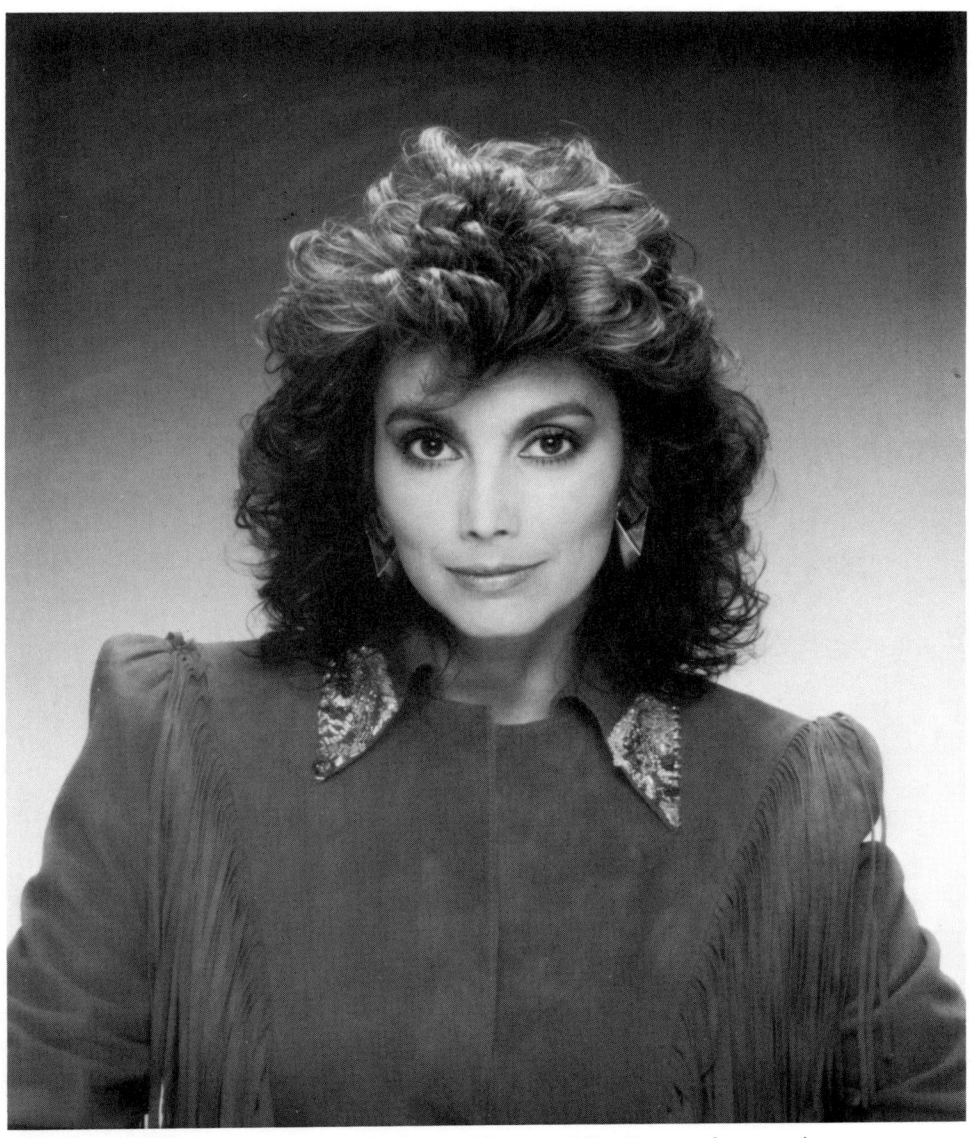

I cut Emmylou's waist-length hair and layered it all over for maximum movement and volume.

TOVAR'S CLASSIC BEAUTY

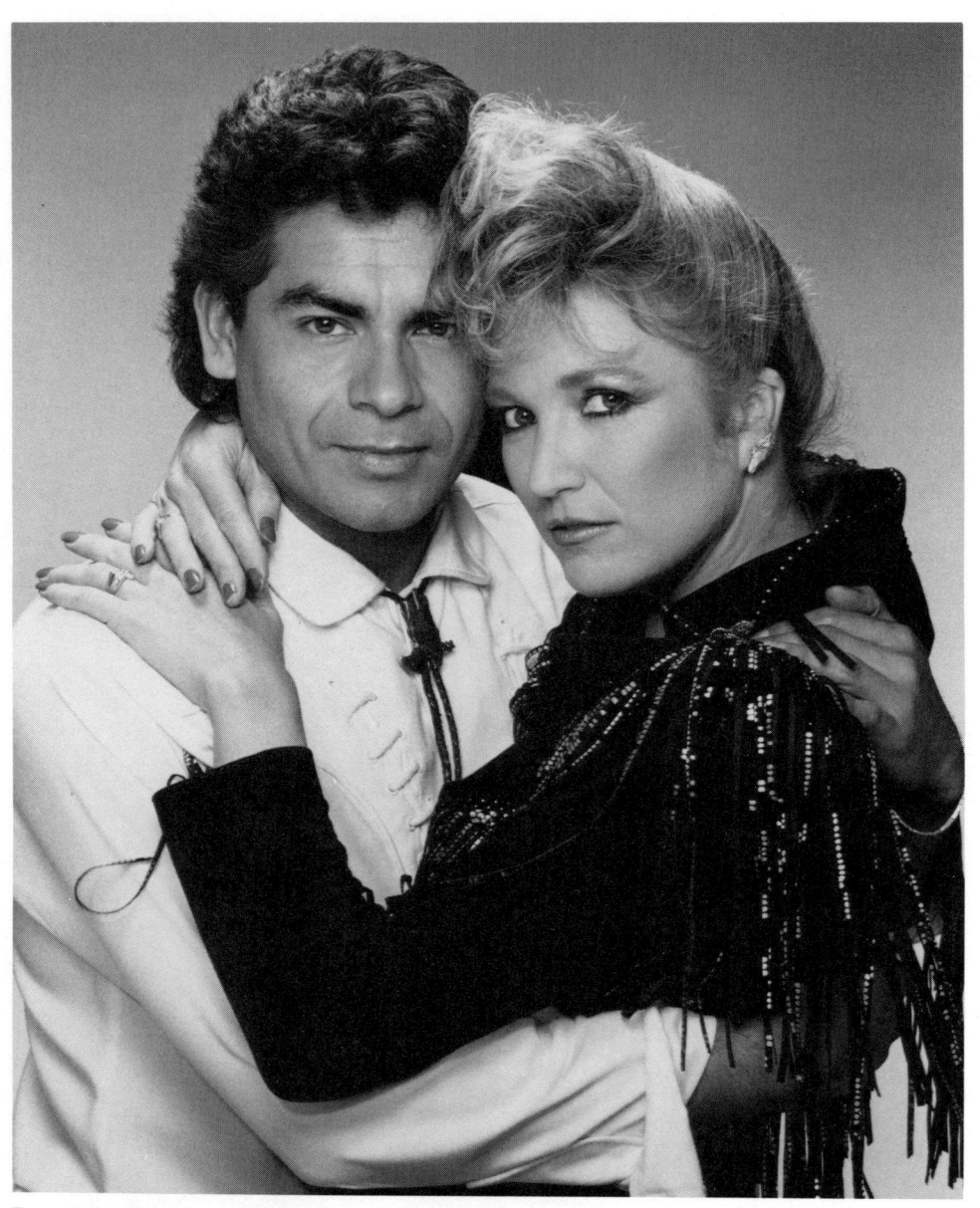

Tanya Tucker's new look is much more controlled and she can wear her hair beautifully up or down.

My very first star was Tanya Tucker, back in the days when I worked for Allen Edwards. One day Tanya burst into the salon in her usual rambunctious way and said, "Gimme somebody," and I was available. When Tanya first came to me, she was 18 or 19 and wore her hair in a style that was too old-looking for her. This was a very aging look; hair not worn right can be very, very aging. But look at Tanya now—her hair is shorter, softer, windblown, and carefree.

I am trying to get all my clients—stars and nonstars alike—away from the battered, damaged look. There is nothing classic about faddish looks. Mousse abuse is gone; hair is calming down; you can still wear it loose, carefree, windblown, but not wild and woolly. Remember, classic beauty doesn't have to mean one look. The new classic beauty has many more choices available to her today.

It was through Tanya Tucker that I got all my country-and-western star clients. Tanya brought Glen Campbell (whom she was then dating) for a haircut, and Glen brought Emmylou Harris, and Emmylou brought Dolly Parton, and through Dolly came some of her brothers and sisters, including Rachel Dennison, who starred in the TV series "Nine to Five," playing the part Dolly played in the film.

Dolly Parton is a classic beauty I haven't discussed yet, and she is a true classic, even with all those wigs and bouffants that she has worn through the years. But that look is Dolly; she is known for it; it has made her famous. She looks very soft and petite, but her look is very individual. She does wear wigs all the time, but she also wears her own hair in front for a natural-looking hairline, with the wig cascading down the back. Wigs are Dolly's trademark, she has worn them forever, yet her look is very traditional. Not all the women who are known for their wigs wear traditional looks, and that is why they select wigs. Look at Tina Turner and Cher. They both are very different types of classic beauties.

TOVAR'S STYLING PHILOSOPHY

What I am trying to prove here is that all women can look different, yet look great. Any haircut can be versatile, and versatility is what makes a hairstyle fun. You wouldn't wear the same clothes day after day, so why bore yourself with a hairstyle that doesn't allow for change?

Hair can be your best fashion accessory. You can dress it up or dress it down. Wear it long, medium, or short—whatever suits your style and personality best. However you wear your hair, wear it in a way that is individual. You don't need long hair to wear it many different ways. Even the shortest haircut, like the one Abby Dalton wears, can be worn slicked back, in a riotous "rockabilly" pompadour

TOVAR'S CLASSIC BEAUTY

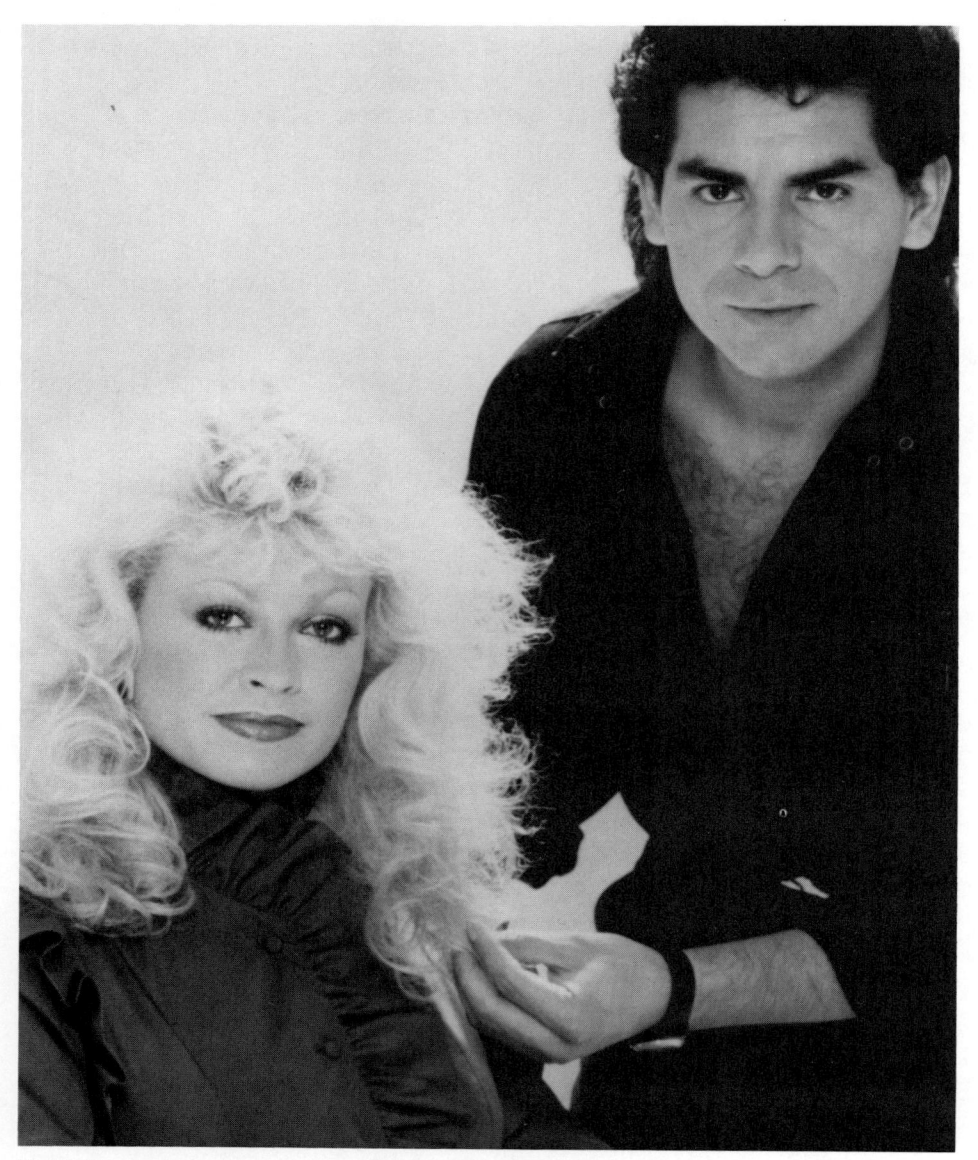

Dolly Parton and her sister Rachel Dennison (shown here) are two of my special star clients.

How You Can Become a Classic Beauty

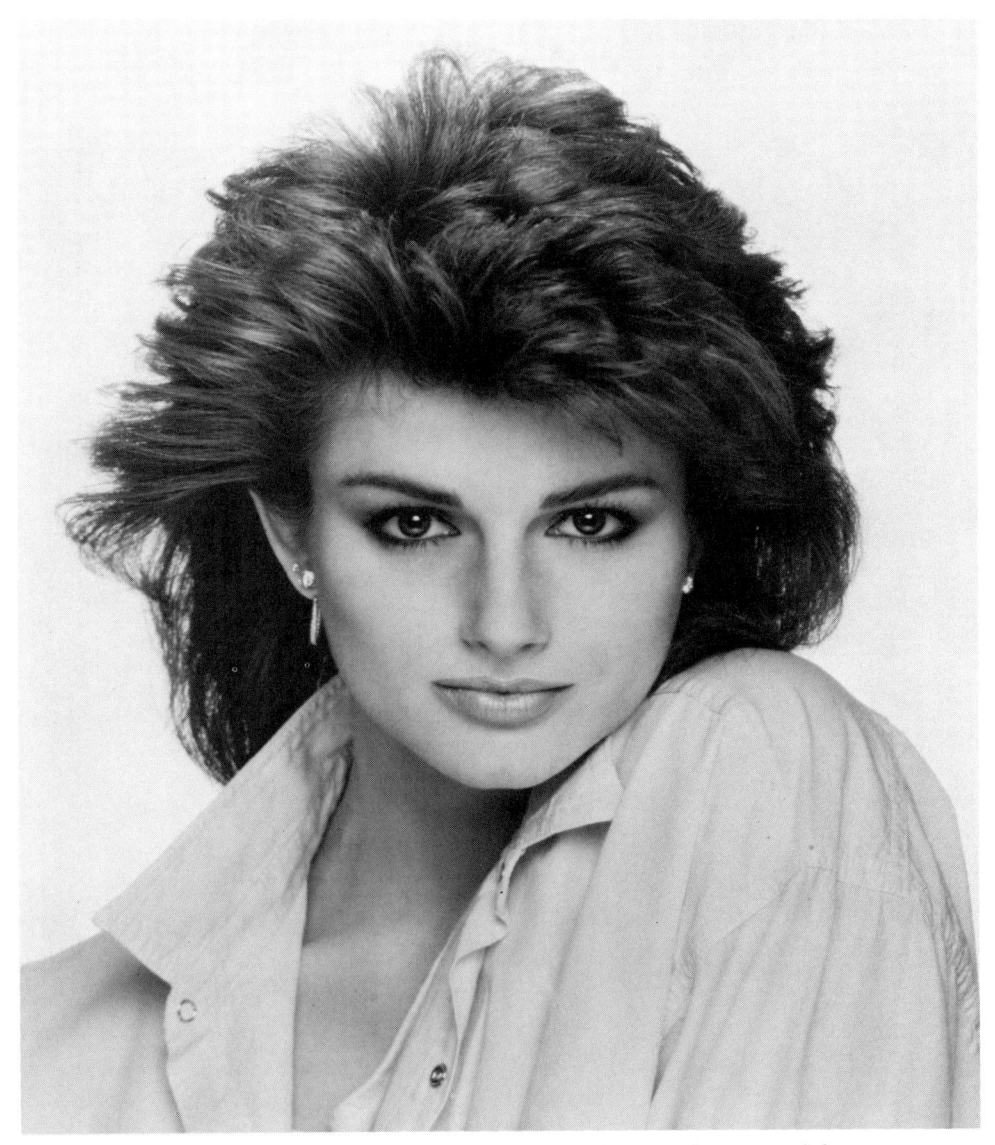

Sylvia is another of my country music stars and one of my most famous makeovers. Sylvia's hair used to be long enough to sit on. It was also straight and limp. I cut Sylvia's hair into this layered, windblown look with bangs and graduated sides for lots of styling versatility.

top, with wispy bangs, with spiky bangs. Learn to play with your hair. Remember that it is a fashion accessory.

Your hair is like a jewel, an ornament. It is a celebration—make it have fun. I think of myself as a doctor of hair, a magician, somebody who creates illusions—somebody who makes your hair celebrate.

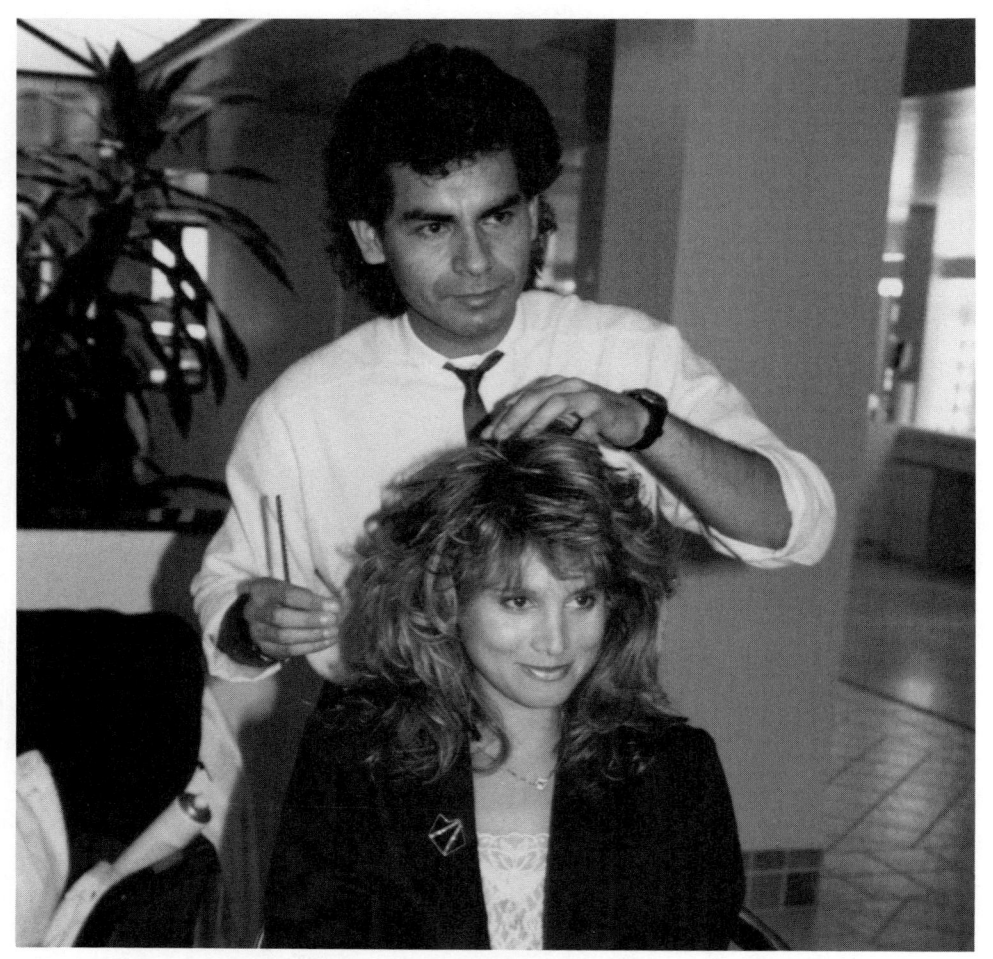

Hillary Kanter, country music star, wears her hair long and layered. A body perm and highlights give added volume and body to her naturally thin hair.

ADAPTING THE CLASSIC BEAUTY LOOK TO YOUR INDIVIDUAL NEEDS

The famous beauties in this book—Barbara Carrera, Dolly Parton, Tina Turner, Heather Locklear, Jayne Kennedy, Erin Gray, Abby Dalton, Merete Van Kamp, Season Hubley, Rosalind Chao, Nia

How You Can Become a Classic Beauty

Peeples, Roxie Roker, and all of the others—have learned to personalize their beauty routines. You can do it, too, by applying the advice in these chapters to your needs. Heather and Barbara like simple hair, yet they can wear something slightly wilder for a special occasion. Barbara will wear her hair up (as she is wearing it on the cover). Heather likes hers scrunched, for lots of volume without much curl.

Jayne Kennedy Overton and Debi Richter have tons of very heavy hair, yet they know how to break the rules and wear their hair very long. They both look great with long hair, and make use of hair accessories to keep the hair off the face so it is not overpowering.

Melody Anderson and Ellen Bry have very similar hair types, one blond, the other brunette. Their hair is so curly that it tends to frizz. So they both keep it at a very workable medium length. They can wear their hair blown dry to control the frizz, slicked and braided, or just wild when they feel like it.

Rosalind Chao has typical Oriental hair—very straight, coarse, and heavy. Yet she doesn't wear it in a typical way. Her bangs are cut in chunks (a great cut for coarse hair), and the rest of her hair is layered for natural volume and fullness. Rosalind can wear her hair straight or scrunched for volume with lots of bend to it.

Merete Van Kamp has baby-fine hair. She could have opted for a perm for more volume, but Merete likes the sleek and straight look. Its almost severe lines make the most of her marvelous facial features. So Merete wears her hair silky, straight, and very close to the head. When she wants a change, she can always braid it or scrunch it for some volume with bend that will wash away.

When adapting popular looks to your own style, keep in mind what you look good in and what you like. If bangs are in but your forehead is too low, try side-swept bangs. If long hair is in but your neck is too short, try wearing it up. If short hair is in and you want to keep yours long, an up-do gives the look of short hair.

Finally, study all the classic looks—the bob, the braids, and the chignons. Apply new hairstyling techniques to the classic looks. A bob can be layered, shorter or longer, with or without bangs. Braids can run the gamut from skinny and sleek to wild and fanciful, depending on your type of hair or look. Chignons and twists can be worn just sleek and smooth at the nape, or you can add wavy bangs, side tendrils, and hair ornaments for a more elaborate look.

Whatever you decide to do with your hair, be creative with it. Remember, your hair is the ultimate fashion accessory and ornament. Make it as exciting as you can.

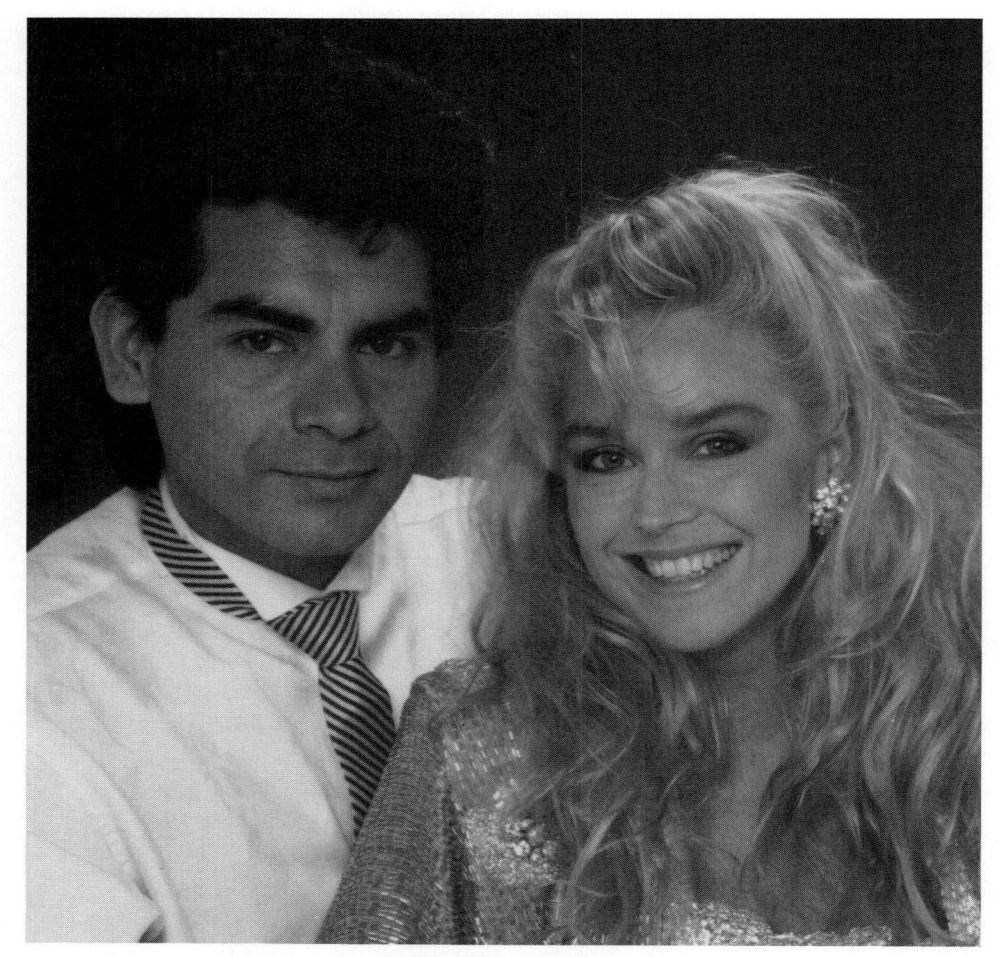

Catherine Hickland

2
STYLES FOR YOUR LIFESTYLE

When I see a client for the first time, I have to find out as much as possible about her in order to design a style that is going to suit her looks and her lifestyle. This involves give and take between the client and me. She has to communicate her likes and dislikes to me, what her hair will and will not do. I have to educate her about all the possibilities available to her with haircutting, styling, and chemical treatments.

Yet she has to tell me exactly what she wants out of the style. Is she a career woman who needs to look crisp and positive all the time? Is she a housewife with small children who has little time to fuss with her hair? Is she a society matron who needs many different looks for different occasions? Or is she a star who is in the public eye and considers her hair to be part of her image?

Other things come into consideration, too. Does she want a look that is really "wash 'n wear," or does she like to fuss with her hair, perhaps setting it on rollers? Does she like a style that needs hair spray, or does she hate spray? Does she like long hair or short hair? A lot of women love long hair until they find out how time-consuming it is to maintain.

Many hairstylist/client disaster stories have to do with lack of communication. Perhaps one of the worst cases happens when a woman "of a certain age" walks into the salon with a picture of a young model clipped from a magazine and asks you to make her look like that.

TOVAR'S CLASSIC BEAUTY

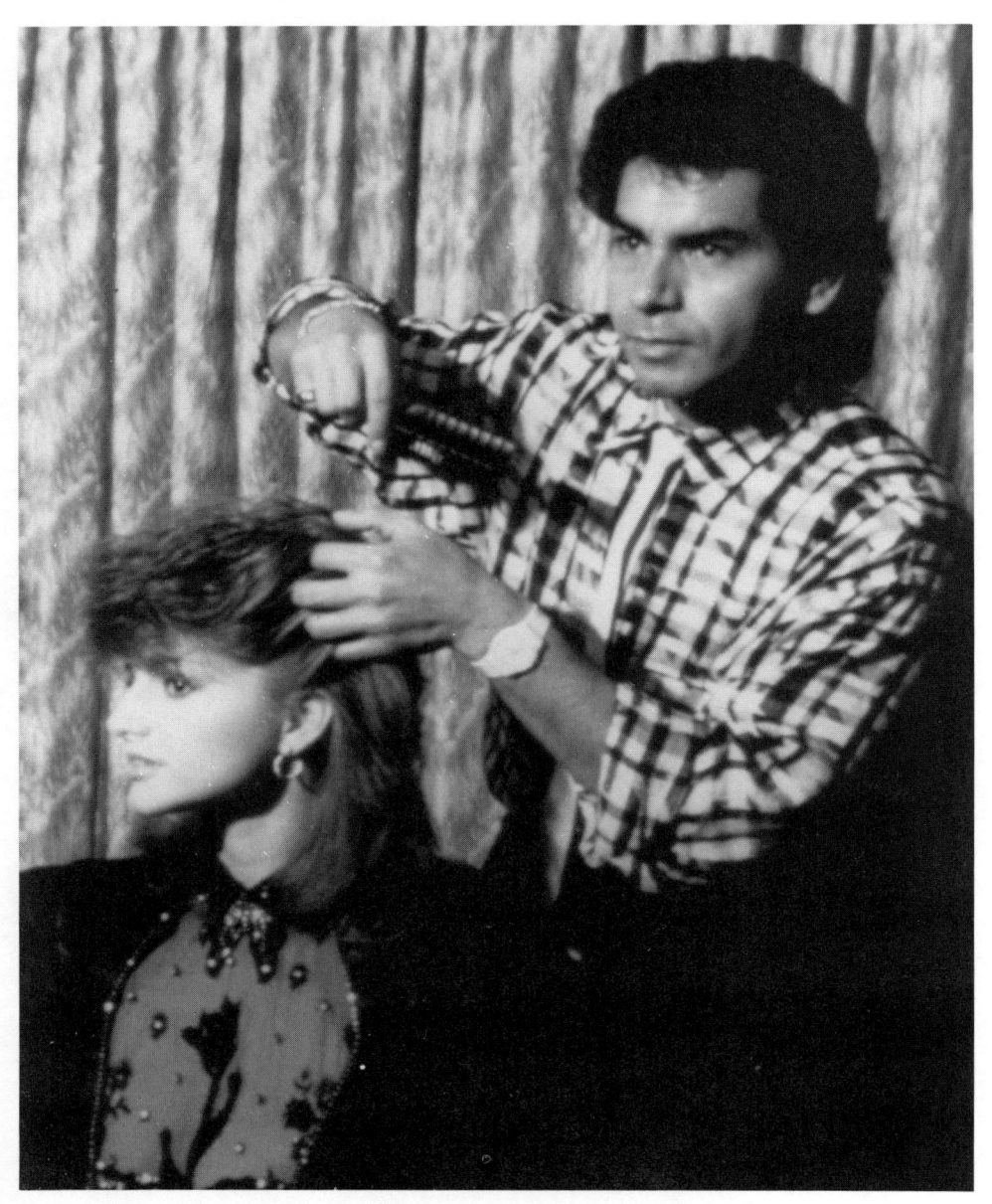

Here I am putting the finishing touches on Sylvia's new look.

Styles for Your Lifestyle

It is the stylist's job to tell the woman why that look won't be suitable for her. First of all, the model in the picture is perhaps 20 years younger and can wear her hair differently from an older woman. Second, does the client know the amount of "faking" that goes on for a magazine shoot? That style may look great from the angle the picture was taken, but it may be pinned and propped in back to make the hair look just right from a particular angle.

Very few clients will insist on your doing something when you tell them it is not going to end up looking the way they want it to look.

Another area where good communication comes into play is in suggesting what chemical treatments are necessary to achieve the look both of you have agreed on.

If you say that you want lots of volume and fullness in your hairstyle, and your hair is fine and limp, the stylist knows that you need a body wave and perhaps some highlights to create that volume. Be sure that the stylist explains what is going to be necessary to achieve that look. Most of the time, a cut alone won't be enough to achieve the hairstyle look you want.

My personal approach with a new client begins the moment she sits in my chair. First, I study the hair, its texture, density, and type. Does she color her hair? Does she have a perm now? If not, can a perm add more body and volume? Is it too short or too long for her now? Is its shape all wrong for her facial structure? How about more or less layering? Is her hair in good condition, or does she need treatments?

Then I start asking the questions. What brought her to me in the first place? What is she looking for, a complete change or just a slightly different look? Does she like to play with her hair, or does she want a style that is maintenance-free? What does she do for a living? Does she like short hair or long hair? Does she like a trendy look, or does she feel safer with a more traditional look? All these questions and many more that come up as I talk to the client must be answered before I decide what to do about her hair.

The most difficult part of giving a woman a new hairstyle is making her change. We all get used to that face, that image that we see in the mirror day after day. We feel safe with it. A new hairstyle is going to change that image.

Some of my celebrity clients are notorious for resisting change. Take Dolly Parton, for example. She is famous for her wigs, and for a long, long time she wore her hair (or her wig) styled in the same way. Dolly sees herself with those masses of curls and waves. Her own hair is baby-fine; if she was going to wear a style that used only her own hair, it would have to be very short. Short hair is not Dolly's image; it is not her look. But Dolly now is beginning to experiment with different wigs, and they are getting less bouffant, prettier, softer, and not as overdone.

TOVAR'S CLASSIC BEAUTY

Change is essential for most women, even those who are concerned about a public image. The changes can be very subtle, or they can be major, like my famous makeovers for Sylvia and Emmylou Harris. Both changes were traumatic in a sense. It is difficult for a woman to part with all that hair. But the changes were really for the better, and Emmylou and Sylvia have never looked better.

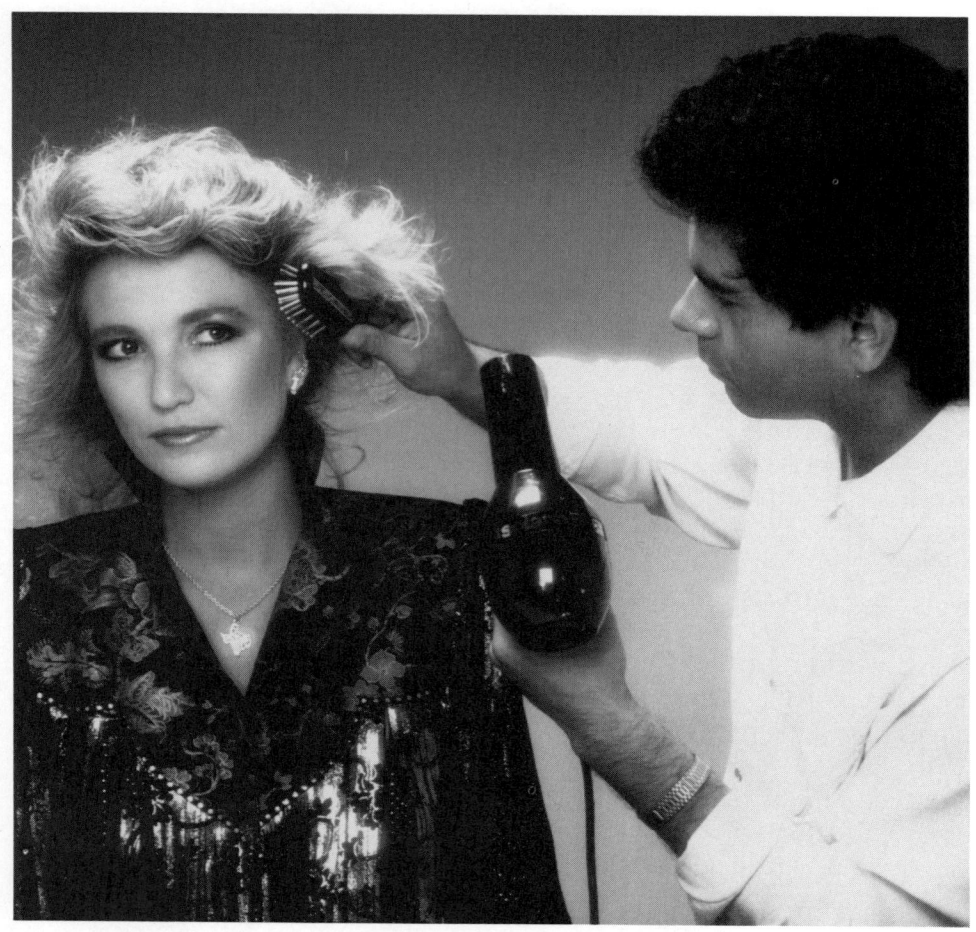

It is important to work with your chosen hairstylist to get the right style to suit your looks and lifestyle.

A lot of women are afraid to get their hair cut. They are afraid of the unknown. They have become used to that hairstyle. It is like insurance: it makes them feel safe. But as with a lot of safe things, you get into a rut. You get bored. And when you wear the same look for too long, suddenly you find yourself behind the times, old-fashioned. You need to educate and to trust your hairstylist to feel secure enough about that change.

Even stars have a problem making changes. Barbara Carrera needed a drastic change. She was looking the same as she had since her days as a top cover girl. She had worn that long, long hair for years. So I suggested that she cut it to just below the shoulders. I trimmed off about four inches, I gave her a one-length bob with wispy bangs, and brightened her color.

Before that her hair was too long, and it looked skimpy. I like long hair, but only when it can look lush and full. Barbara now looks younger. Her hair has a sparkle with the red tones I suggested. She is very happy with it, and I don't think she will ever let it grow that long again.

Abby Dalton is another celebrity who opted for a drastic change. Abby had worn her hair in a medium-length, layered bob for years, but she works out for about two and a half hours a day and needed more of a wash 'n' wear look. So Abby had her hair cut short, very short, but with enough movement and length at the crown to allow her the greatest styling versatility.

Some of my clients know instinctively how to wear their hair. Debbie Mullowney, for example, knows that her fine hair looks best in a layered style. Because she likes the one-length look, I cut her hair in a modified bob with layering, but with the look of a one-length style. Using the right cutting technique, a layered hairstyle can appear one length.

Merete Van Kamp is one of those clients who need a little coaxing. She likes to wear her hair long, but because it is so baby-fine, it looks skimpy around the ends. So we compromise, and sometimes Merete wears her hair up in a braided style. If she wants to wear it down, it is scrunched with a little bit of mousse for volume.

Barbara Stock is blessed with a magnificent head of hair, and she knows exactly how to wear it. It is cut shoulder length, layered, and with heavy bangs. She doesn't have to do much with it. She can wear it up or down. Her cut allows for great styling versatility.

When I first meet a new client, after I study all the qualities of her hair, I group her into one of the four basic lifestyle groups. This is done to achieve a hairstyle that is truly becoming and manageable for her. However, some women overlap one or two of the four categories and certain adjustments must be done in order to obtain the right look for her. Whatever the finished style I achieve, the most important category in my mind is her individuality. Giving her a look that is totally unique and her very own is my first goal. Following is a description of each of the lifestyle groups most of my clients fall into.

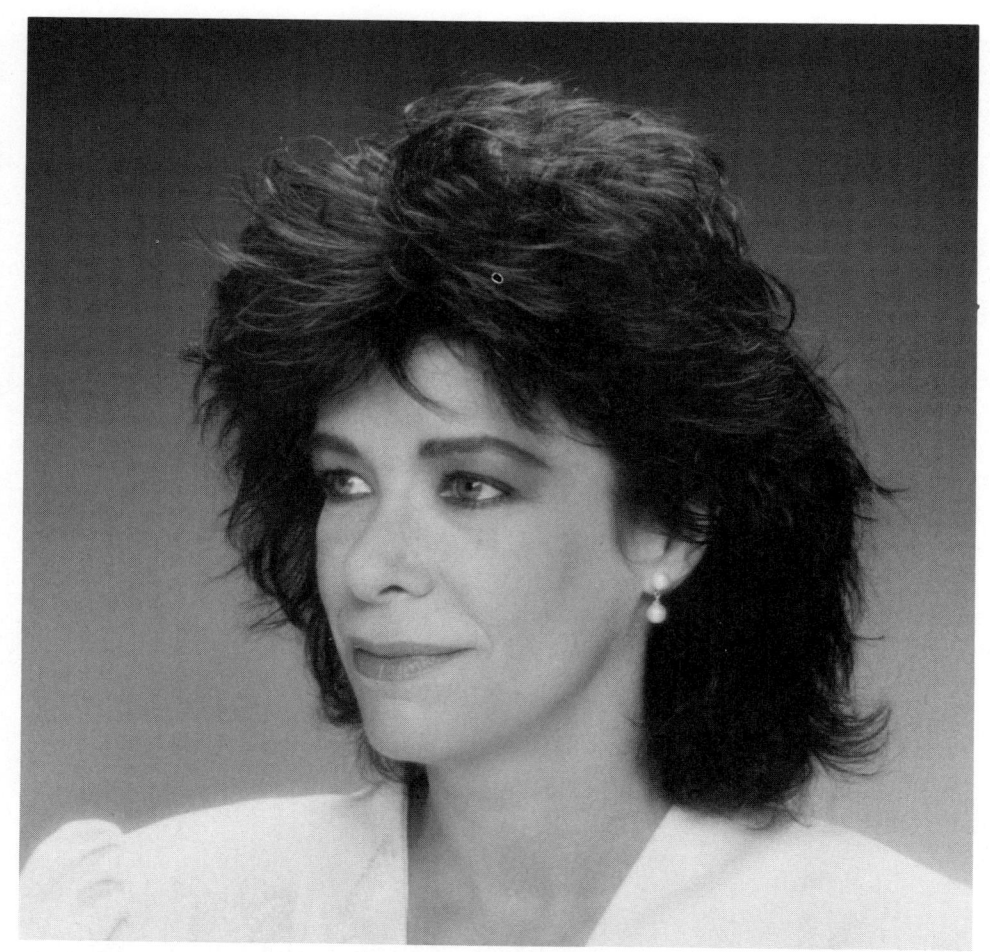

Joan Green, the high-powered personal manager, wears a truly simple, becoming style. Suit by Jeran Designs, Los Angeles.

CAREER WOMEN

My clients come from a wide variety of fields. I do the hair of some high-powered women in town like Susan DePas, who is the head of Motown Records and one of the most powerful women in Hollywood. My two career women models for the book are Joan Green, a personal manager who owns Joan Green Management and has among her clients some of the hottest names in the business, and Marilyn Heston, a celebrity publicist with a client roster as impressive as Joan's.

Both of these women, and my other career woman clients, are constantly on the go. Their days usually start with breakfast appointments and end with business dinners and other after-work

Styles for Your Lifestyle

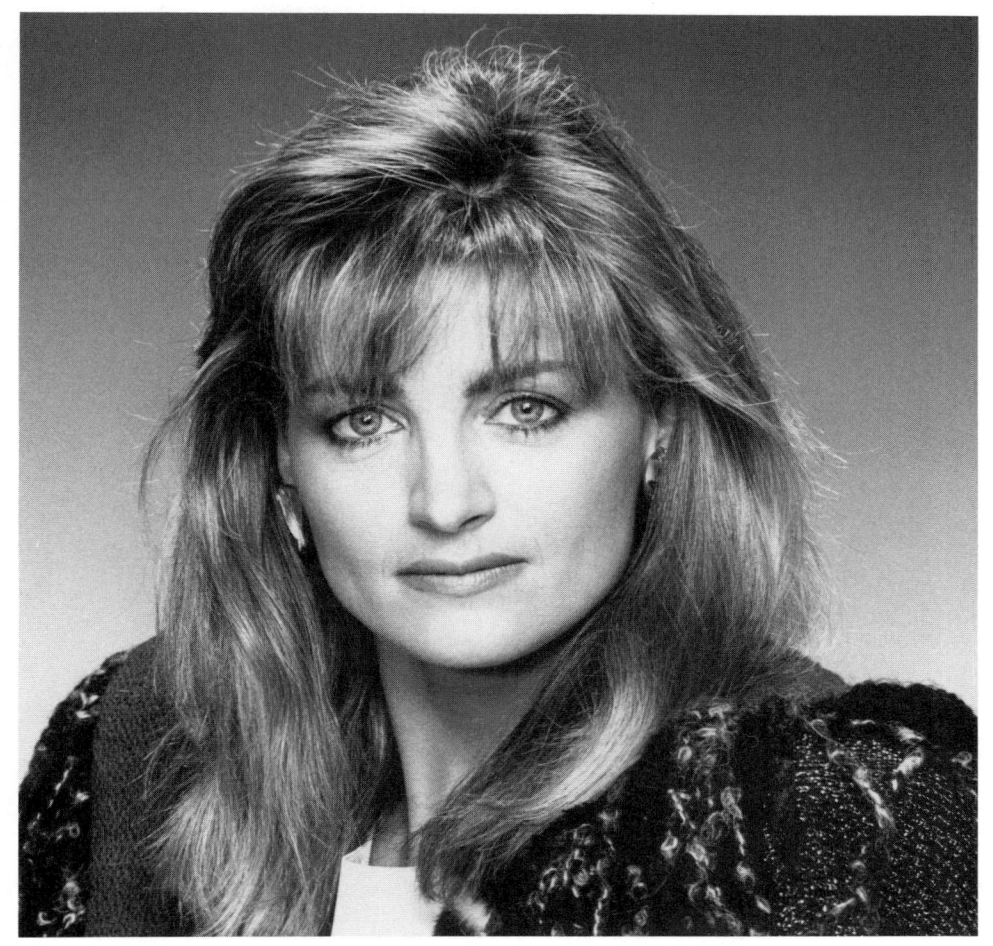

Marilyn Heston, the personal celebrity publicist, looks stunning in a smooth and sleek style with airy bangs. Suit by Margi Kent, Los Angeles.

affairs. Both Joan's and Marilyn's styles are very simple, based on excellent cuts and a number of support treatments to make these styles as maintenance-free as possible.

Joan's dark hair is layered all over and cut very short at the crown for lots of fullness and volume. Her bangs are cut chunky and airy, and she can wear as much or as little of them on her forehead as she likes. The rest of her hair is left longer, to touch the nape and balance her long, thin neck.

Marilyn has a strong, square face with angular edges. She looks best in just-below-the-shoulder hair, a slightly parted crown with a little height, and straight, piecey bangs slightly parted off center, to play a sort of peekaboo effect that emphasizes her great eyes.

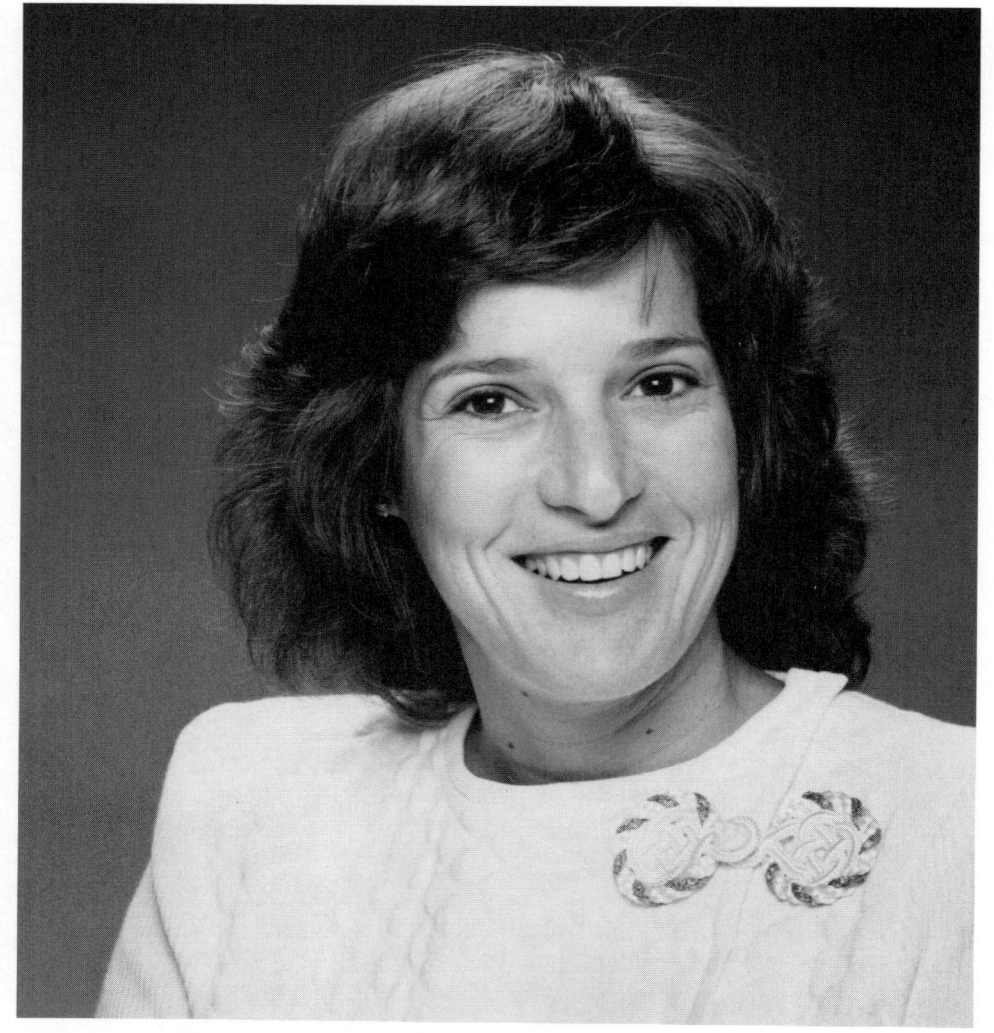

BEFORE: Susan Jannick, my housewife model, with a shapeless, bulky style.

HOUSEWIVES

I have many housewife clients, and they range from the wealthy Beverly Hills and Bel Air housewives who come in two or three times a week to the middle-class housewives who come in every six weeks for a cut. What I have noticed most about my housewife clients is that they all appear to prefer simpler hairstyles.

No matter where they come from, they all ask for the type of maintenance-free, no-hassle, no-fuss, styles that wash 'n' wear. This request is more in evidence when the client has children.

My housewife model, Susan Jannick, had just had a baby, and she needed a new look. In her *before* picture above, her hair is shapeless

Styles for Your Lifestyle

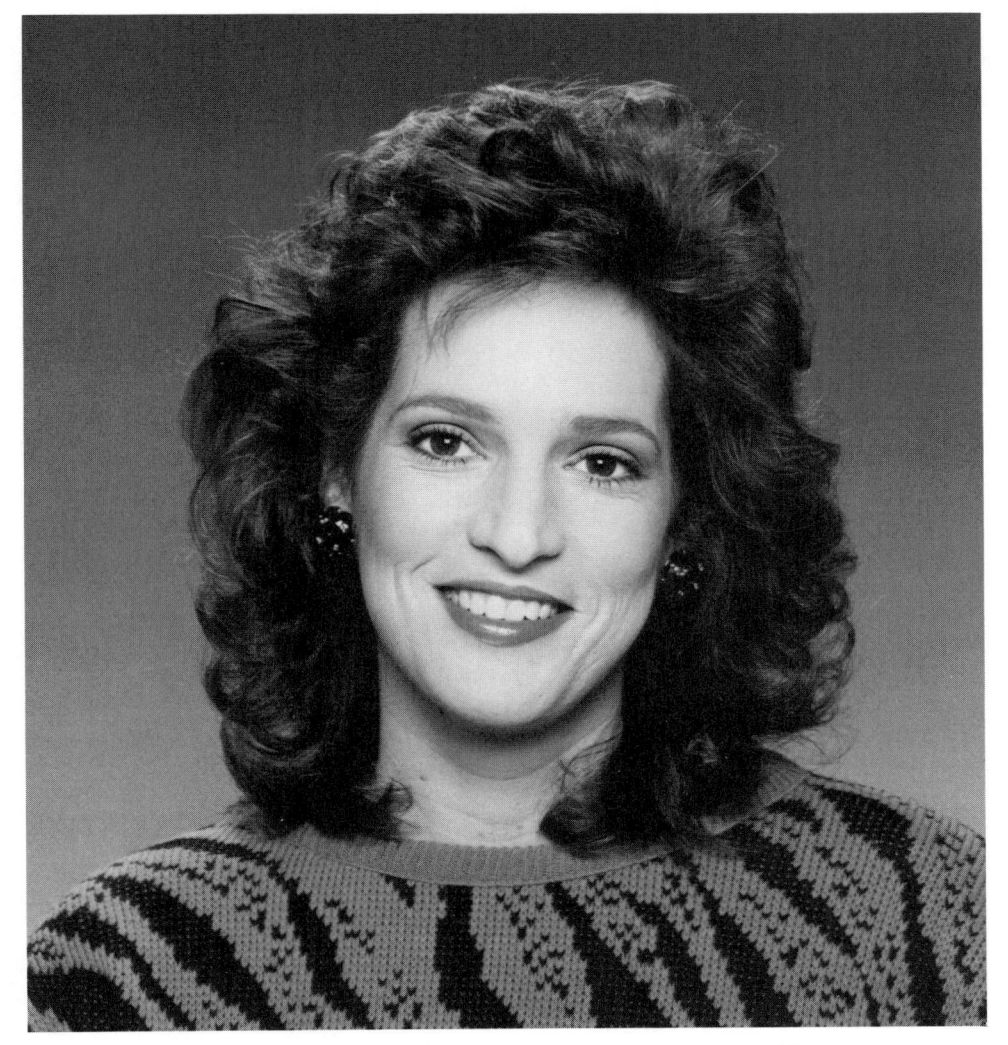

AFTER: A big difference, with a style that bares the face and has some fullness at the sides and crown. Sweaters by Knit Maven.

and too bulky at the bottom. She also needed some makeup. For her *after* picture, I layered her hair all over, leaving length at the bottom, which she needs to balance her long face and long neck. I got rid of her bangs, which were too heavy over her narrow forehead. Also, by sweeping her front hair back, I gave her more height in front and at the crown. This is the type of hairstyle that doesn't require lots of maintenance. Susan's naturally curly hair provides enough body (if it had been straight, I would have suggested a body wave). All she has to do is shampoo, put on a little mousse, and blow-dry upside down first, then add the finishing touches and a couple of curls with a curling iron.

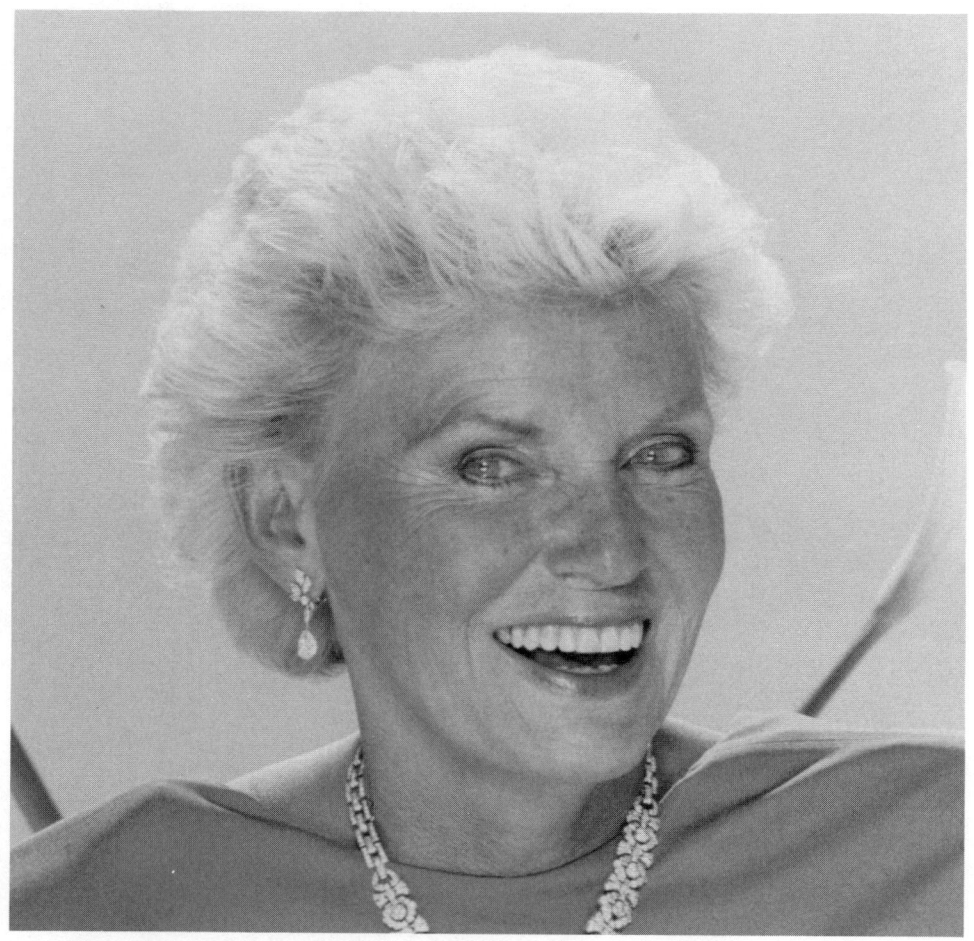

Jane Morgan Weintraub, my society matron model, in her signature short, platinum-blonde style, brushed back from the face for a very elegant feeling.

SOCIETY MATRONS

The society matron model in this book is Jane Morgan Weintraub, who has been my client for many years and who later became my backer along with her husband. Jane is the perfect example of the society lady with a super-packed schedule. Her husband is one of the most powerful men in Hollywood, and they are always going somewhere, from all types of Hollywood parties to galas at the White House.

Jane's hair is basically a wash 'n' wear style. She has the kind of very curly hair that is easy to handle and that does a lot of things. Jane lives in Malibu most of the year, and her hair looks as good

Styles for Your Lifestyle

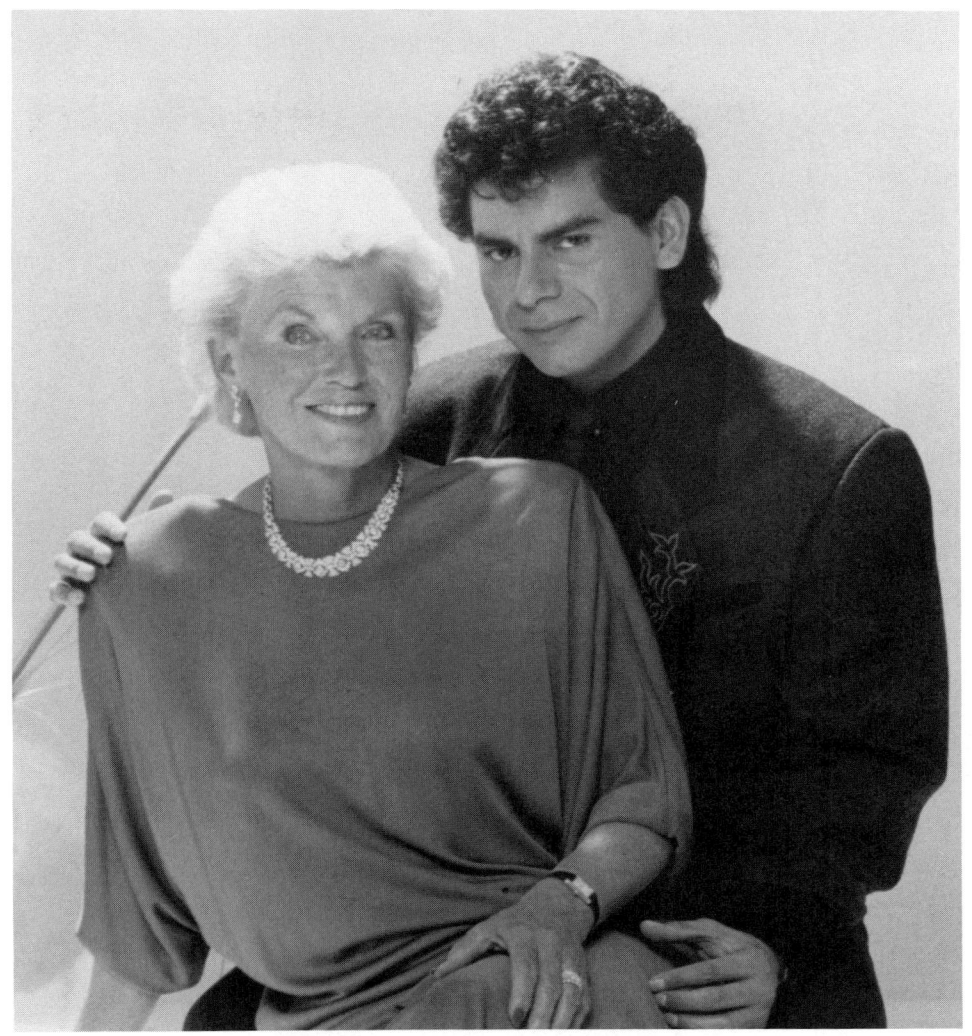

A final pose for Jane Morgan Weintraub and me at my Beverly Hills salon.

when wet as when dry. All she has to do is shake those curls and she is ready to go.

For more festive occasions, Jane's hair can be blown dry, making it very full and sweeping it off her face for a very elegant, chic look. Jane's hairstyle is short, yet it offers the multitude of styling possibilities that Jane needs for the many occasions that make up her average day.

Also, short hair is a better choice for most women after they reach a certain age. Short hair is youthful and very becoming. I recommend it to all my mature clients. But I never force anything on anyone, so an up-do serves the same purpose by "uplifting" the face, just like a natural face-lift.

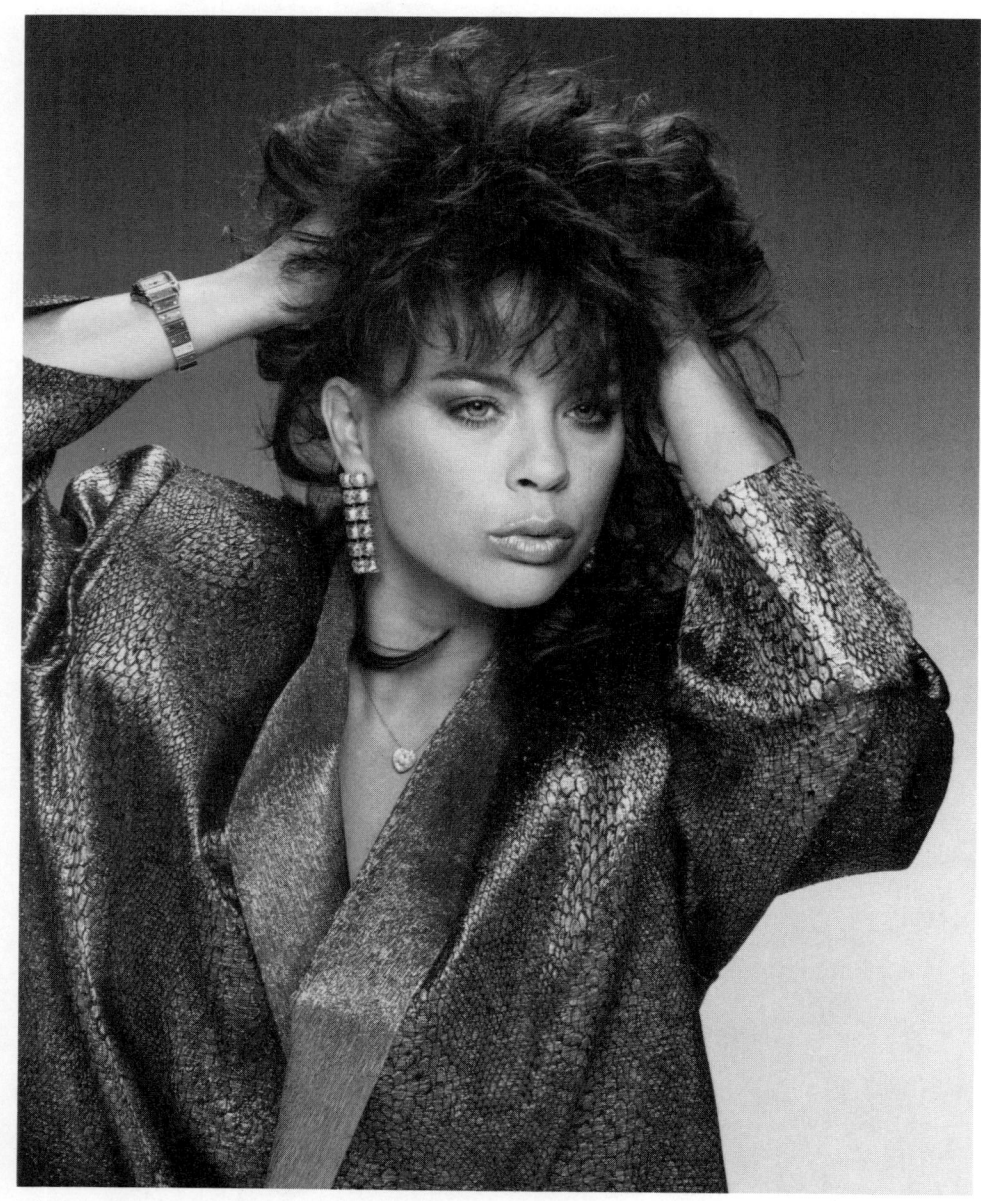

Many of my star clients, such as Brogan Lane, prefer long hair because it allows them a greater choice of day and evening looks.

Styles for Your Lifestyle

STARS

My last group is the stars. Most of them are going to prefer long hair because it allows them the versatility that their many roles demand. Barbara Carrera is the perfect example of the star look. Her hair is simple, straight, one length, yet it can do a million things. She can wear it up, down, half up and half down, under hats, any way she needs to.

Jayne Kennedy Overton's style is basically low-maintenance. Her long hair is almost all one length, cut with some long layers in the front for movement. This length is perfect for Jayne because all that heavy hair weighs it down and keeps it in control.

Heather Locklear looks great in her long, layered bob. The cut gives the illusion of long hair, and it is truly versatile. Heather can wear it pulled back, up, half up and half down, scrunched with some mousse for fullness, simple, or dramatic.

Erin Gray is a perfect example of a classic beauty. Her look is pure and simple, yet she can wear it many ways. Her basic bob with bangs can be swept up, sideways, or simply worn as is.

Claire Yarlett has beautiful hair with natural body and wave, cut in long layers to the shoulders. It is a look that suits her very well, and she can wear it up or down, depending on her mood or the demands of her career.

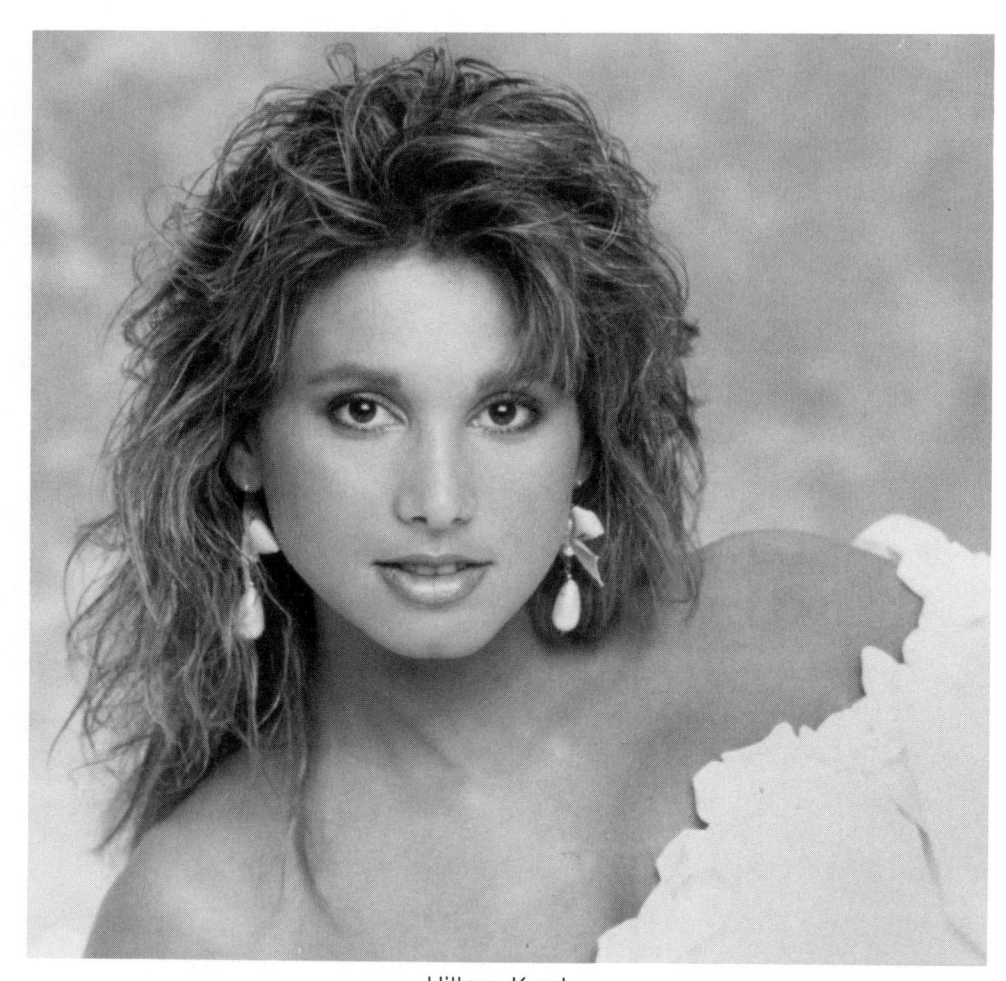

Hillary Kanter

3
MAKING THE BEST OF YOUR HAIR

Not everyone is born with a great head of hair, but whatever you were given, there are a number of ways to make it look great. Before I proceed to tell you how to do so, however, you must determine your hair type.

As I said in the introduction to this book, hair is the ultimate fashion and beauty accessory. And, like any fine accessory, it should be cared for properly. However, in order to do this, you must know what hair is, how it is structured, and how those qualities affect the care and handling of hair.

Hair is a fiber that contains a certain degree of elasticity. It is most elastic when wet, less when dry. It is this elasticity that allows hair to be styled in many different ways—curly, wavy, straight, up, or down. Hair is made of a protein substance called *keratin*, which is also what nails are made of.

The condition of the hair also determines its degree of elasticity. Hair that is in good condition will have the most, allowing it to be stretched (for styling purposes) to the maximum degree without damage or breakage. When the hair is in poor condition, either from overprocessing with chemical treatments (perms, color, etc.) or from exposure to the elements (chlorine, sun, or salt water), it loses a lot of elasticity and begins to break easily. So the condition your hair is in also plays a part in how it is styled.

Although all hair looks similar to the naked eye, it is all very different when you look at it under a microscope.

Most hair contains three layers:

The Cuticle: This transparent outer layer protects the inner layers. It is made up of scale-like cells that grow pointing away from the scalp to the hair ends.

The Cortex: This middle layer is what gives elasticity and strength to the hair. It is made up of fibrous, elongated cells that are bundled together. This layer contains the pigment that determines hair color.

The Medulla: This is the innermost layer, and it is made up of round cells in a row pattern. This layer can be partly or totally absent in thin hair, which is what makes it limp.

When hair is exposed to chemical treatments, these penetrate the cuticle or outer layer to deposit the chemicals on the cortex and change the structure or color of the hair. Overuse of chemicals can damage the cuticle severely, in some cases making it break and disappear from whole sections of the hair. This not only causes hair to break, but also makes it dull and dry. When used improperly, hair appliances like blow dryers, hot rollers, and curling irons can have the same effect. So can overexposure of the hair—especially if it has been chemically treated—to sun, salt, and chlorinated water. All this can lead to dull, brittle hair and split ends.

The thickness of the cortex is what determines the thickness of the hair. Thin hair has a thinner cortex; coarse hair has a heavier cortex. Because the thickness of the hair is what makes it behave in certain ways, you will note that lightweight, thin hair can be hard to handle and flyaway, and some types of very coarse or wiry hair always look bushy and wild.

ALL ABOUT YOUR HAIR

All hair shows the same characteristics, and these determine how it's worn. These are texture, which determines the thickness; formation, which determines the curl or lack of it; density, which determines the amount; and color, which works to enhance skin tones.

Texture

Fine Hair: This type of hair falls into two categories: fine hair and baby-fine hair. When fine hair is in good condition, it will feel soft and silky, almost slippery to the touch. Baby-fine hair is sometimes

Making the Best of Your Hair

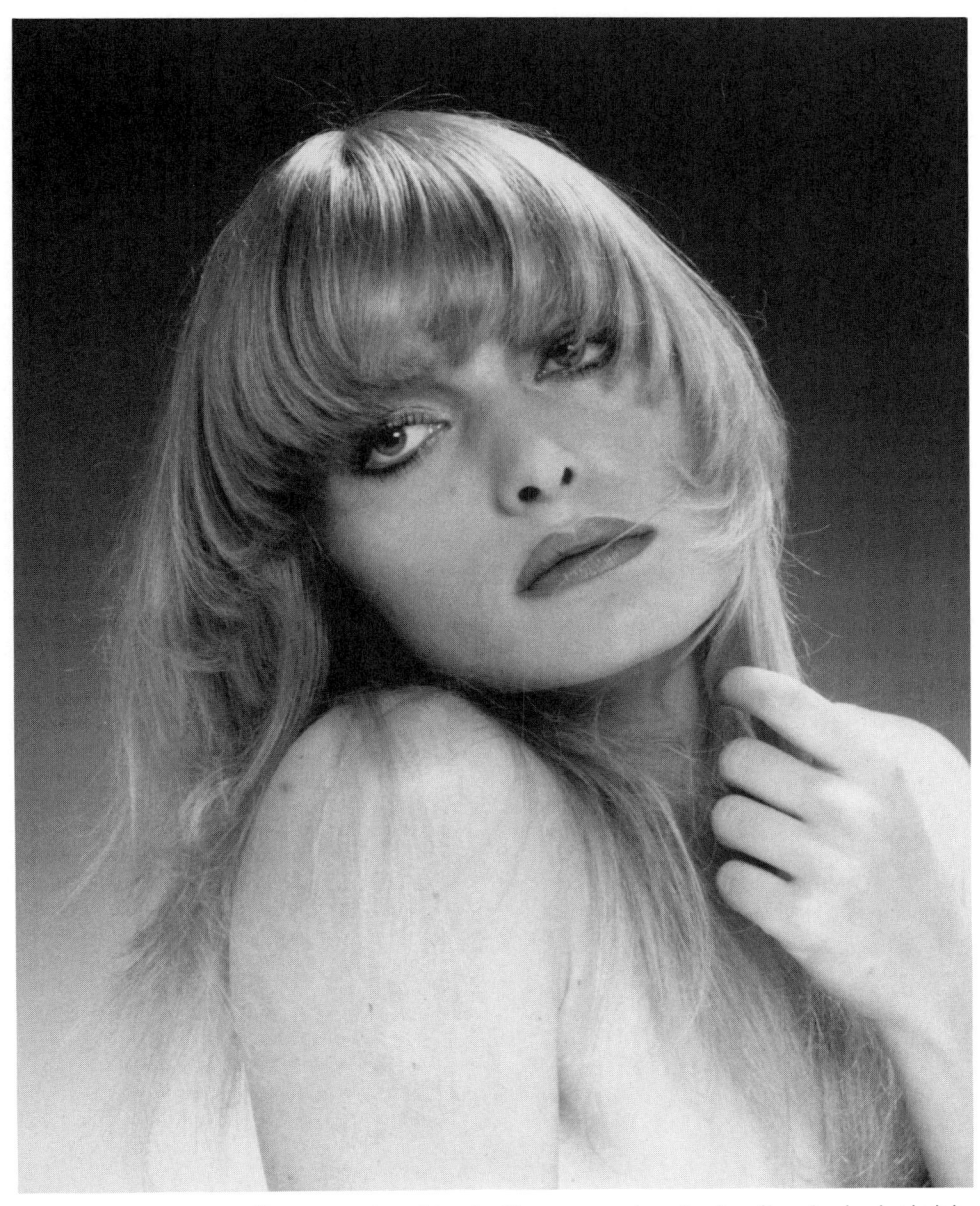

Merete Van Kamp likes a natural look. She wears her baby-fine hair straight and down. Added highlights give her hair extra body and volume.

sparse and tends to be delicate, flyaway, and hard to manage. Many women with fine hair have lots of it, which is one of the ways nature compensates for the thinness.

Dealing with Fine Hair: Adding body and adding volume are the most important things you can do for fine hair. There are several ways of doing this:

1. Chemical treatments—perms and color. Body waves, root perms, and partial perms (only the crown, for example) are great ways to add body to fine hair. Color also makes hair thicker by making it porous; both tinting and highlights achieve the same thickness effect.

2. Styling aids—blow-drying, curling irons, hot rollers, pin curl sets, mousses, gels, and spray. Blow-dry upside down for added volume. Curl areas where fullness is desired (crown, front, sides) with curling iron or hot rollers. Beware of mousses and gels and use only a very small amount, as they can coat the hair, making it heavy and limp. The best way to apply mousse and gel is *to the roots* for volume from within.

3. Cutting—the right cut is the foundation of any style, especially when you have problem hair. Thin hair can be worn in a variety of lengths, depending on how thin or limp it is, but it should always be blunt-cut at the ends, and layered around the face and crown for movement and volume.

4. Conditioning—thin hair must be kept in excellent condition. Thin hair tends to be delicate and fragile and sometimes breaks easily. Choose the right shampoo and conditioners and be careful to stay away from products that have heavy formulas. These tend to make the hair go limp and flat.

Normal Hair: This is medium-textured hair with lots of body and bounce; it holds the style and curl well. This type of hair can be straight, wavy, or curly. If either of the latter two, weather conditions can affect it, making it frizz in hot and humid weather. Straight hair can go limp for the same reason. However, overall this is the easiest type of hair to work with.

Dealing with Normal Hair: There are two ways to deal with this type of hair. One is to bring out and emphasize its natural properties—for example, the way Erin Gray wears her medium-thick hair in a blunt-cut classic bob. The other way is to change the natural formation (curl or lack of it) with the help of a body perm or straightener. Color treatments work well with this type of hair, enhancing it and adding to its manageability.

Making the Best of Your Hair

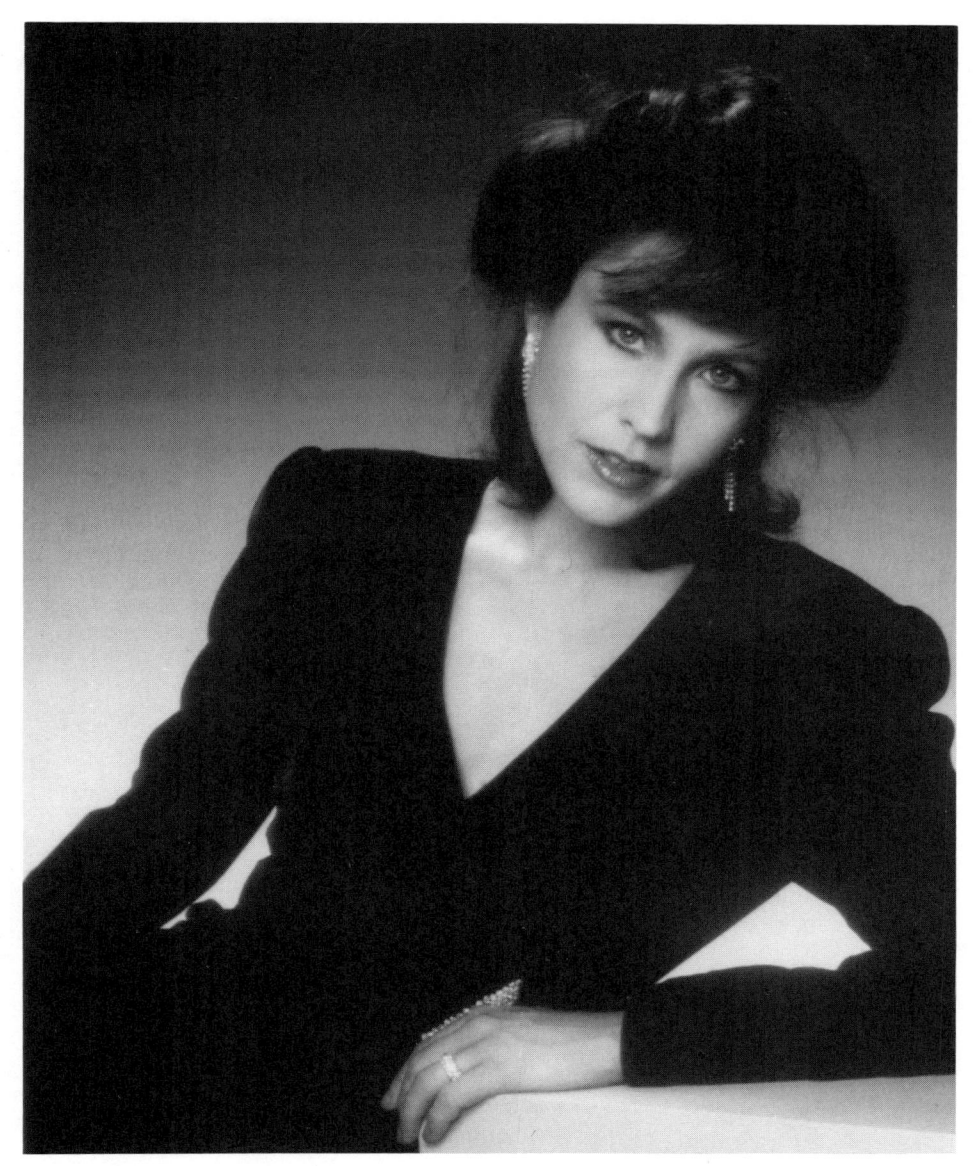

Erin Gray's best style for her medium-thick normal hair is a blunt-cut classic bob, which she can dress up for evening by pulling the sides and front back and up.

TOVAR'S CLASSIC BEAUTY

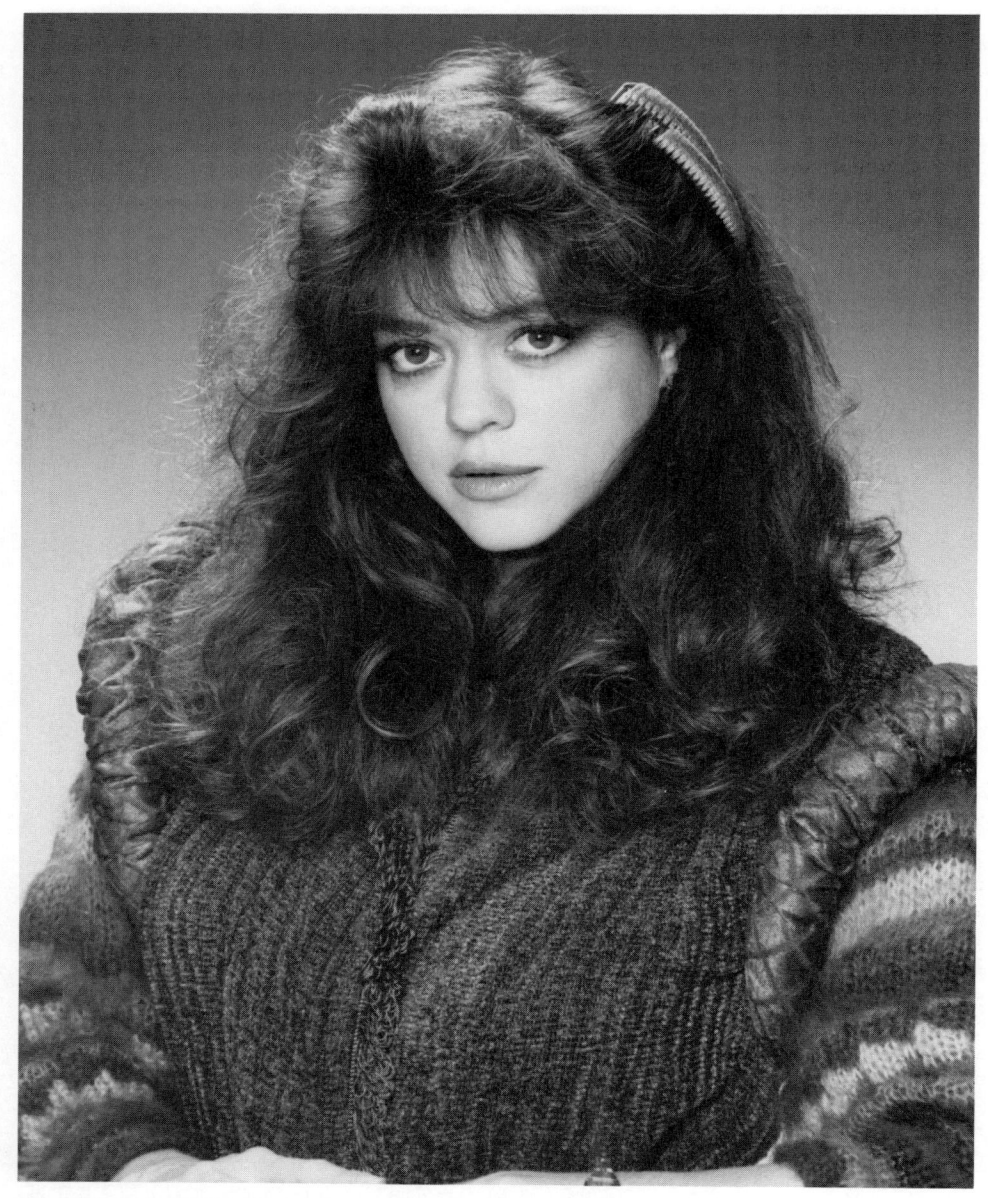

Very thick hair like Debi Richter's can be worn long, but use hair ornaments (as shown here) to pin it off the face, so it doesn't look overpowering.

Making the Best of Your Hair

1. Keep medium-textured hair blunt-cut at the ends. Some layering around the face and crown can be added for styling versatility.

2. If you wish to add curl to your straight, medium-textured hair, it will be relatively easy, as this type of hair takes a perm well. However, stay away from too curly looks that will have a tendency to look bushy because they will add too much volume to the hair.

3. Any type of color treatment will be a plus for this type of hair. Cellophanes and other semipermanent coloring methods also work very well, adding shine and bounce.

4. When conditioning this type of hair, be careful not to overcondition. If the hair begins to feel heavy and limp after treatments, it means you are using too much of a product or using it too frequently.

Thick Hair: This type of hair often feels coarse and wiry. Weather conditions play havoc with the way it looks, making it too bushy and wild. The same effect also can result from the wrong cut. When this type of hair has a tight curl formation, it is often dull, lacking shine. Very often, when people with other hair types begin to get their first gray hair, it grows out coarse and wiry.

Dealing with Thick Hair: The proper cut is essential to making this type of hair manageable and attractive. You can wear this type of hair long, medium, or short, depending on styling preference, as long as it is cut properly. If you like to wear it long (as Debi Richter does), be sure to keep it off the face with combs or style it in braids; otherwise the thickness of the hair will overpower and cover the face.

1. Keep thick or coarse hair cut in layers. Be aware, however, that too much layering can make it look wild and woolly, which is just the effect you want to stay away from. Blunt-cutting is also a no-no for this type of hair.

2. Frequent trims are essential to keep the line and shape of the style.

3. This type of hair can be blown dry almost straight, resulting in a style with lots of body and volume. Just a small touch of mousse will help the blow dryer do its job.

4. If you are the daring type, like Brogan Lane, select a style that makes the best of all the curl and volume in your hair. This is a classic case of flaunting what you have.

5. Learn how to use mousses, gels, and hair spray to keep hair tamed and in place. Also learn how to braid your hair and put it up in many different ways. Braids and up-dos are great hot weather hairdos for this type of hair.

TOVAR'S CLASSIC BEAUTY

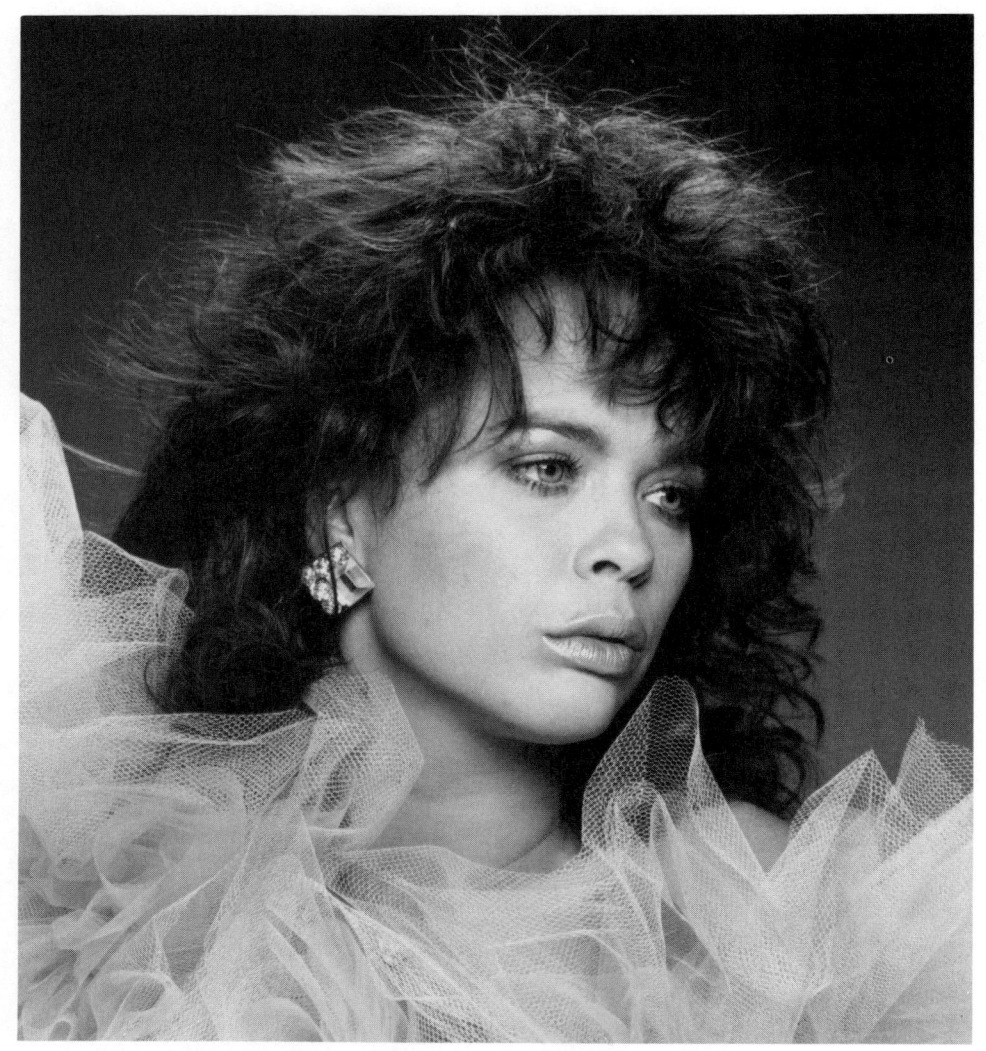

Brogan Lane is another one of those stunning ladies who breaks all the beauty rules—not doing it would make her look boring. I cut Brogan's hair shorter on one side, longer on the other. The front is brought forward into wild bangs.

Making the Best of Your Hair

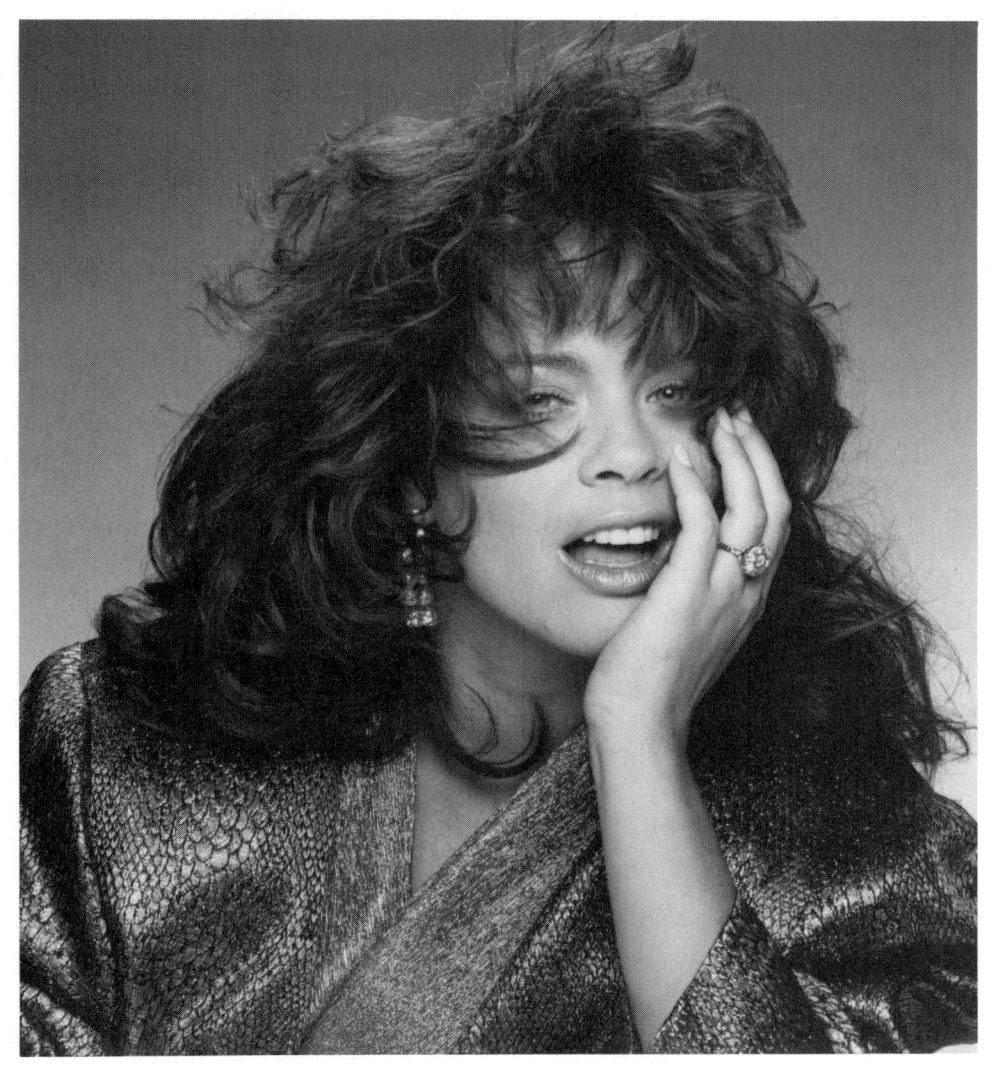

I did two styles with Brogan here—the one on page 40 is soft, curly, and very romantic; this one is wilder, untamed, and unique.

Formation

Formation refers to how much or how little the hair curls. There are three types in this category: straight, wavy, and curly.

The shape of the hair shaft is what determines its formation. Straight hair is round, wavy hair is oval, and curly hair is flat. Some heads of hair combine two or three formations, while others are just one type. It's not uncommon for some people to have a combination of straight and wavy hair, or wavy and curly, or all three.

Curl or lack of curl in the hair is a key factor in selecting a style. A logical and easy way to do it is to tailor the style to the amount of curl in the hair. This will make the style easier to maintain, and you won't have to deal with regrowth problems caused by perms or straighteners growing out. Most of these treatments have to be repeated every three or four months, depending on how quickly hair grows—with very short hairstyles sometimes sooner because the hair is cut more frequently.

You also can select a styling method that requires a body perm or chemical straightener. New product formulas are mild enough not to damage your hair, even though the treatments have to be repeated with some frequency to maintain the style you have selected. I really oppose home treatment products for this purpose, because it takes the skill and experience of a professional to apply and time the product correctly to prevent hair damage.

If you want to achieve this type of result at home, I recommend that you work with nonpermanent methods like setting lotions, gels, mousses, blow dryers, electric rollers, and curling iron. Keep in mind that anything you do with this type of method *will wash off* with your next shampoo. The type of permanent chemical treatment described above takes several months of professional corrective treatments that are costly and require time. So my advice is to leave the chemical treatments to the professionals and stay with the semipermanent treatments for do-it-yourself care.

In this book you will learn hundreds of trade secrets that will enable you to achieve these home tricks with hair aids and appliances. You can dry curly hair straight or add curl and bend to straight hair. You can achieve all kinds of styles with curling irons, hot rollers, mousses, gels, and hair spray. You can wear your hair "wet" and slick, or "wet" and curly. You can look punk or carefree. Whatever effect you want to achieve, you will find a product among the many available on the market to make the task easy. The possibilities are endless, and you will learn all about them in "Styling—The Look That's Right for You," Chapter 6 of this book.

Making the Best of Your Hair

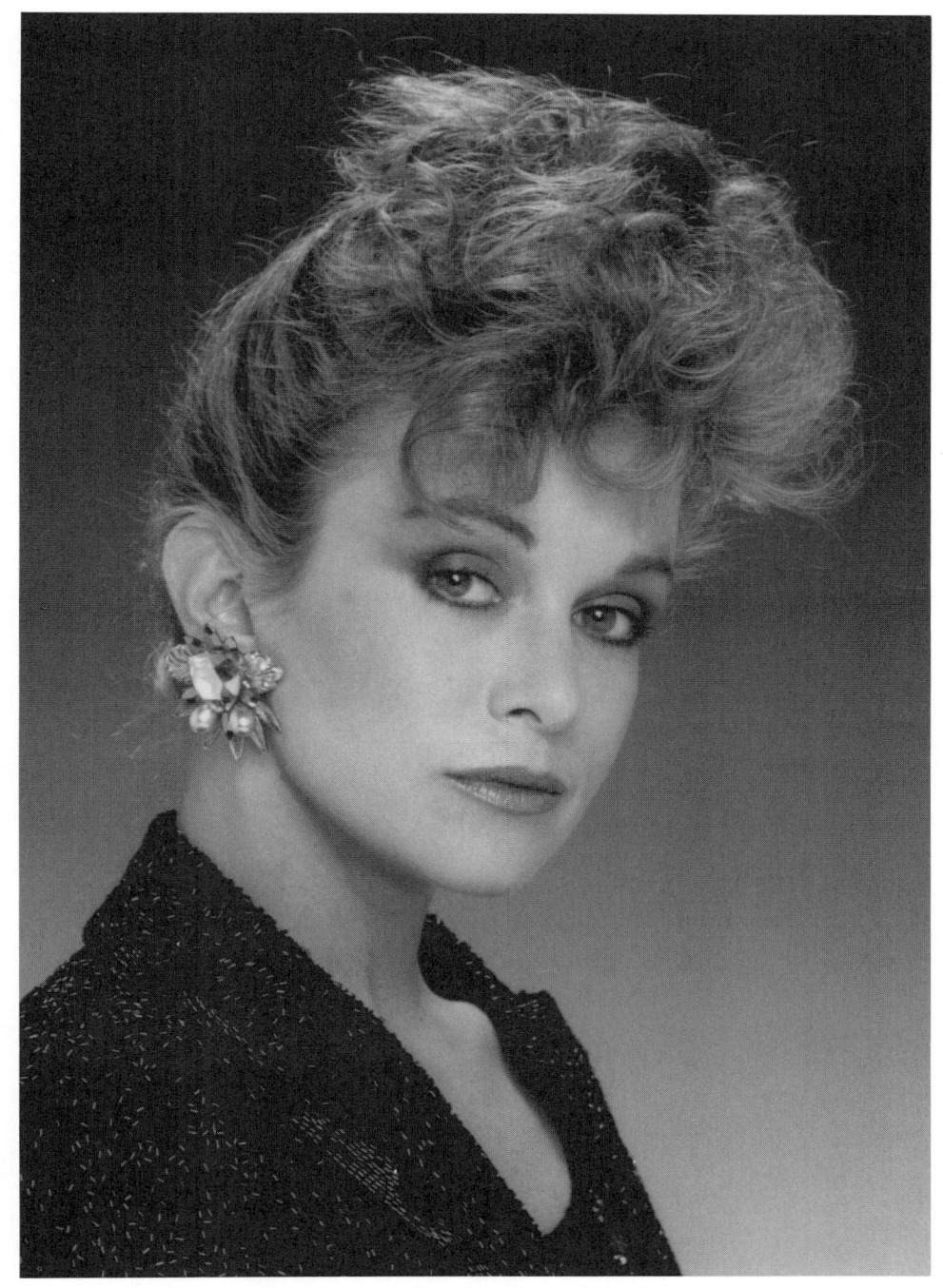

Season Hubley has fine hair, but the density is thin. She needs a layered cut and color highlights to add thickness. Season also looks better with her hair up.

Density

Density describes the volume of hair on your head. This is also taken into consideration when styling. The best way to determine the density of your hair is to examine it when it's wet.

Thin Hair: If your hair density falls into this group, the scalp will show through, in severe cases even when the hair is dry. This type of hair can be straight or have some degree of curl; if curly, it tends to look like the curls on a baby's head. Conditioners, mousses, and gels can make this type of hair flat because the formulas coat the hair with a very heavy film. Sometimes this type of hair density is caused by illness, medication or stress.

Medium Hair: When your hair completely covers your scalp, you have medium density hair. This type of hair, curly or straight, holds any style well and never looks too bushy or too sparse.

Thick Hair: This type of hair looks like a "cap" that covers the entire head, wet or dry. Sometimes, especially when your hair is overdue for a trim or you have the wrong cut, it has a tendency to look bushy and wild. This type of hair requires the proper cut, meticulous maintenance, and the use of styling aids like gel, mousse, or hair spray for control.

Sometimes the same head of hair shows different densities, but many times this is due either to overprocessing with chemical treatments or to the effects of illness and medication. If this condition is related to natural causes, it can be corrected chemically with perms or straighteners. But if it is due to treatment abuse or illness, cutting and conditioning is the prescription until it returns to a manageable state.

Hair Color

Hair color, whether natural or chemical, also determines how you style your hair. As we all know, the hair color we are born with doesn't stay with us forever. Some people have several natural changes of hair color from their birth to their late teens. This usually happens to people born with light hair, which turns darker as they grow older. But people born with dark hair can have the opposite happen: their natural hair color tends to fade with age and as the gray begins to grow in.

Hair color is determined by the same pigment that regulates skin color, and it is called *melanin*. How much melanin is packed into each hair determines the intensity of the color. Hair color not only loses this pigment and turns gray with age; it also fades in the same manner that skin color fades with age. That is why when your first strands of gray hair begin to grow in it is not a good idea to go back to the hair color you had when you were 18 or 20. Older skin no longer has the glow of younger skin, so the new hair color will look harsh and will age instead of enhance skin tones.

It is well known that we don't have to accept for life the hair color we were born with. Natural hair color can be changed in many ways: tinting, a one-process method, lightens or darkens the hair just a few shades by removing the melanin from the cortex and depositing new color. Semipermanent and vegetable dyes deposit color on the surface of the hair and wash off with one or several shampoos. The color change is very minor; it only brightens or intensifies the natural color. Highlights are achieved by bleaching some of the hair several shades lighter and weaving the lighter-color highlights to enhance hair color.

When selecting hair color to enhance your personal style, it is best to stay within a reasonable range. For example, if you are a natural brunette, your skin coloring probably won't look right with very pale blond hair. When adding highlights, keep in mind that they must look natural and believable, so going only four or five shades lighter than the overall color is the best choice. Avoid the old-fashioned and fake-looking striped light and dark look. The purpose of hair color is to enhance your personal style and to help you look natural and believable.

MAKING THE MOST OF YOUR HAIR

All the stars that were photographed for this book are following my advice to make the most of their hair. These women are constantly in the public eye, and I am not always around to do their hair, so they must be able to do it themselves and always look the same.

Also, they all have different types of hair—as different as their looks and styles. Some are blonds with baby-fine hair; others are blonds with very wavy, coarse hair. Some of the brunettes have coarse and curly hair, while others have abundant thin hair. There are also black women with different types of hair textures and Oriental women. Yet they all have one thing in common—they all have great-looking, manageable, wearable hairstyles.

There are a number of hair aids and helpers that can work miracles with your hair. Some of these are temporary measures like mousse, gel, sculpting lotion, and hair spray. Others—like perms, cutting, and hair color—offer more permanent results. We will discuss each one, what it does, and how to use it in the styling chapter (Chapter 6).

Wigs and hairpieces are other great style aids that are regaining their popularity. As you will see throughout this book, some of my most famous clients sport looks that are their trademark and that are achieved with wigs and hairpieces.

Dolly Parton's signature blond waves are wigs that she wears with her own hair coming out in front, so her own hair line shows. Dolly strives for a glitzy show biz look that is natural and believable. The shimmering cascade of blond waves and curls could easily be Dolly's own hair. Wigs make it easier for her to maintain her look, especially on the road, when I'm not around to do her hair for every performance.

Tina Turner is just the opposite. I designed her wig for the video "We Don't Need Another Hero," and she liked it so much that she decided to keep it for a while. Tina's silver-blond wig ends just below her hips, and the sides of her hair were shaved in a semicircular pattern. Tina is a daring lady, and she wears this truly amazing look like a champ. It is the kind of look that only she can wear.

Barbara Carrera is a brunette with lots of fine hair. A blunt cut works best for her type of hair; layering all over would only accentuate her hair's thinness and make it look sparse when it really is not. Barbara's personal style is also extremely classic; I designed the one-length bob for Barbara to give her the greatest styling versatility. Having one-length hair, she can wear it pulled back, half up and half down, rolled into a "rat" in front, pinned back at the sides with combs and other accessories, or just down and simple in the manner of a classic beauty. I also brightened Barbara's naturally dark hair to a berrywood red to bring out her Latin good looks. The effect is simply magnificent.

Season Hubley has the type of hair that has been given body with the proper cut and color highlights. Season's hair is slightly layered to look like a bob, but the layers add body, movement, and volume and keep the hair from lying flat. The golden highlights on Season's honey-blond hair add thickness and accentuate the movement. Season looks great when she wears her hair up. The upward lines of the up-do "lift" her face and make her look younger.

Erin Gray has a wonderful head of coarse, coffee-brown hair with lots of weight and body. Erin is known for her classic looks. Her bob style with just a dash of soft, piecey bangs is the perfect complement to her good looks. The bangs were added for styling versatility, and she wears them swept to one side or parted most of the time to show off her magnificent face and bone structure. Erin keeps her hair long enough to be able to wear it up or down, as her mood and needs require.

Making the Best of Your Hair

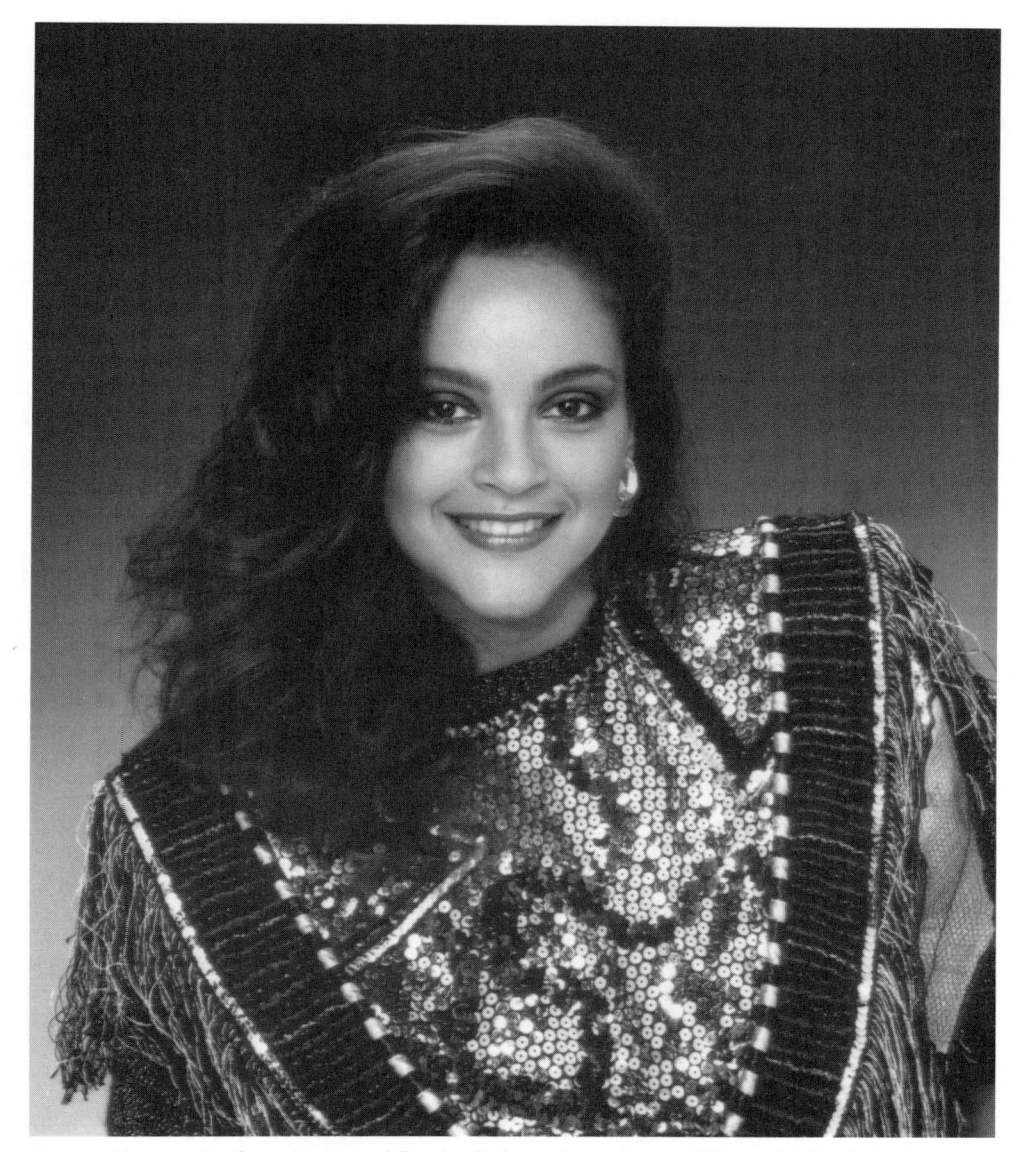

Jayne Kennedy Overton and Roxie Roker show how different black hair can be. Jayne's is silky, full, and heavy. It looks great worn in the loose, long look she prefers.

TOVAR'S CLASSIC BEAUTY

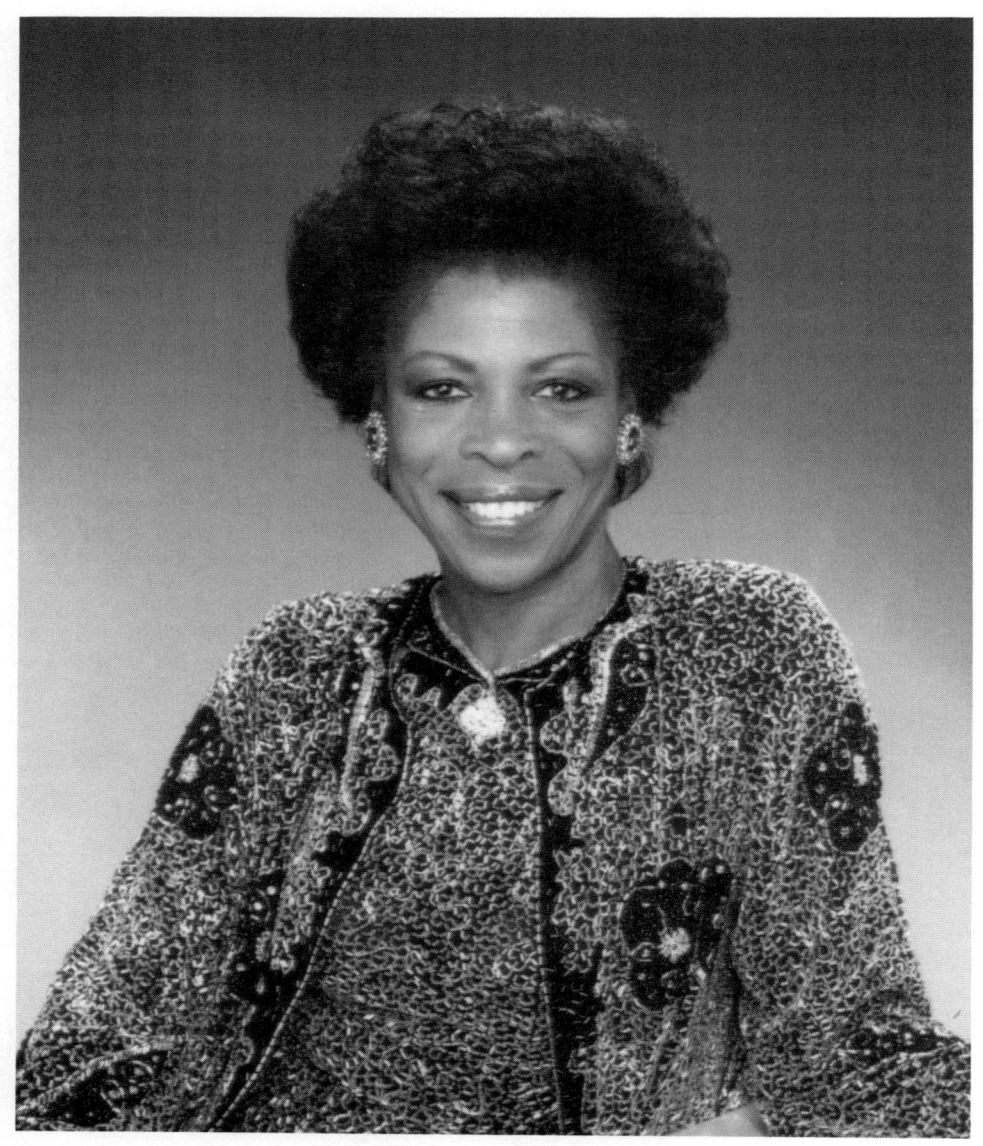

Roxie's hair is coarse, with a very tight curl formation. It looks better short and curly.

Making the Best of Your Hair

Heather Locklear has lots of medium-coarse blond hair, the type of hair I love to work with and can style in a number of different ways. Heather doesn't like the "doey" look, and she prefers to wear her straight hair that way most of the time. Heather's hair must be layered; otherwise, it will look too flat and skimpy. The layers add volume and fullness to her style. Because of the quality of Heather's hair, she can easily go from straight to wavy. All it takes is a quick twisted pin curl set with a touch of mousse added before making pin curls, some squeezing and blow-drying, and . . . presto! Heather has a lovely, wavy mane.

Jayne Kennedy Overton is a perfect example of how good lovely, long hair can look. Long hair is one of the things I am promoting in this book, and many of my star clients have long hair because of the styling versatility it offers. Jayne's hair just cascades down, soft and shining. Her hair is coarse, full, and heavy, yet it is not the typical black hair that is very wiry and curly. Jayne is a very tall woman who needs all that hair to compensate for her height. She is a lovely lady who is very well proportioned and knows exactly what looks good on her. Jayne's hair looks best as she wears it in this book, long and loose.

Roxie Roker is another one of my famous black clients, yet Roxie's hair is as different from Jayne's as their looks are. Roxie has very coarse hair, with a very tight curl formation—what is known as kinky hair. Roxie's hair is chemically straightened periodically, and a short haircut works best for her. Roxie also wears wigs when she wants a different look. For her photos for this book she wore her own hair styled in a softly curled natural wave, then changed to a short bob wig for a totally different look. The moral here: if your own look is limited in styling versatility, don't be afraid to experiment with wigs and hairpieces.

Merete Van Kamp has the type of baby-fine blond hair that is very difficult to handle. Merete prefers to wear her hair straight, so although I think her hair would be easier to handle with a body wave, it is out of the question because she likes wearing voluminous hair. Merete's hair is highlighted, which does add some body. Merete's classic bone structure makes it possible for her to wear her hair either dead-straight and down or in many of the simple up-dos she prefers for evenings.

Brogan Lane has a naturally wild, full head of hair that enhances her incredible good looks. Brogan's vital, bubbly personality and looks are the perfect foil for her very layered cut. Her style is very tousled, almost messy, and she wears it very well. It goes perfectly with her young, almost-wild look.

At my salon I work with women with all types of hair. Regardless of their hair types and limitations, they all expect to come out looking great. It is my job to make that happen; my job is to create that illusion with a combination of haircut, styling, and color and to achieve the effect my client deserves—the very best.

A successful look is a combination of factors, but it is the styling that is very, very important since that is what leaves the lasting impression. No matter how precise my cut and how beautiful the colorist's job, if the style leaves something to be desired, or if my client doesn't like it, she won't like the rest.

I have developed the following chart as a quick, foolproof guide to making the most of your hair. Follow it and you will be very pleased with the results.

TOVAR'S FOOLPROOF GUIDE

Type: Baby-Fine

Cut: Very layered, especially around the crown. The more layers, the more volume. Short on top, but good at all lengths.

Helpers: If the hair is virgin, add perm or color. Virgin hair is very difficult to work with if there is no porosity. Baby-fine hair looks best with highlights or perm.

Color/Perm: Brunettes will most likely have more hair than blonds. Dark hair will also be coarser than light hair. Add color or perm.

Hair Aids: Mousse, hair spray, or anything else that gives hair volume is a must.

Type: Fine

Cut: Not as layered as baby-fine, but still shorter on the crown for volume. Long layers are possible.

Helpers: Same as for baby-fine.

Color/Perm: Same as for baby-fine.

Hair Aids: Same as for baby-fine.

Type: Medium Straight

Cut: Since hair is straight, there are two excellent cutting possibilities: very short hair or one-length hair, with or without bangs.

Helpers: If hair is medium straight and damaged, cut it off. It is better to have short or very short hair that doesn't look damaged than longer damaged hair. If the hair is healthy, leave it as long as you want. A bob is a good cut for this type of hair.

Color/Perm: Medium straight hair will look good in any shade, as long as it complements skin coloring. A body perm is a good idea if you want a style with more excitement.

Hair Aids: Mousse for body. Gel or sculpting lotion for special effects. Straight hair will also look great in braids.

Type: Medium Curly

Cut: All lengths. Hair with body and bounce looks best with layers to bring out natural wave.

Helpers: Medium curly hair that is dry has a tendency to look frizzy. Cut off damaged ends and condition well with a deep-penetrating product. If hair is in good condition, leave it long.

Color/Perm: No perm is necessary for this type of hair. Highlights woven through the hair will bring out the curl.

Hair Aids: Mousse will give it the most volume and bring out the curl. Don't abuse the mousse, or hair will be flattened.

Type: Coarse Curly

Cut: Short, medium, or long length. Can be layered; the amount of layering depends on how much curl—the more curl, the less the layering. The weight of the hair will tame it down.

Helpers: Same as for medium curly hair. Very coarse, curly hair must be conditioned more often than other hair types.

Color/Perm: Do not use more chemicals than are absolutely necessary on this type of hair; it will look overprocessed and dry.

Hair Aids: Gel to control the frizz, or any other type of product that will control the frizz.

Type: Coarse Straight

Cut: All lengths will look great, layered or not. A body perm is possible for those looking for styling excitement.

Helpers: Same as for baby-fine hair.

Color/Perm: Same as for medium straight.

Hair Aids: Depending on the style desired, all hair aids will work well on this type of hair. Play with them, experiment, make your hair a celebration.

Type: Black

Cut: Depending on hair type and styling requirements. If you prefer to wear your hair curly and natural, or as close to its natural stage as possible, then have it layered. If your hair is fairly straight or you have it chemically straightened, you can wear a blunt cut.

Color/Perm: All types of chemical straighteners. One-process coloring, henna, cellophanes, and other types of semipermanent colors.

Helpers: Conditioners that put moisture back in the hair. They should be the deep-penetrating type used with the aid of a hair dryer or other heat source, like a heated cap.

Hair Aids: Mousses, gels, sculpting lotions, anything that will help tame the hair and keep the style.

Type: Oriental

Cut: One-length cuts look best on Oriental hair. Long and silky styles are most becoming.

Helpers: Most Oriental hair has plenty of natural oils to keep it silky and shining. Do not overcondition.

Color/Perm: Stay in the brunette family. Highlights can look harsh and artificial. Keep hair color dark, soft, and natural. If hair is limp, a light body perm is suggested.

Hair Aids: Add a bit of mousse or spray for soft fullness.

HAIRCARE BASICS

No hairstyle will look good if the hair is not in good condition. No matter how creative your hairstyle and how well it looks on you, if your hair is not glossy and shiny, the style will lose most of its appeal. The following are the most important basics for beautiful, healthy hair.

Shampoo

It all begins with clean hair. Most people should wash their hair every day. Only those with extremely dry, brittle hair and black hair should not shampoo daily.

Selecting the shampoo that is right for your hair is as important as selecting the right hairstyle. Shampoos come in formulas for dry, normal, and oily hair. There are also conditioning shampoos, body-building shampoos, color-enhancer shampoos, dandruff shampoos, stripping shampoos, shampoos for everyday users, and shampoos for color-treated and permed hair.

To shampoo properly, you should lather twice. The first wash removes buildup from mousses, gels, hair spray, oils, and pollution. The second finishes the cleansing process. It is not uncommon for your shampoo to suds less during the first wash. At this point most people make the mistake of adding more shampoo. Avoid doing this, because the shampoo won't cleanse any better and because all that soap will be difficult to rinse out, sometimes leaving a film that dulls the hair and makes it hard to manage. Many gentle shampoos are formulated *not to suds* much.

Your hair begins to build a tolerance to one type of shampoo, and it is a good idea to alternate shampoos to get the best benefits from the formula you are using. There are two ways of doing this—One is to alternate every day—use one brand of shampoo one day and another one the following day. Alternate between these two, making sure that both brands are for your hair type. The other way is to finish one bottle of one brand, then start with your alternate brand. Both methods work well. The one to choose should be the one you find easier.

Shampoo your hair with a moderately vigorous scalp massage. This will encourage the blood circulation in the scalp area and be very beneficial to the hair. It also will remove oil and hair products deposited on the scalp.

Conditioning

Conditioning follows shampooing, but a common mistake is to follow every shampoo with a conditioning treatment. If your hair is damaged to the point that only a conditioner will untangle it, you should consider a series of deep conditioning treatments to repair the damage.

There are as many types of conditioners as there are shampoos. You can select from instant conditioners that work in a few minutes, body-building conditioners, conditioners for oily hair, those for permed or color-treated hair, moisturizing conditioners, deep-penetrating conditioners, and products containing all types of natural herbs and moisturizers like aloe.

   Conditioners fall into three categories: instant, which are applied after a shampoo and rinsed out after one to five minutes; deep-penetrating, which are applied to the hair and left on for 10 to 30 minutes and used with a hair dryer; and ampoules, that are applied to the hair and left on. The type you use depends on the condition of your hair.

If Your Hair Is Normal: Use an instant conditioner once or twice a month, especially after a color or perm treatment. To keep your hair in good condition, have a professional deep-penetrating treatment about every six months. At the end of summer and in the spring are good times to do it.

If Your Hair Is Oily: There are conditioners for oily hair, and once-a-month applications are fine. Be careful not to use too much product; it can only weigh your hair down and make it limp. And apply the product only to the ends. Avoid the roots, since they have enough natural oils to keep them in good condition.

If You Have Chemically Treated Hair: Color and perms rob the hair of natural oils and can sometimes make it look dull. Condition hair regularly, maybe twice a week, with a specially formulated conditioner. Use a detangler after shampoos. Professional deep-penetrating conditioners should be applied once a month, more often (follow beautician's advice) if the hair has been overprocessed, until it's back in good health.

If You Have Fine Hair: If your hair is in good condition, follow the same advice as for oily hair. If it is dry and damaged, apply conditioner at home, but only twice a week and only to the ends. Be sure not to use too much product and to rinse off well, so hair is not weighed down and appearing limp. Follow a prescribed routine of salon treatments.

If You Have Black Hair: If your hair is chemically treated, use a very oily conditioner with fatty amino acids to put moisture back into your hair. Condition hair three times a week. Also follow a regular program of salon treatments as prescribed by your beautician.

Special Treatments

I recommend special stripping treatments at the salon every three to four months to remove all the buildup—from mousses, gels, hair spray, and other hair preparations—that regular shampooing doesn't remove. These treatments should be done professionally. Just before a perm or a coloring process is an ideal time as the treatments prepare the hair for better absorption of the chemical treatments.

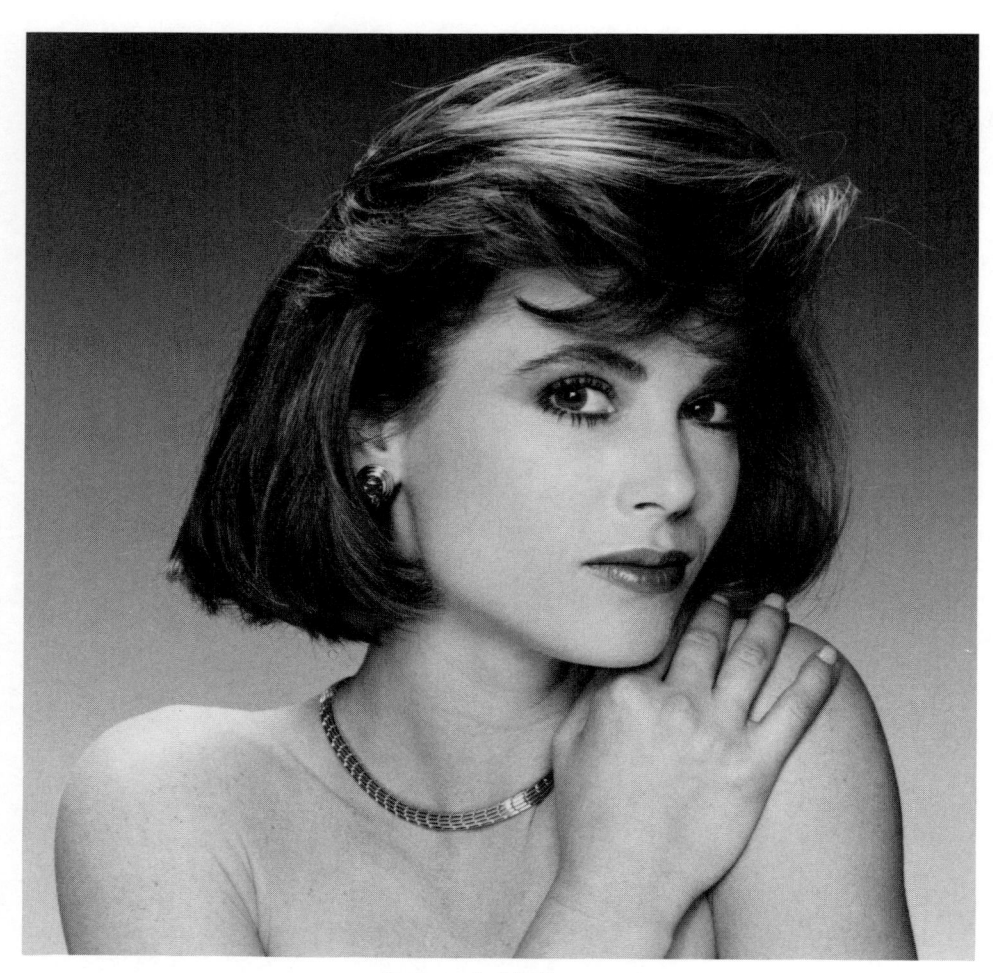

Deborah Mullowney

4
THE CUT

A great haircut is what makes a hairstyle look great. The right haircut makes the hair fall right into place as the style is finished. The right haircut makes it easy for you to maintain between salon appointments the style your hairdresser designed. And the right haircut must be tailored to the type of hair, face, and lifestyle—hence my philosophy of tailoring every haircut individually to the client.

The haircut is the foundation of any style. The way your hair is cut determines the finished results. If you like to wear your hair with some fullness, it should be cut in layers. If you like to wear a sleek bob, your hair would probably look best if it is cut blunt. Whatever your hairstyle preference, the right haircut is necessary for the best results.

Hair that is cut properly always looks good—even when wet or after not much fussing with a blow dryer. A haircut is something that should be left to a professional—it is not a do-it-yourself project. Haircutting is the most difficult subject for me to explain. I believe that one has to be born with the creative ability to be able to cut hair. Either you are a good haircutter or you are not—it is possible for one to learn how to do a particular haircut or a new technique, but one can't learn to be creative.

I am a creative haircutter, and when I cut a woman's hair, I feel that cut. One of my clients whose hair is always cut in a one-length blunt bob asked me how could I get her hair even on both sides. She was surprised when I told her that it wasn't by measuring, because you can't measure hair using the face as a guide as most faces are not the same on both sides. So I explained to her that I feel the length of the hair and that I just can see when the length is perfect.

Those mirrors in front of the cutting areas are not for the woman to look at herself. They are for the hairstylist to look at her and keep control of the outcome of the haircut or style. I cut hair in the same way experienced chefs cook—a pinch of this and a dash of that. I just feel what I am doing and look in the mirror to see the hair taking shape and form, enhancing the bone structure and bringing out the features.

The best haircut for you depends on your hair type. There are many ways to cut hair, using different techniques and tools. Some hairstylists prefer to cut the hair wet, others when it is dry. All methods work as long as your stylist uses the one that is best for you. There is a successful way to cut every type of hair, and that is why it takes a trained professional to do it.

CUTTING TOOLS

The most important tool for a haircut is the scissors. I do most of my cutting with smaller scissors, four to five inches long. This is a matter of personal preference. Other haircutters may prefer to work with larger scissors, six to seven inches long. I prefer the smaller ones because I use a very precise cutting technique, and I find this size just right for my needs.

I have developed my own method of cutting hair. One of the things I don't do is section the hair before cutting. I do all the sectioning in my mind, and I know exactly what I will be doing with that hair. As I said before, I feel my cuts.

I finish a lot of haircuts with thinning shears or tapering shears (as they are known in the trade). These shears have one smooth blade and one grooved blade that does the thinning. I use this technique to finish the ends of a blunt cut on fine hair because this gives extra volume to the ends. This cutting technique gives extra oomph to the hairstyle; it literally makes the hair explode with fullness. I also use these shears for very short cuts, because by cutting the hair in this manner I get that extra pop—that fullness that adds volume to the style. I use the same technique to cut wispy bangs.

TYPES OF HAIRCUTS

Here is a quick description of the different types of haircuts and the types of hair they are suitable for.

The Cut

Blunt Cut: All one length or layer, depending on the type of hair. Heavier hair can be cut either way, but fine hair should be layered. The hair is cut with scissors and can be finished with thinning shears for added volume.

Feathered or Thinner Cut: Some types of coarse and wiry hair have to be cut this way to remove the bulk. All feathered cuts should be layered.

Tapered Cut: The hair is layered and graduated in thinness to remove the bulk and control the lines of the style. I use a lot of tapering at the crown, especially when I am doing a very short haircut. This is ideal to give movement to a style.

Thinning: I usually apply this technique when cutting the bang area for a lighter, airier look. But thinning is also a good way to help control the thickness of very wiry or curly hair.

WHICH TYPE IS BEST FOR YOU?

Fine and Abundant Hair: A blunt or semiblunt cut with tapered ends will add more body and volume to fine, abundant hair. The layering also achieves the same effect. If you let this type of hair grow too long, it will look stringy.

Fine and Sparse Hair: Blunt-cut the ends for an illusion of thickness. Baby-fine hair should not be allowed to get too long, as the ends will tend to look skimpy. Layering is also recommended for adding volume and fullness.

Medium Straight Hair: One-length or layered blunt cuts. This is the type of hair that looks good in almost any haircut.

Medium Curly Hair: Layered cuts are best. How much layering depends on the curliness of the hair. The less the curl, the more the layering. Too much layering on very curly hair can give it too wild a look.

Coarse and Curly Hair: A controlled, layered cut works best for this type of hair. The ends should be layered and thinned to remove the bulk. Regular trimmings are essential to keep the shape of the style.

Coarse and Wiry Hair: A tapered and layered cut is best for this type of hair. The bulk can be reduced by thinning with the proper shears. A short cut or a longer style both work well. With a longer style, the weight of the hair pulls it straight.

BANGS

Cutting Techniques

Bumper Bangs: Full, heavy bangs that are blunt-cut. They look good only on those with very classic or very unusual features.

Wispy Bangs: The hair is thinned or slithered, section by section, to remove fullness and bulk in an uneven manner. Some sections of the hair should be shorter than others. These bangs look great on almost everyone, except those with low foreheads.

Who Looks Great with Bangs

Heather Locklear: Hers are the most versatile bangs. Heather looks great with either straight or scrunched bangs. I cut her bangs so they are full and chunky to obtain the greatest number of styling possibilities.

Abby Dalton: Perfect proof that bangs can be youthful—she looks great in those "rockabilly" pompadour bangs she wears with her silver outfit.

Rosalind Chao: The updated "China Doll" look—nothing boring or traditional about her look. She wears pointy, piecey bangs that look very hot and new.

Merete Van Kamp: The beauty that breaks all the rules and gets away with it because of her magnificent looks. Merete's classic features allow her to wear full, generous bumper bangs. And she looks great with them off her face, too.

Deborah Mullowney: Her bangs are used to correct facial flaws, a very high forehead here. But this look is fashionable and elegant—a true classic beauty.

THE CUT: HOW LONG OR SHORT?

I like extremes—either very short or very long hair. By long hair, I mean anywhere from shoulder length to about four inches below. Long hair is coming back into the hair fashion scene, although it has always been the trademark or signature style of most classic beauties. But you should be free to use a length that suits you. Here are the best lengths:

The Cut

Jayne Kennedy Overton: She is very tall and has tons of wonderful, thick hair. She needs that length to balance her height; she has the kind of presence that can carry off all that hair.

Claire Yarlett: She has a fabulous face, almost perfect and flawless. Claire is a true natural beauty. All that luxurious, natural blond hair is just perfect for her look. She just looks magnificent.

Debi Richter: She proves that thick, wavy hair can be worn long if it is styled correctly. In this case, either pinned off at the sides, if worn loose, or braided for a neat, smaller-head look. Both are just great looks for Debi.

Barbara Carrera: Going shorter doesn't have to mean a drastic change. I recently shortened Barbara's hair by about four inches to update her look—and she looks better than ever!

Brogan Lane: Wild hair can look wonderful if it goes with your own personal style, as in Brogan's case. She is a young, exciting beauty, yet she is a classic in her very own and unique wild way. Her look is just like her—young, exciting, and very beautiful.

Priscilla Barnes: Why fight nature? This is the way she feels, and she loves her slightly layered, sleek look—a classic, blunt-cut bob. Priscilla likes to show off her delicate silvery blond hair color, achieved by weaving soft highlights through her hair. This type of coloring requires a totally simple style.

Ellen Bry: Thick, curly hair doesn't have to be cut very short to be controlled. It is all in the cut and style. Ellen's hair could be wild and uncontrollable if cut improperly. I use the thinning technique on the ends of her layered cut, and her hair behaves any way she wants.

Roxie Roker: Typical black hair looks best in a short, layered cut that makes the best of the natural curl. Roxie switches to wigs and hairpieces when she wants to wear a sleeker, straight look. This also helps prevent hair damage caused by using hot appliances on this type of fragile hair.

Abby Dalton: Short hair can take years off, and this over-40 beauty looks really hot with any of her short-short cuts. Another point emphasized here is that when hair is styled properly, even women "of a certain age" can go for severe, trendy looks.

Emmylou Harris: Here is proof that the right hairstyle can almost work miracles. Emmylou's "old" look was too long, plain, and straight. Now she looks wonderful with her layered haircut, which gets added support from a body perm and highlights.

TOVAR'S CLASSIC BEAUTY

A HAIRCUT MAKEOVER

Model Jessica Norman Pappas is a young woman with good-quality, thick blond hair. Jessica's hair is basically straight, but it holds the curl well because it has some natural bend to it. Jessica came to me for a haircut but wanted to keep the basic lines of her classic bob. Her style was badly in need of shaping and movement.

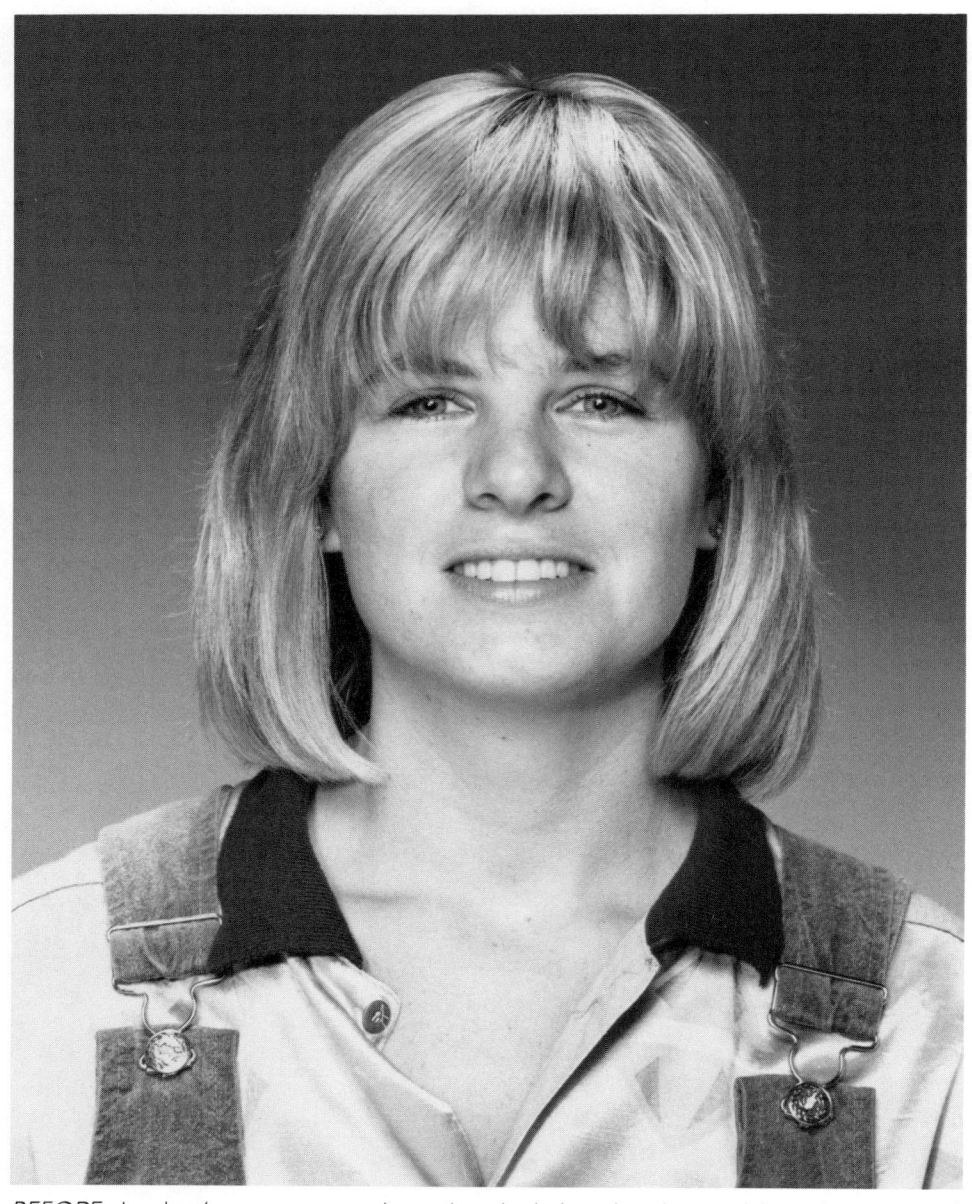

BEFORE: Jessica's overgrown, shapeless bob has too-long, stringy bangs and is too bulky and shapeless at the ends.

The Cut

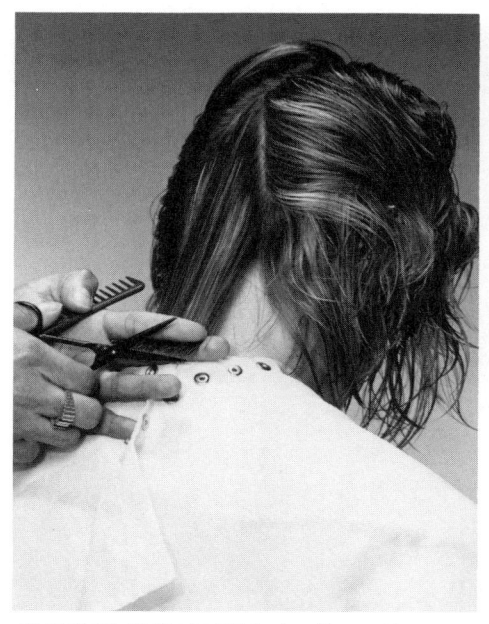

CUTTING THE NAPE: I don't section the hair on the customer's head as many stylists do; I keep the sectioning in my head. It is easier for me to visualize the cut this way.

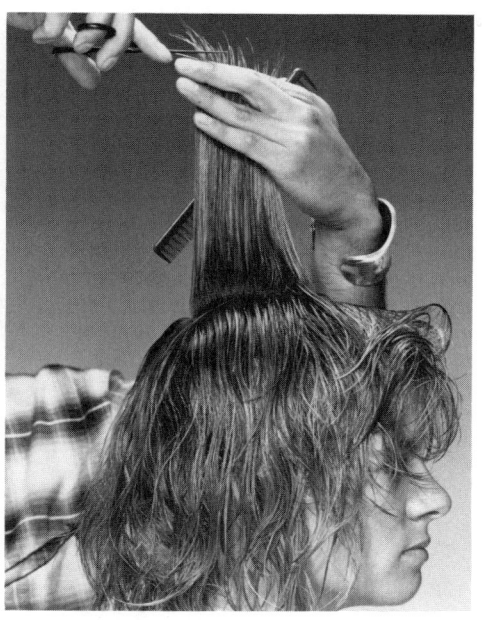

THINNING THE ENDS: Here is how I do my famous finishing technique. It adds volume and fullness to the ends when the hair is dried.

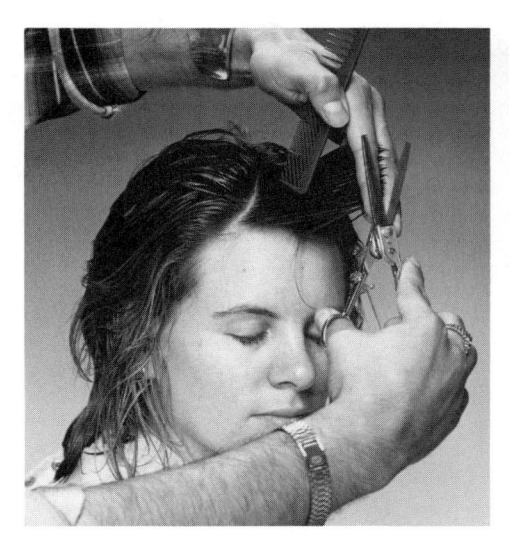

THINNING THE BANGS: This technique is essential to add versatility to the bangs.

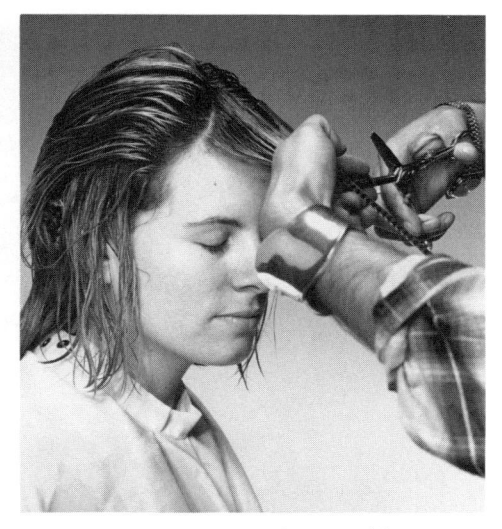

If the bangs are too full and heavy, she won't be able to wear them in different ways.

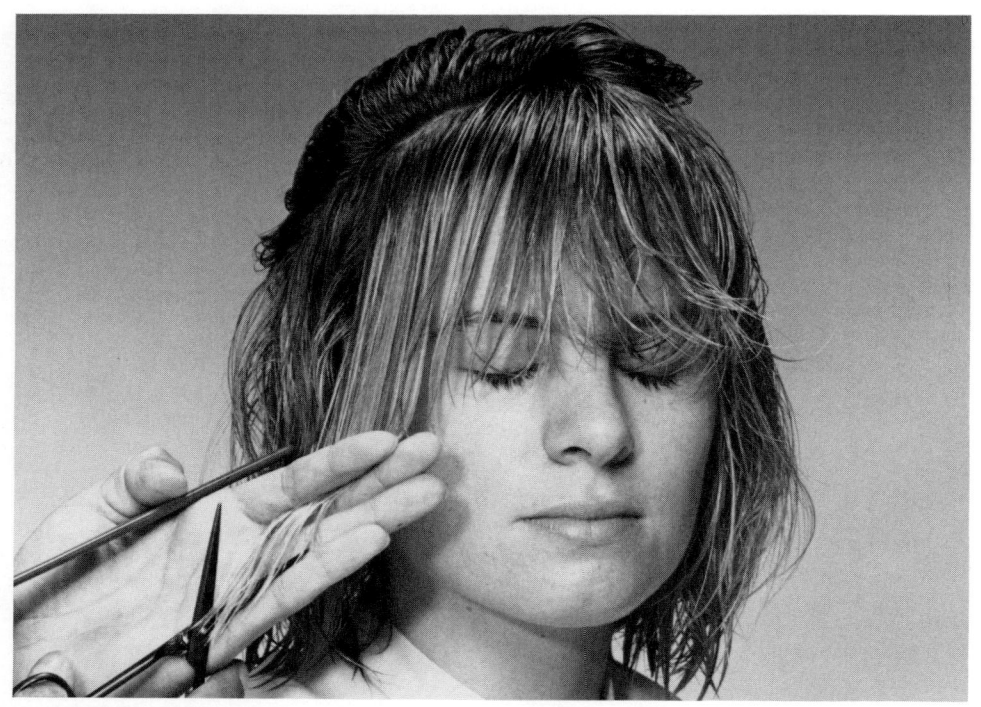

LAYERING THE SIDES: This part is important to keep the style from emphasizing the parts of the face it should not emphasize.

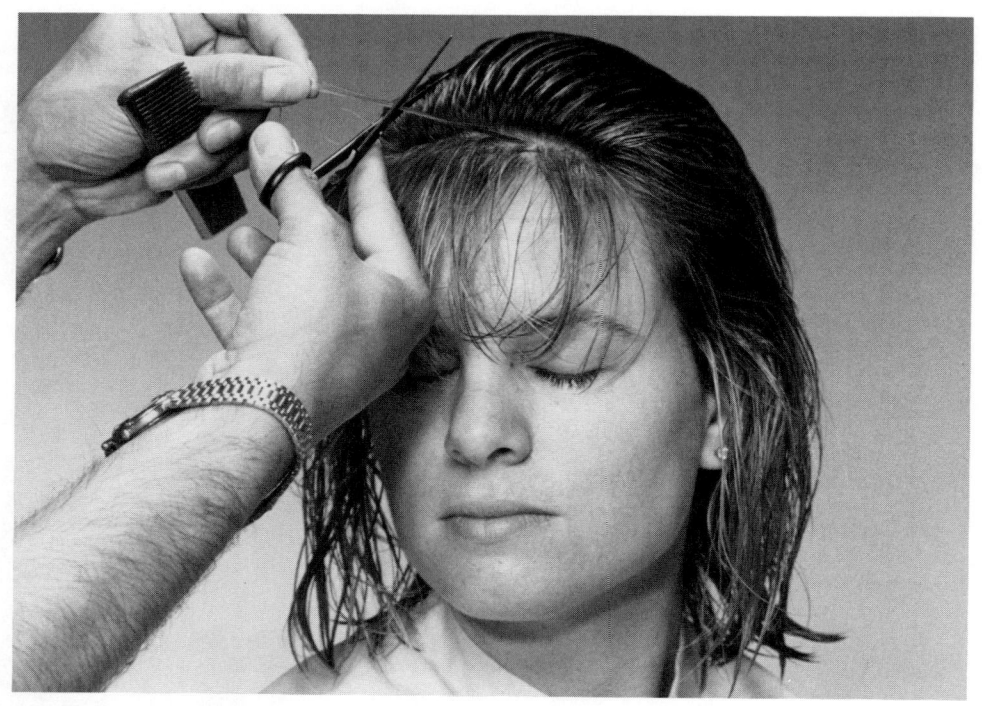

SLITHERING THE BANGS: This technique is essential to obtain that wispy look that allows for the greatest styling versatility. It is very becoming to most faces.

The Cut

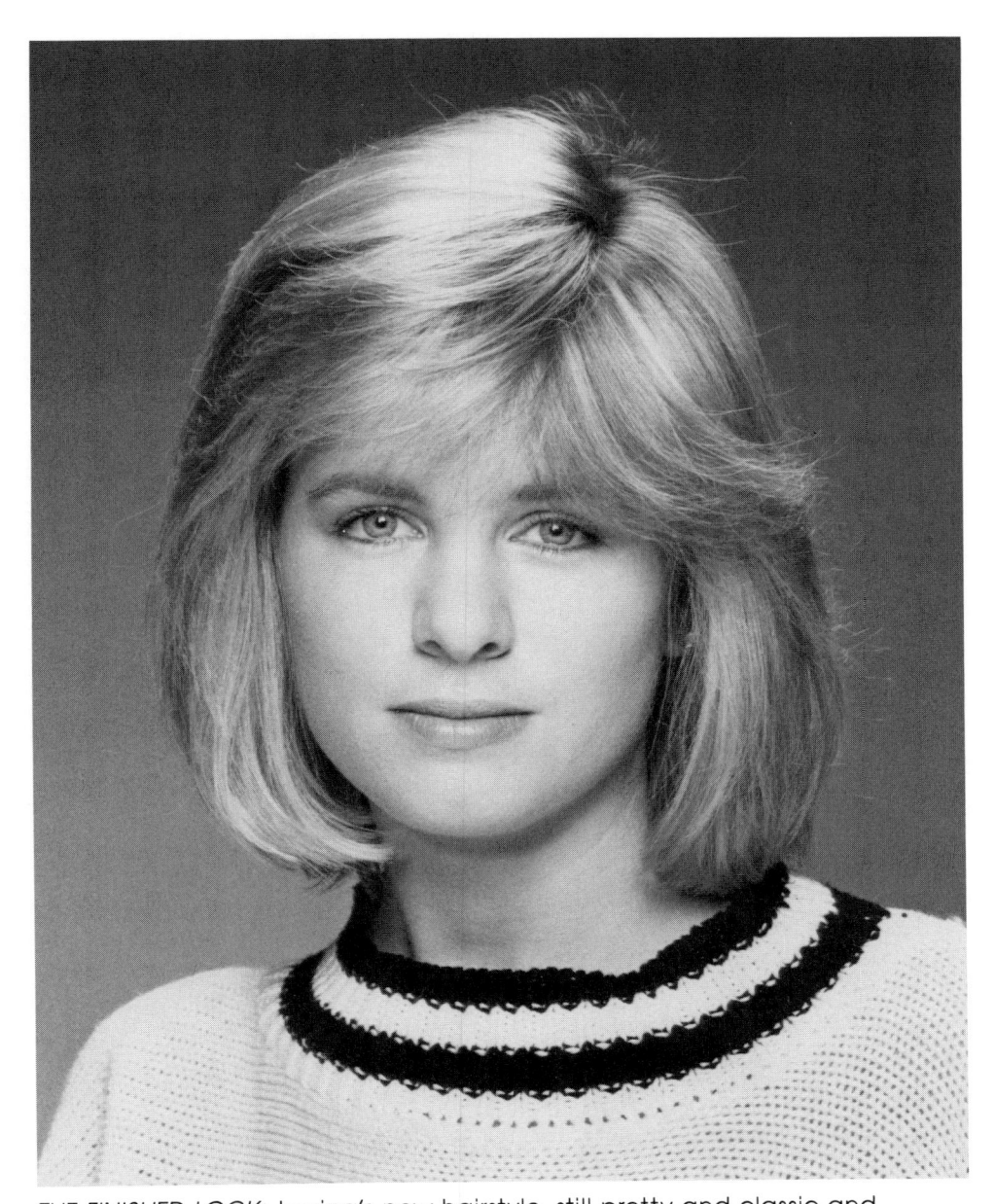

THE FINISHED LOOK: Jessica's new hairstyle, still pretty and classic and perfect for her. Yet note the subtle changes and their effects. A side part instead of a center part gives better balance to her features (only perfect features can get away with center parts); the thinner, side-swept bangs with new movement emphasize her pretty eyes; the overall smooth, round style presents a very becoming look.

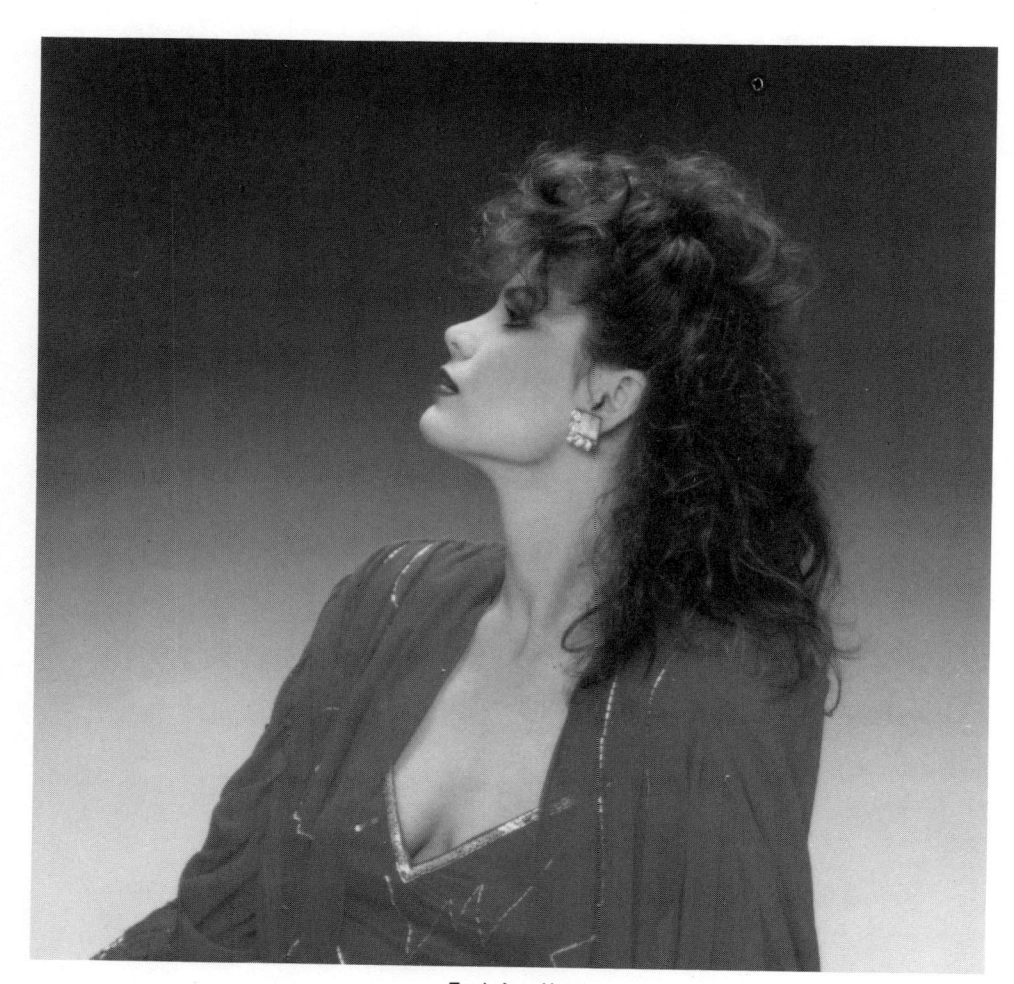

Teri Austin

5
COLOR AND PERMS

Today's hair treatment science has advanced by leaps and bounds. Years ago, chemical treatments—color and perms—were for the very daring. Those were the days when a woman could be called a "bleached blond" and when the results of a wave left a lot to be desired.

New technology takes the guesswork out of chemical treatments, and most preparations produce great results if used at the salon or at home according to directions. While there are certain types of chemical treatments (some types of color) that can be used safely at home, others (like perms and straighteners) require the skill and training of a professional and should be done only in the salon.

HAIR COLOR

Hair color is used like makeup for the hair. It is used to enhance and correct, and it can change the texture and behavior of the hair. The right hair color can brighten dull or faded hair, add shine and volume, bring out the eyes, and correct skin tones.

The best color changes are subtle and natural. Color should never be a drastic change, for only in very few instances are drastic color changes going to look natural. A natural look should be the principal goal of any chemical treatment.

The following is a recap of the latest in hair color:

Chemical Color

Permanent Tints: Available in cream, lotion, or shampoo-in formulas (usually for home use). The products are designed to work when mixed with peroxide (an oxidizing agent) that allows the color formula to penetrate the hair shaft to the cortex layer, strip the natural hair color, and deposit the new color. The color results with this method are permanent, but new growth at the roots requires touch-ups every four to six weeks. If doing this type of coloring method at home, be sure to follow instructions strictly, to apply color to the roots only to avoid overlapping, and to remember the patch test.

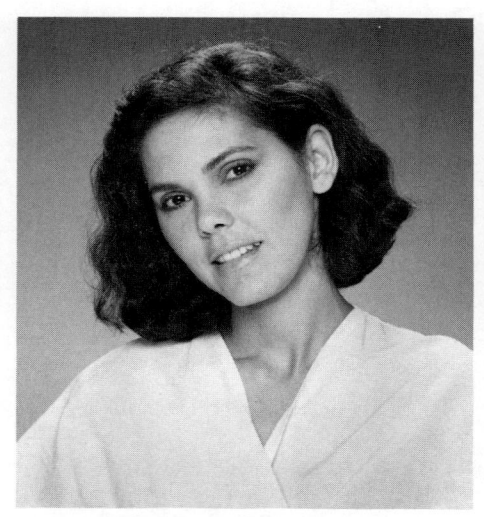

TINTING: Model Nastassia Henson's roots show the regrowth.

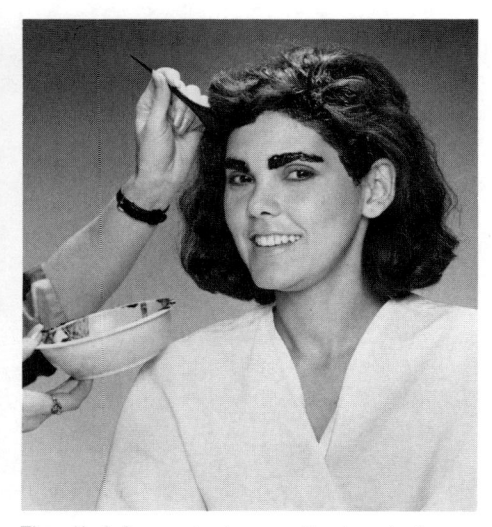

The tint formula is applied only to the roots for a touch-up.

A note of caution: if you are changing shades after using a permanent tint—e.g., going from a reddish brown to a golden brown—be sure to have it done professionally for best color results. Never use any type of hair color formula to tint lashes and brows.

Semipermanent Tints: These formulas contain no peroxide, and they are used without mixing. This type of product works by depositing the color on the transparent cortex layer of the hair. The best results from this method occur when going to a darker shade or brightening dull hair. Cellophanes fall into this product category. Color lasts from four to six shampoos, and it fades without leaving a regrowth line. If processing at home, remember to use the product as directed and to do the patch test.

Color and Perms

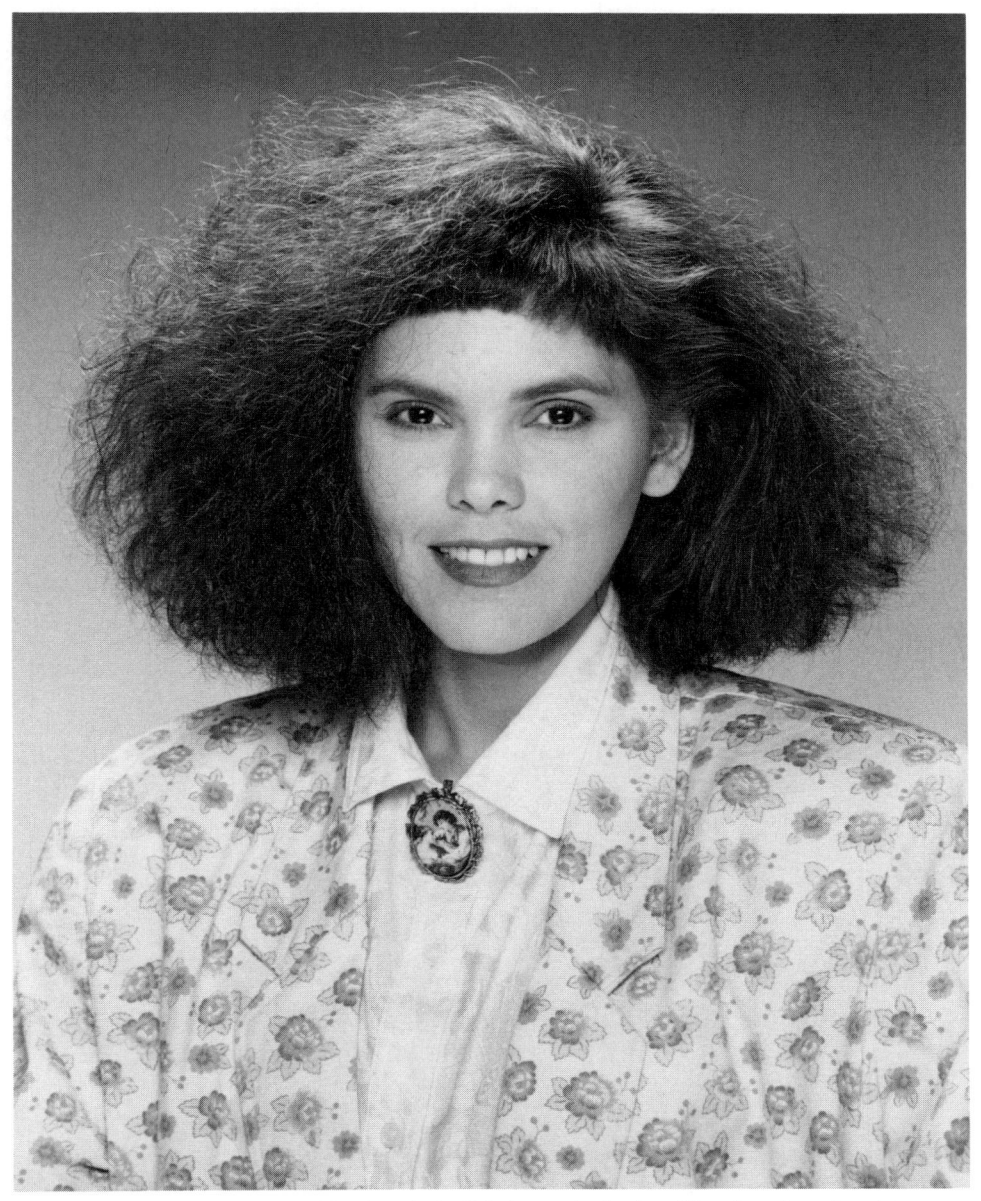

THE FINISHED STYLE: I cut Nastassia's thick, curly hair with chunky, short bangs and a blunt cut. Then the hair is scrunched with some mousse for lots of fullness.

Temporary Rinses: This type of hair color product coats the hair without penetrating the hair shaft. There are two types of temporary rinses: the natural color enhancers that brighten hair color and cover gray and the fun colors (pinks, reds, purples, blues, and greens) that are used on light hair for a festive effect. These colors last only until the hair is shampooed. If using them at home, follow directions carefully, being careful not to overuse the product, which can cause dull hair.

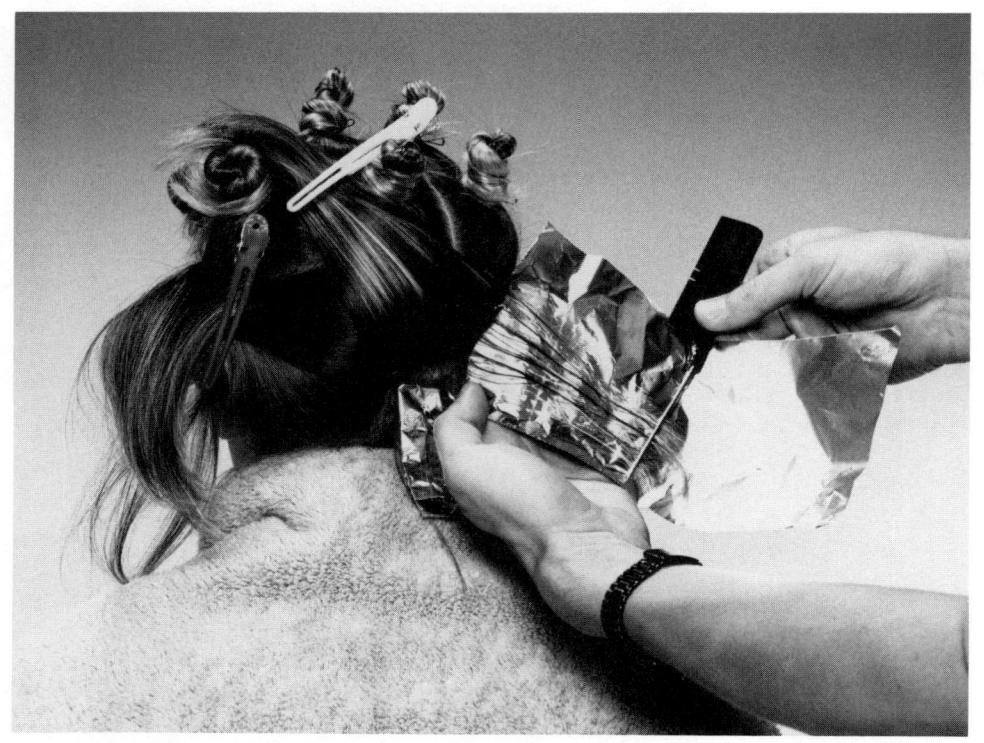

HIGHLIGHTS: Very thin strands of hair are selected, covered with coloring formula, and wrapped in foil for processing.

Highlights and Lowlights: Peroxide and ammonia-based color formulas are applied to predetermined strands of hair to create color depth. This coloring method is ideal for adding body and volume to the hair, which happens because the color treatment makes the hair porous. Highlights look best on blonds whose hair is getting darker or gray and on those with red or brown hair that is beginning to look dull. Highlights should never be more than five or six shades lighter than the base color of the hair. Highlights should never be a do-it-yourself project.

Metallic Colors: Hair color sprays make up this color group. They coat the hair with color. Color sprays come in metallic shades of gold and silver. The effect is most attractive on lighter hair shades. Don't use this type of color if you have tinted hair, as it can turn green (light shades) or brassy. Color lasts until shampooed or brushed out, but invisible metallic residue can remain on the hair, so have a colorist do a strand test if you've been using this kind of product and are considering a color treatment.

Vegetable (Natural) Colors

Henna: A natural red staining product of plant origin that coats the cuticle or the transparent layer of the hair with color. Henna comes in red or neutral (no-color) shades, and it can be mixed with other natural substances for color variations—e.g., black coffee for brown or red wine for a light mahogany. But no-color henna also can be used as a conditioner and to make hair shiny without changing the color. Henna is a permanent color change, and the roots need touching up every six to eight weeks.

Henna should not be used by anyone with light colored or gray hair, as the color result will be a carrot-top red. Because henna is a natural substance, it is very difficult to control the color results. Thus it should be applied professionally. Henna is a metal-based hair color, so an improper color application can cause severe damage to the hair. Because of its metallic base, henna also remains on the hair long after the color is gone; this is another reason to have it applied professionally. Never apply a chemical hair tint to hair that has been colored with henna, as the combination can cause severe hair breakage. A professional colorist can perform a strand test to make sure there is no invisible henna buildup on the hair.

Chamomile: To be used only on natural blond hair as a brightener. Chamomile can be mixed with other natural ingredients for different effects, such as a light bleaching action or the addition of a golden hue. The color change produced is permanent.

Marigold: Best results are obtained when used on blond or white hair. When applied to blond hair, the color obtained is a rich golden shade. On white it is a soft, golden yellow.

Dark "Teas": These formulas are obtained by boiling a number of natural substances to darken medium to dark or gray hair. These strong infusions, very much like teas, can be combined with ground cloves, ground walnuts, sage, or the bark of dark wood trees like oak to obtain different color results. Let your colorist advise you on the best formula for your hair's needs.

Rhubarb Root: This is one of the most effective of all the herbal lighteners. It works on all shades of hair to lighten and add highlights.

A note of caution: Natural hair colors are fun to use, but they can be very tricky and the results unpredictable. Therefore, they are best left to the expertise of a professional.

CARE OF COLORED HAIR

Although color is probably the mildest of all chemical treatments, any type of hair that has been chemically treated is fragile hair that requires lots of TLC.

- Don't overshampoo colored hair, and be sure to use preparations formulated specially for this type of hair. Shampoo hair with a gentle finger massage. Never rub the hair, since any type of chemical treatment makes the hair somewhat porous, which can make the hair tangle if handled roughly.

- Condition hair, following your stylist's advice. Use an instant conditioner after every shampoo to make detangling easy. Condition with a deep-penetrating product once a month, or more often if your hair is dry or damaged.

- Follow other dos and don'ts for colored hair as part of your hair care regimen.

Color Dos and Don'ts

Do . . .

keep up your touch-ups. Nothing can make a head of hair look worse than roots growing out. Tinted hair requires monthly touch-ups. Highlight touch-ups should be repeated three or four times a year.

Do . . .

protect your hair at all times. Wear swimcaps in the pool or ocean, beach hats or scarves under the sun. Select hair products that contain sunscreens for extra protection.

Do . . .

when covering gray, select a shade only a few shades lighter than your natural color. Never go darker, or the results will look fake.

Color and Perms

Do...

condition regularly. Once a week, have deep conditioning salon treatments. Two or three times a week, use an instant conditioner after your shampoo.

Do...

wait at least one week after a perm to have your hair colored or touched up.

Do...

have perms and other chemical treatments done by a professional in the salon. It takes special skill and knowledge to handle all the different chemicals and their reactions to each other.

Do...

keep up hair trims to get rid of split or damaged ends caused by chemical treatments.

Don't...

use shampoos, such as dandruff shampoos, that have a strong detergent content. They strip the color off the hair and make the hair dry.

Don't...

use a hair-coloring product if there are open wounds or abrasions on the scalp or any feeling of soreness.

Don't...

try to let your natural color grow out naturally. Nothing is more dreadful than two-tone hair. If you want to let your natural color grow out, tint it. Or, in the case of damaged hair, use a nonperoxide, semipermanent product. And have it done professionally for best results.

Don't . . .

rely for shade selection on the colors shown on the front of packages or on color charts. These show how colors look on pure white hair.

Don't . . .

overshampoo your hair. Colored hair should be washed two or three times a week, not daily. Be sure to select a mild shampoo formulated specially for tinted hair.

Don't . . .

get light blond highlights if you have very dark hair. You will end up with a striped effect that is too fake. And *don't* use a bleach to lighten hair. It will leave it dull, lifeless, and dry!

PERMS

Once upon a time, perms used to curl the hair, most of the time not very successfully. The curl of the old perms was usually too tight or didn't "take" at all. Today's perms can offer a variety of options, curls being just one of them. Now a perm can give body, volume, and shape; make thin hair look thicker; and straighten very curly hair.

Perm waving lotion breaks the bonds in straight hair, changing the structure to add curl, wave, or bend. A benefit of this process is that chemically treated hair is not at the whim of heat and humidity, and your style will remain perfect without drooping (if your hair is limp and thin) or frizzing (if your hair is curly).

A Perm Is a Perm . . . or Is It?

Perms have evolved from the old-fashioned cold waves, to the frizzy looks of the 1970s to the wide range of perms available today. Today there is a perm for everyone. The following is a listing of perm choices with explanations of how they work.

Body Wave: Now that hairstyles have gotten away from that "wild" look, this is the most popular type of perm. Hair is wound on large rods for a looser wave (rather than a tight curl), and the waving solution is timed to produce the looser, wavier results. A body wave is perfect for thin, limp hair; it adds fullness and bend without adding curl. Short hair can be dried naturally or blown dry. Longer hair requires blow-drying.

Color and Perms

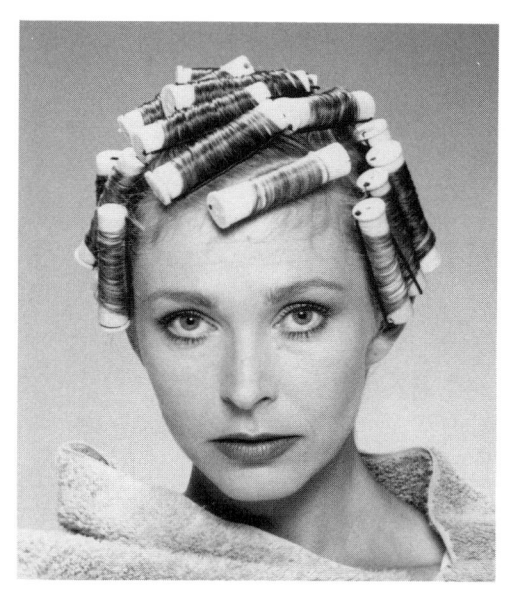

A BODY WAVE: All of model Alana Persson's hair is wrapped in large-size rods for a loose wave with lots of fullness and volume.

Root Perm: The hair at the roots is wound on perm rods to give the finished hairstyle volume without curls. Root perms are perfect for touching up a perm that is growing out or to add fullness to very short, layered hair. Only a skilled professional should handle this process.

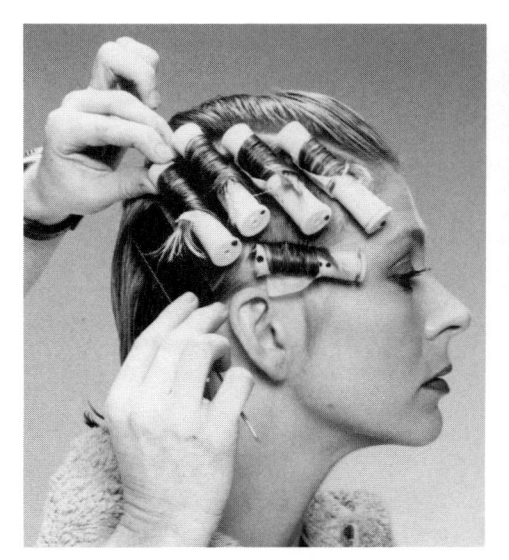

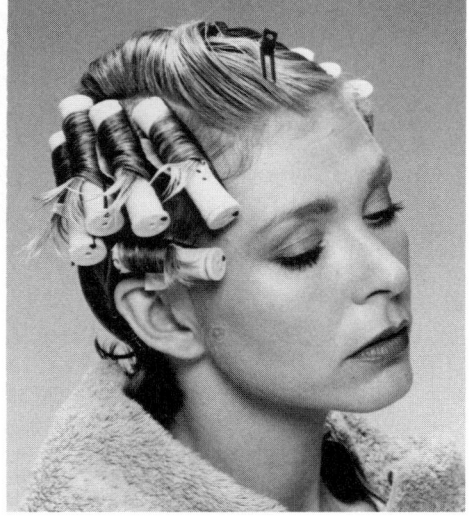

A ROOT PERM: The hair is wrapped around medium rods. Note how the ends are left loose to keep them from curling.

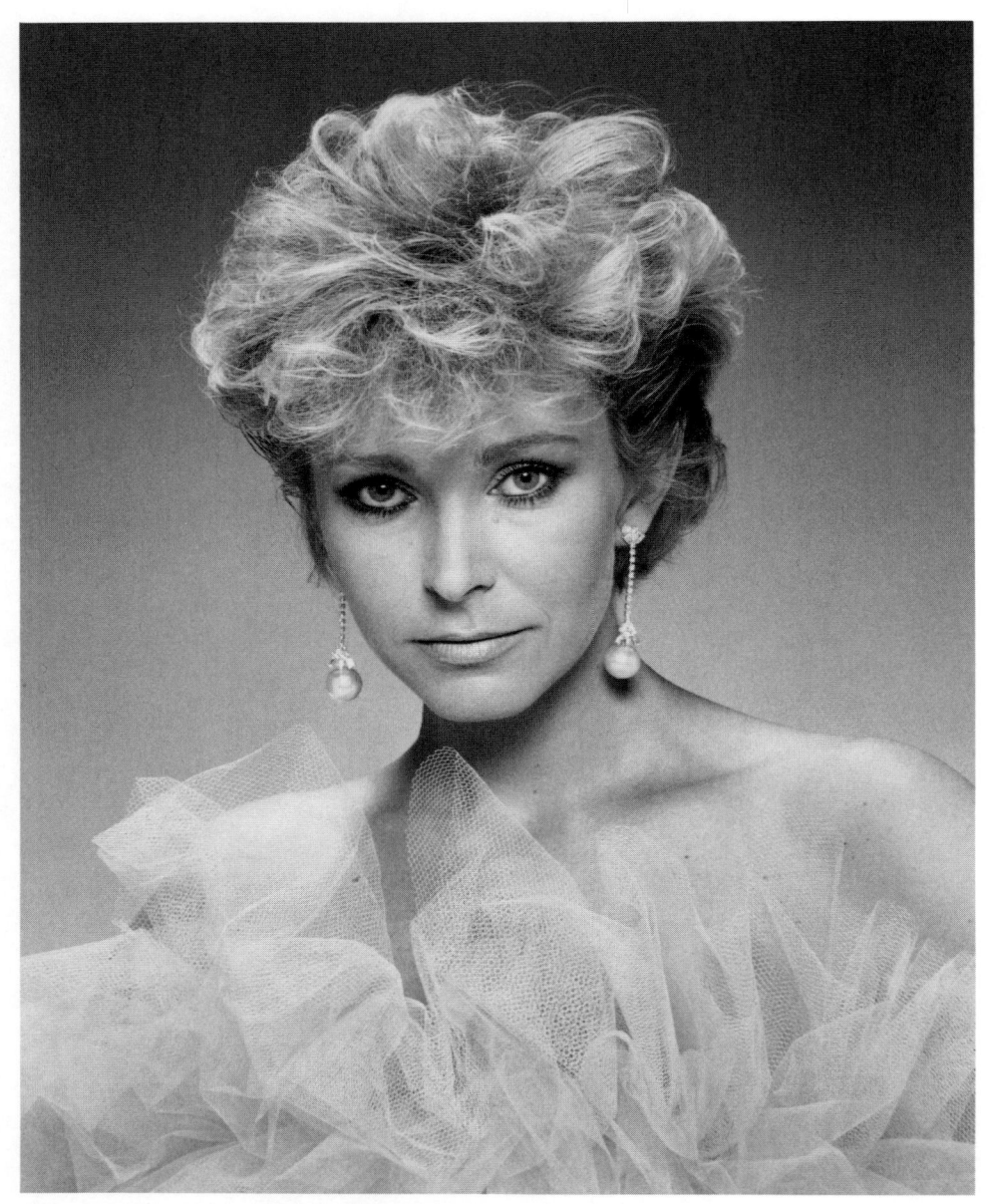

STYLING VERSATILITY WITH A PERM: Alana's crown hair is styled in loose curls coming forward over the forehead. The sides are slicked back with gel.

Color and Perms

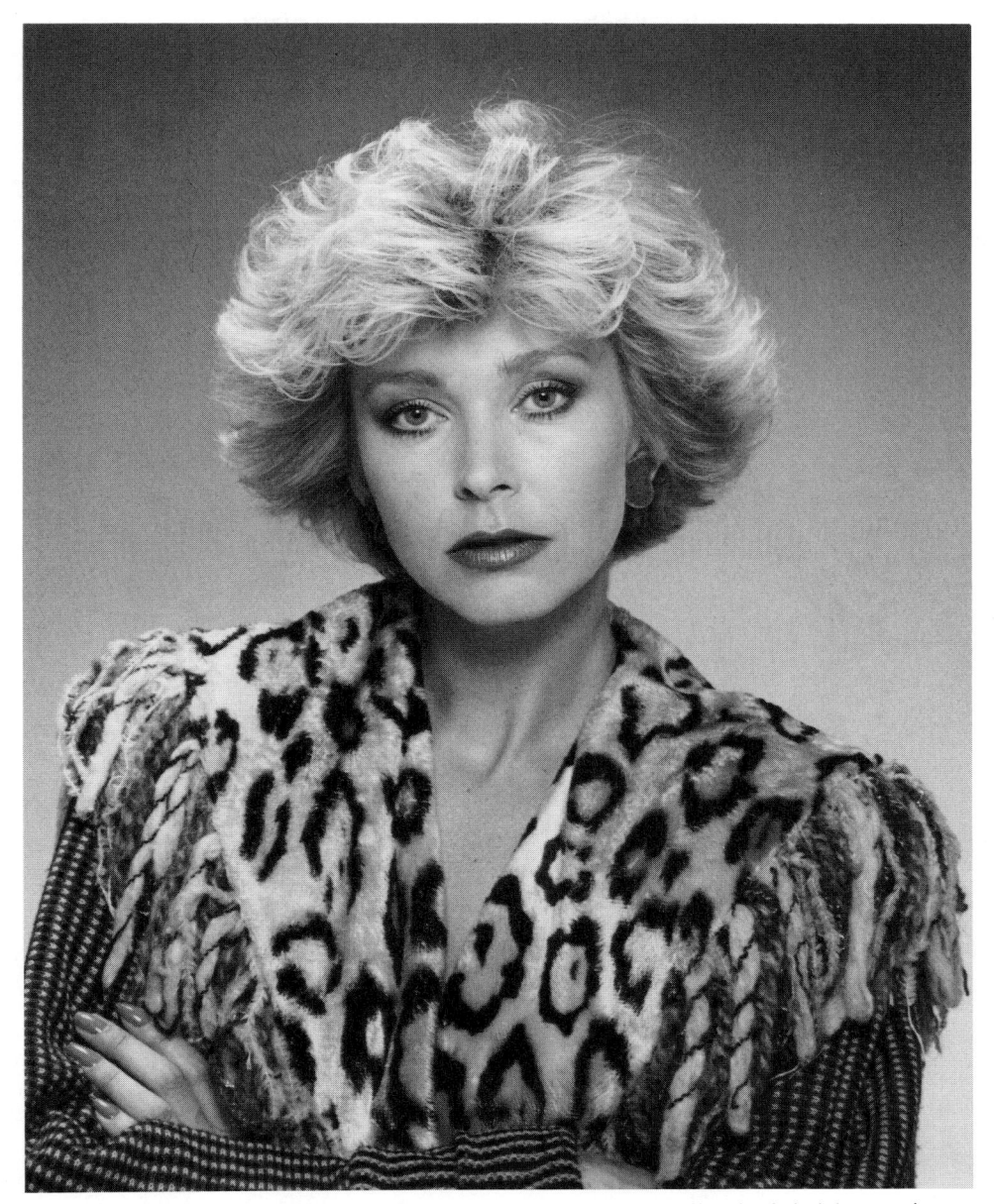

STYLING VERSATILITY WITH A PERM: For a second style, the hair is blown dry and shaped with a round brush for a very soft, feathery style with lots of fullness all around.

Curly Wave: This type of perm is a style rather than a styling aid. The hair is wound on smaller rods. Curly perms can be worn air-dried or lamp-dried and fluffed with fingers or a pick for a natural look. Or they can be blown dry with a round brush (just as you would do with naturally curly hair). You can also blow-dry curly hair, but be sure to use a diffuser (a blower attachment that regulates the air flow) to avoid disturbing the curl.

Directional Perm: This is achieved by placing the rods in the direction you want the hair to go; e.g., all back and away from the face. This method is also good to tame troublesome spots like cowlicks. This process is for salon use only.

Support Perm: Especially successful for longer, blunt-cut hair that needs some volume and fullness at the sides and bottom. Only the hair from the top of the ears down is permed. Hair is wound on large rods, and a mild waving lotion is used (just like a body wave).

Spot Perm: Only for those who want volume or curl at a specific place; e.g., at the crown to add height. The hair in the section to be treated is wound according to the effect desired—body wave or curly perm.

Reverse Perm: This process removes the tight curl from the hair. The stylist rolls the hair on very wide rods to rearrange the curl pattern to a looser version. This process should be done only on naturally curly hair that has not been chemically treated.

Perm Wave Formulas

The variety of perms available today is very wide. The following is a list of the different types.

The Cold Wave: An ammonia-based formula that does not require heat to set the curl. This is the most commonly used salon wave today. This type of perm lasts until the hair is cut; roots grow out straight.

Hair Type Formula: These formulas are specially designed to treat colored hair, hard-to-curl hair, dry hair, and a number of other special conditions. Let your perm professional select the one that will work best for your own individual needs.

Acid Perm: A milder formula than those described above, these work more slowly and with the help of heat from a hair dryer. Acid perms achieve a softer effect and loosen up quite a bit during the first week. This perm is ideal for fragile hair.

PERM TOOLS

Rod size and shape is as important to the finished results as the type of perm formula. Here is a guide.

Large Rod: For a body wave or a loose wave

Medium Rod: For medium-sized curls

Small Rods: For very tight curls

Concave Rod: For curlier ends, smoother roots

Straight Rod: For the same degree of curl all over

Flexible Tubes: For soft waves

Plastic Clips: For very tight curls

Caring for Your Perm

Permed hair, like any chemically treated hair, is fragile and requires lots of TLC.

• Shampoo with a gentle, low-pH product designed specially for permed hair. Most permed hair is very porous, and a low pH helps prevent its soaking up too much water and becoming difficult to comb out.

• Use an instant conditioner after every shampoo to make detangling easy. Use a wide-tooth comb to detangle wet hair.

• Handle permed hair gently. When washing and drying, never rub the hair with fingers or towels to keep the hair from tangling. Try using fingers for combing hair as much as possible.

• Use hairstyling preparations like mousses, gels, sprays, and styling lotions formulated for permed hair.

Perm Dos and Don'ts

Do . . .

get a haircut before a perm to remove dry and split ends and shape the hair.

Do . . .

let your perm stylist know about other chemical treatments on your hair and when you had them, to prevent damaged, overprocessed hair.

Do...

precondition hair before a perm and use a special type of conditioner as prescribed by your stylist.

Do...

get a perm before coloring, if you color your hair. Perm solution will lighten the color, changing the shade if the color application is fresh. Wait at least one week between perm and color treatments.

Do...

tell your stylist exactly what you want from your perm and what you don't like. Lack of communication is the culprit when you get results you don't want.

Don't...

have any type of perm treatment, even the mildest kind, on hair that is damaged or in bad condition. Healthy hair is a must for a perm.

Don't...

shampoo your hair for 48 hours after your perm. This will help "set" your perm.

Don't...

abuse permed hair with too much use of heated appliances. Permed hair is fragile. Use a blow dryer at medium setting and keep it at least six inches from the hair. Try to avoid curling irons. If you must use one, select an iron with a coated barrel. Apply a thermal setting spray to hair for additional protection.

Don't...

be afraid to change. Most types of hair can benefit from some type of perm procedure.

REVIVING A PERM

Everyone who has ever had a perm has had the same problem— the time comes when it is too early to get another perm, yet the old perm has seen better days. Here is what to do:

- Keep hair trimmed—nothing looks worse than an out-of-shape haircut and perm.
- Side-part hair and sculpt waves on top and sides with setting lotion or sculpting gel.
- Apply mousse or gel to the roots only and make pin curls just with root hair (leaving ends loose). Dry and fluff with fingers.
- If you wear long hair and the new growth is more than four inches, consider a root perm.

Relaxing the Curl

A chemical straightener has the opposite effect of a wave; it penetrates the hair shaft and changes the curl formation to remove it. Of all the chemical treatments, this is the strongest and the most likely to cause damage to the hair. For best results, hair should be in great condition before this type of treatment.

The effects of a chemical relaxer are permanent. Only the roots growing out will need to be touched up about every six weeks. It is very important to apply the relaxer formula only to the new hair growth. Applying it over already relaxed hair can cause the hair to break and be severely damaged.

Chemical relaxing is a complicated process that should be done professionally. Be sure the stylist does a strand test before applying the solution to your hair to be sure the chemicals and your hair are compatible. If the hair feels sticky after the test, that formula shouldn't be used; it is too strong for that particular type of hair.

As with other salon treatments, communicating with the stylist is essential for best results. Be sure to tell the stylist how straight or wavy you would like your hair to be. As with a perm, hair should be relaxed before a color treatment, and at least one week should elapse between relaxing and coloring.

Follow the same haircare guidelines as for permed hair—even more so, since relaxed hair is the most fragile of all chemically treated hair. Be sure to select products that are formulated for relaxed hair, too.

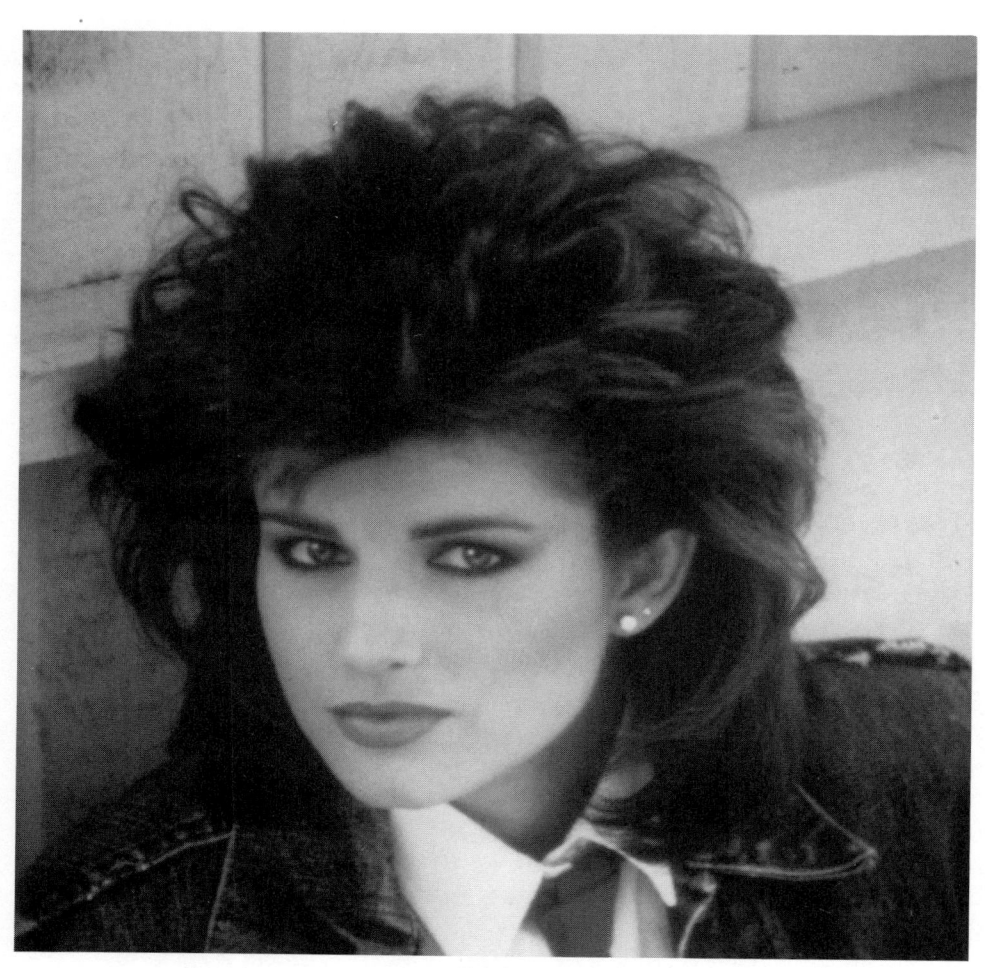

Sylvia

6
STYLING—THE LOOK THAT'S RIGHT FOR YOU

Selecting the right styles means more than following the current fashion trends. The latest hairdos may look great on a model, your friend, or an actress, but they may not work with your individual characteristics. However, selecting the right style and one that is in fashion should not be too difficult now that you know how to make the best of your beauty assets.

As a hairstylist, I am very much against the type of trendy look that makes every woman look the same. It just doesn't work. The most becoming styles should bring out a woman's best features. So if bangs are in this year and you have the type of great face that looks best without bangs, you should not feel forced to wear them no matter what the style trends say. I believe that this "cookie cutter" approach is what makes a lot of women afraid to change their hairstyle. One bad experience with a trendy hairstyle is all that it really takes to make many women reluctant to change.

Owning a top Beverly Hills salon lets me see all types of women. Of course my star clientele is one group, but we do get women coming into the salon from all walks of life. And one of the worst problems I see with many of these women is their reluctance to change their hairstyle.

I see a lot of young women in their mid twenties and early thirties who walk in with the same hairdo they wore for their high school yearbook picture. I see a lot of older women who come in still wearing those horrendous lacquered 1950s bubbles. Not too long ago, the wife of a very famous man who was being honored at a social event came to me to have her hair done for the evening. I was really shocked when this attractive woman "of a certain age" insisted on wearing her hair in "petals." It took a lot of talking and hand-holding, but I was able to convince her to change her hairstyle.

Many women feel secure with the old styles they have been wearing for years. They have no idea how much better they will look if they change with the times. Most of these women wouldn't dare walk out of the house wearing clothes from the periods of their hairstyle, so why not change the hair too? Change is good for you. Change establishes a positive attitude.

Some of my famous clients have been reluctant to change, too. When I first met Jane Morgan Weintraub (who later became my backer), she had been wearing the same hairstyle for years. Jane came to me recommended by a friend, but she just wanted her hair done—not changed. I convinced her to change her hairstyle. I cut her hair and styled it in a short, breezy look and she realized how much better she looked with her new style.

While Jane wears her hair within certain basic styling parameters (and most people do)—she prefers it short and in a certain shade of blond—I change her hairstyle all the time. These are not radical changes. Jane doesn't get a different hairstyle every week. But the small changes are obvious enough to be noticeable and effective.

Another of my most famous makeovers has been Tanya Tucker. Tanya became a country-and-western star at the age of 13 and first came to me as a client when she was 18. Tanya lives in Nashville, and at 18 she used to wear her hair in one of those big, overblown styles that required a roller set. Her style not only was out of date and unbecoming, but it also made her look a lot older. Tanya came to Los Angeles to make her first appearance on the Merv Griffin show, and she came to me for a new look. I changed Tanya's style from a style that was too old for her to a soft, full, windblown look, and she was a hit on Merv Griffin that evening.

After Tanya's successful makeover, other famous country-and-western stars came to see me for the same reason. Emmylou Harris and Sylvia both had extremely long, straight hair (they could easily sit on it). I gave them both soft, layered haircuts, body waves, and highlights. I turned them from pretty country girls into the glamorous women they are today.

When I meet a new client, whether she is a star or a regular client, I follow the same system to determine which is going to be the best style for her. First I take a good look at her from head to toe. I see how she walks, how she stands, whether she is outgoing or shy. Then I sit her down on my chair and start looking at her hair. I then ask her the questions I mentioned in Chapter 2.

Styling—The Look That's Right for You

Once we discuss a style that is going to suit her hair type, lifestyle, and do-it-yourself expertise, we discuss how we are going to achieve it. Will it require just cutting and styling? Are chemical treatments—perm, color, straightening—going to be necessary? Within reason, anything is possible, but the style selection must fit the client's own needs.

FACTORS IN SELECTING A HAIRSTYLE

There are four factors that determine the selection of the right hairstyle. These are hair type and texture, facial bone structure, lifestyle, and body proportions.

Hair Type and Texture

Fine and Baby-Fine: Usually limp, flyaway, and wispy in its natural state. If too long, it will have a tendency to look skimpy on the ends. Looks best worn in a short, layered look or in a chin-length blunt cut. Color and perm are recommended to add body.

Straight: Holds the set well, sometimes because there is lots of hair. Blunt or layered cuts work best. To add body, apply mousse to almost dry hair and squeeze a little while using a blow dryer. For added volume, blow-dry hair upside down just before finishing. Color and/or perm adds body.

Curly: Moderate layered cuts look best. Too much or too little layering will make the hair look bushy. Longer lengths are good because the weight of the hair pulls it down. Straightening with a blow dryer and wide-diameter brush usually works well, but humid weather puts the curl back in the hair.

Wiry: Can be curly or just coarse and difficult to manage. A moderately layered cut in medium to long length is best. Body waves help keep the shape of the style. Stay away from tight curls that can make the hair look bushy. Frequent trims are advised to keep the lines of the style.

Having dry or oily hair is another factor to be taken into consideration when selecting a hairstyle.

Oily: Shampoo frequently, at least once a day. Extremely oily hair may need twice-a-day shampoos. A style with minimum maintenance is most sensible, unless you have lots of time to spend on your hair. Short to medium lengths are best.

TOVAR'S CLASSIC BEAUTY

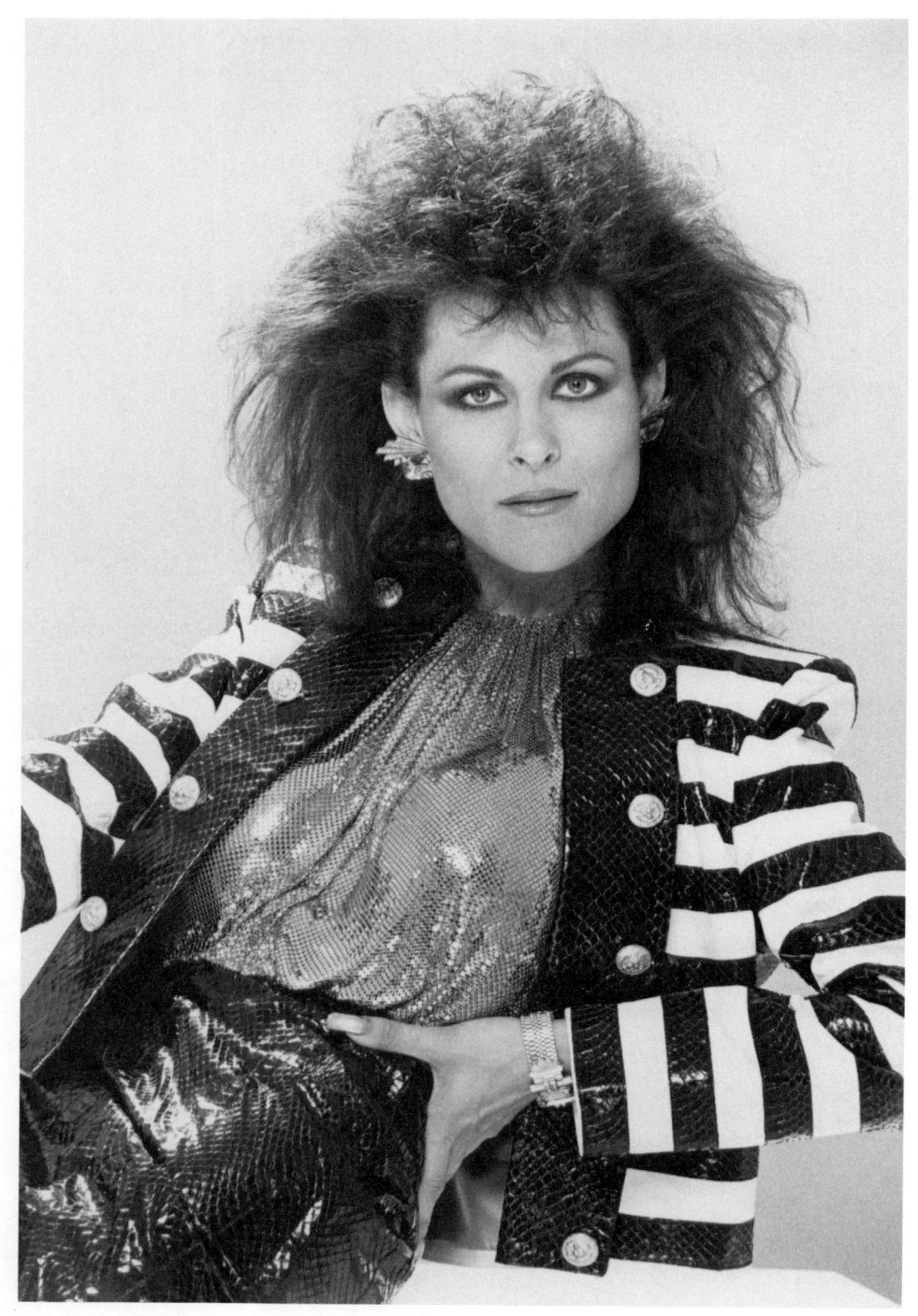

LAYERED LONG HAIR: Actress Wanda Van Kleist wears her hair in the kind of style that lends itself to an almost unlimited number of changes. *STYLE 1 FOR LAYERED LONG HAIR:* Lots of height and movement can be created by layering the crown short. For lots more volume, add mousse and scrunch hair as you use the blow dryer.

Styling—The Look That's Right for You

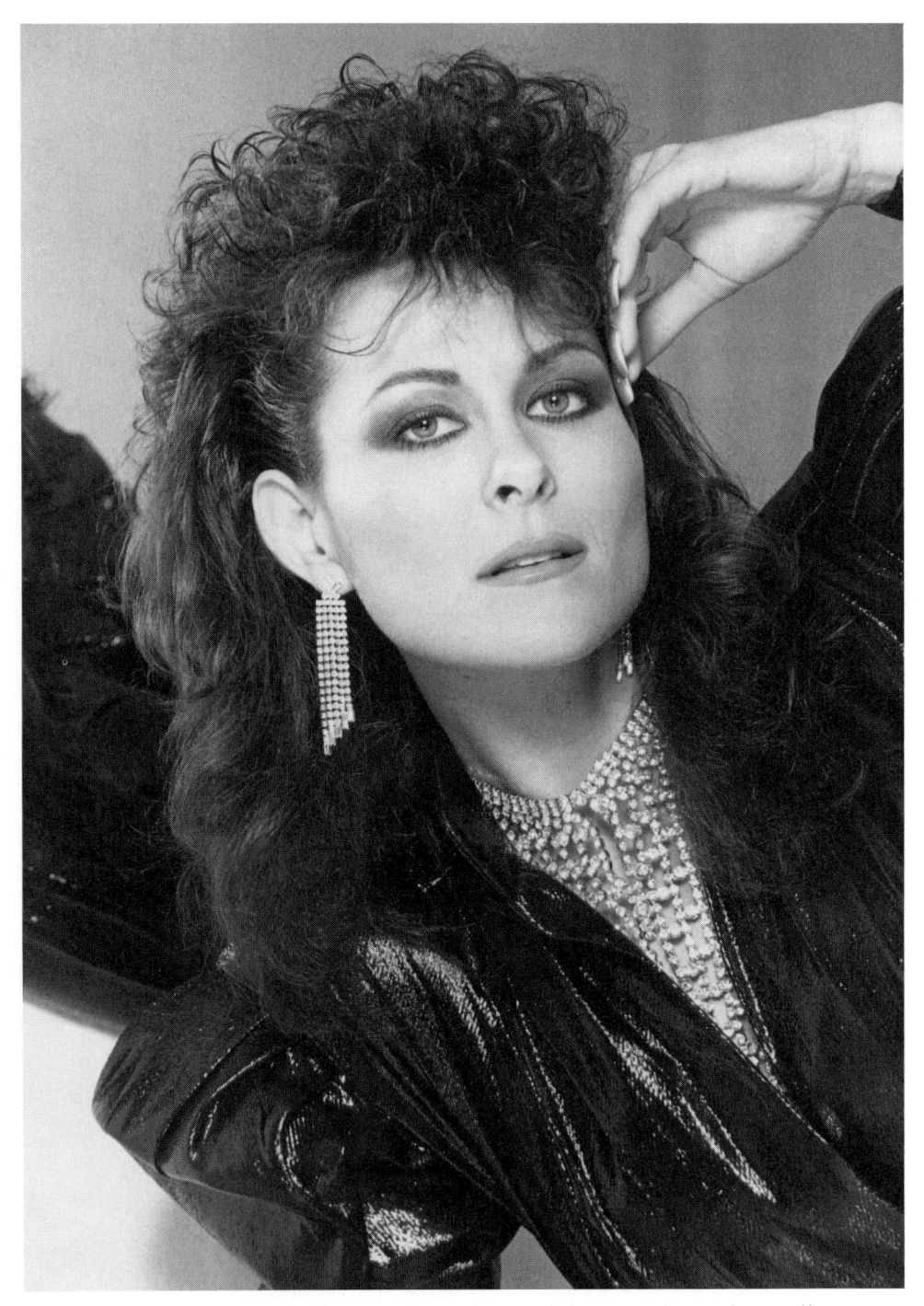

STYLE 2 FOR LAYERED LONG HAIR: A sleeker look is very elegant, sporting long and narrow lines. The top is high and feathery; the sides are slicked back. The rest of the hair is arranged smooth and down.

TOVAR'S CLASSIC BEAUTY

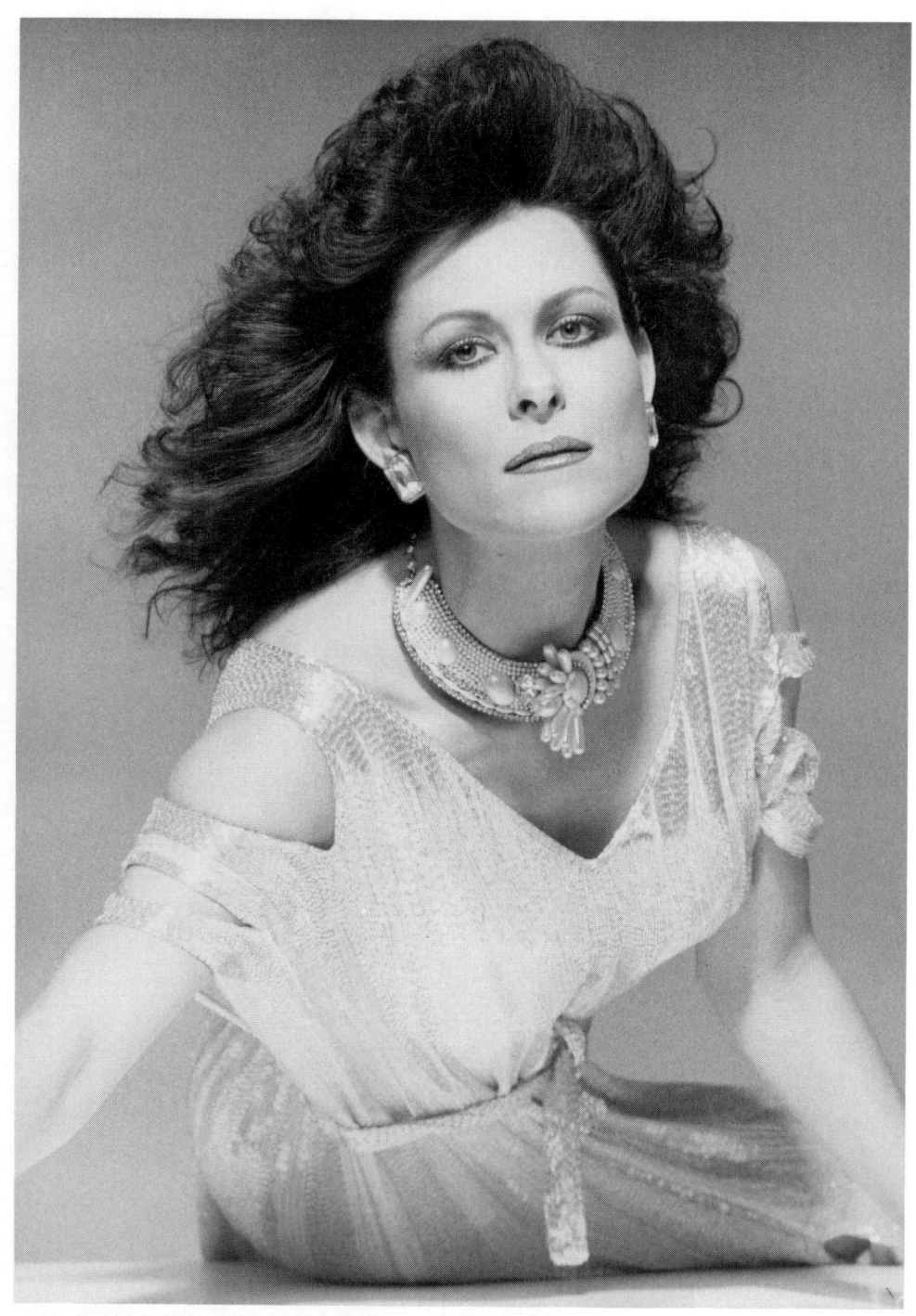

STYLE 3 FOR LAYERED LONG HAIR: The windblown look is not as carefree as it looks. All arranged off the face, high at the crown and very full in back, cascading down to the shoulders.

Styling—The Look That's Right for You

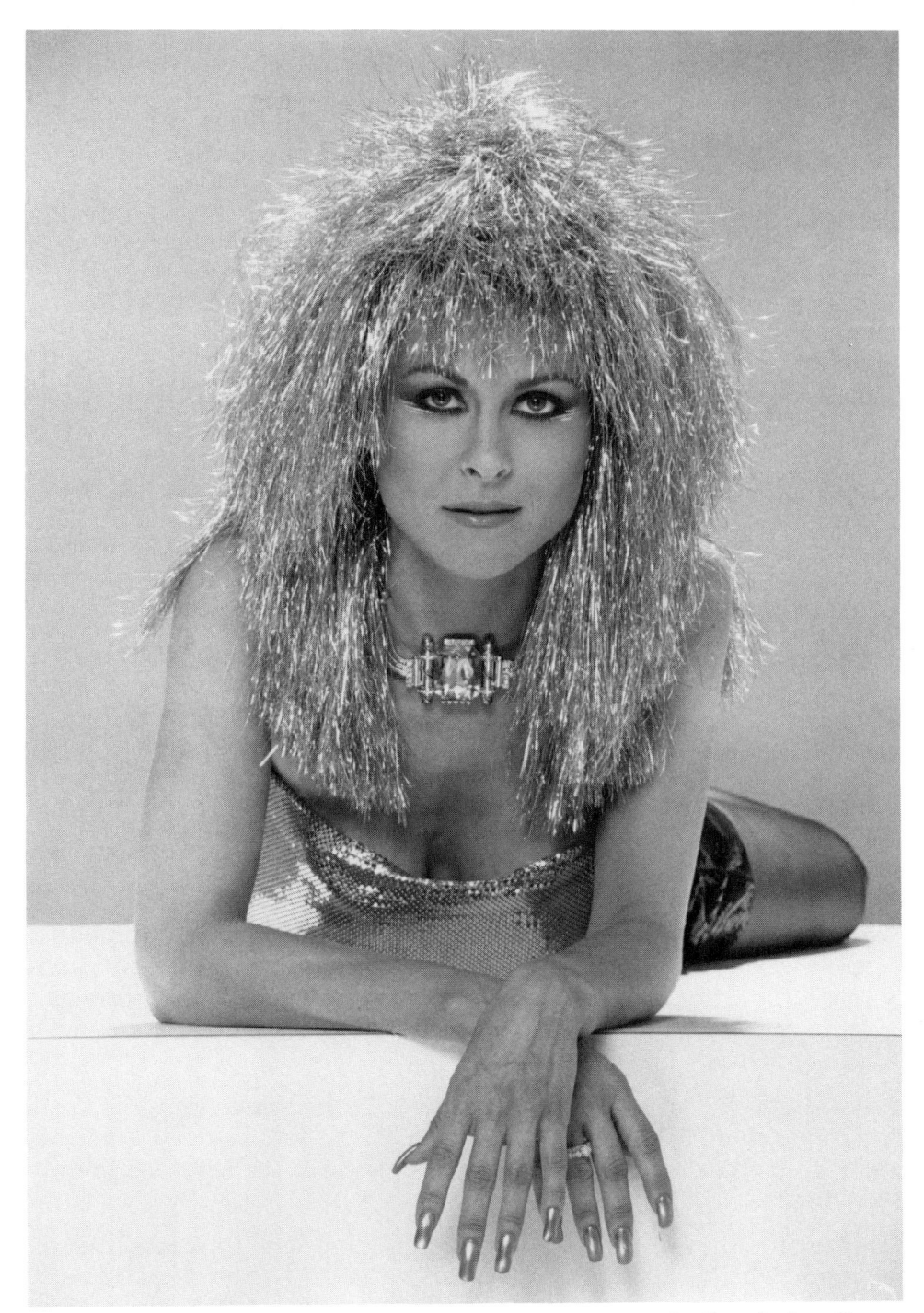

STYLE 4 FOR LAYERED LONG HAIR: The Fun Look . . . Only for the daring. The frankly fake metallic wig is cut short at the crown, with dead-straight bangs and sides. Cleopatra of the disco set, perhaps?

Dry: Dull-looking, sometimes with split ends. Depending on hair texture, also wiry and hard to manage. Avoid styles that require heated appliances like hot rollers and curling irons. Use blow dryer on a medium setting. Let hair air-dry as often as possible. Keep ends well trimmed.

Facial Bone Structure

There are seven basic facial shapes. Hairstyles should emphasize the positive points and distract from the negative ones. A hairstyle should create an optical illusion around the face, to flatter every line and contour. The facial shapes are oval, round, oblong, square, pear-shaped, diamond-shaped, and heart-shaped.

Oval: The ideal face shape. The forehead is slightly wider than the chin and the hairline is gently curved for that oval appearance. The best styles are those that show off the face, although side-swept or airy bangs can be a more attractive choice.

Round: Rounded contours, soft edges, with the appearance of a full circle. Hairstyle should add length. Avoid very short hair or short layers around the crown and top and center parts. Wear medium-length hair with a side part, side-parted bangs, and width from the ears to the chin.

Oblong: Face shape is long, narrow, and angular. The hairstyle should shorten the length to make it appear wider. Layered hair with lots of movement from the crown to the ends and soft bangs will shorten the length and soften the edges.

Square: Straight hairline and square jawline. The hairstyle should create the illusion of length and soften the sharp angles. A short style with width at the sides, fullness at the top, and hair coming forward over the forehead and sides will make this face appear narrower and softer.

Pear-Shaped: Narrow forehead and wide jawline and chin. The hairstyle should add width at the forehead. A short style with height and softness at the crown and forward curls over the jawline achieves this effect.

Diamond-Shaped: Wide across the cheekbones, narrow forehead and chin. The style should reduce the width across the cheekbones. Medium-length hair that is full across the forehead and jawline and close to the scalp at the cheekbones will create the illusion of an oval face.

Heart-Shaped: Wide forehead and narrow chinline. Sometimes this hairline also shows a "widow's peak." The style should make the forehead look narrower and add width at the chin. A medium-length, layered style with short layers at the crown and fullness at the jawline. Side-swept bangs will camouflage the widow's peak. A center part is a good option for an even hairline.

Additional Tips for Corrective Styling

Short Neck: Keep hair short; avoid bulk at the nape.

Long Neck: Keep neck covered with longer hair or, if wearing hair up, with long tendrils.

Plump Features: Keep hair short, with some fullness, wavy sides, soft bangs, and tapered at neckline. Avoid very long or closely cropped hair.

Thin Features: Soft, fluffy styles with lots of height at the crown and fullness at the sides. Keep the nape hair soft and full to balance the thin neck. Avoid flat, too-long, or close-cropped styles.

Uneven Features: Asymmetrical styles with lots of softness around the face. Avoid styles that are severe and bare the face.

Prominent Chin: Short hair with height at the crown, fullness at the sides, and bangs.

High Forehead: Bangs.

Low Forehead: Height at the top, side part.

Lifestyle

How you live and what you do for a living has a strong impact on your hairstyle selection. How much time you have or want to spend on your hair should be the determining factor in your choice of style. Here are some tips for four types of women I often see.

Career Woman: Select styles that require minimum maintenance yet are versatile enough to change from sleek business looks to elegant evening to carefree casual without much fussing. Perms offer great freedom from maintenance. The cut you get should not require very frequent trimming. Very short or very long hair should be avoided, also very trendy looks that would not work with your business personality. The best hair coloring bet is highlights because the regrowth pattern is a lot less obvious than with tinting or bleaching, and touch-ups are not needed that often.

Housewife: Select styles that are attractive and easy to manage. Color and perm suggestions are the same as for the career woman. Since you probably have a little more time for yourself, long hair can be a good choice if it suits you and works well with your hair type.

Society Matron: Hairstyling choices should include a variety of looks for daytime, evening, and casual. The society matron has her hair done either in the salon or by "house call," so she has many more choices. Perm and color choices depend on hair type and age.

Star: A star is constantly in the public eye, and she always wears a look that is her "signature." However, this look has to be versatile enough for a variety of changes. Most stars prefer long hair because it offers much more versatility than short hair.

Body Proportions

Your hairstyle should be part of your total look. A great style that doesn't fit in with the rest of you defeats its purpose. Take into consideration your physical proportions when selecting a hairstyle. Here are the basic rules:

If You Are Small . . .

DO wear short to medium-length styles with some fullness at the crown and sides.

AVOID long hair because it will make you look smaller, or very full styles that will give you a "big head" look.

If You Are Average . . .

DO wear any type of style that works with your hair and facial type.

AVOID any extreme styles.

If You Are Tall . . .

DO wear short, medium, or long styles according to how slender or heavy you are. You can also wear moderately full styles.

Styling—The Look That's Right for You

AVOID very short, closely cropped, or messy-looking styles, spiky or punk looks.

TYPES OF HAIR APPLIANCES

Blow Dryers: The most common type is the pistol. For home use, I recommend a light weight pistol type with three heat settings and two air settings. For best results, dry hair at 1,500 watts and style it at 1,000 to 1,200 watts. To avoid damaging the hair, keep a distance of about six inches between the hair and dryer.

Compact Blow Dryer: If you travel or work out regularly, consider adding one of these to your beauty bag. New models come with as much wattage as the larger kind. A dual-voltage dryer is also available.

Curling Iron: Curling irons come in a large variety. Barrel diameter should be selected according to needs—wide for long to medium hair, loose curls, or straightening; narrow for short hair, tight curls, and bangs. To avoid hair damage, select one that has a nonstick coating around the barrel. Some irons come with brushlike prongs and are meant to give body and fullness (be careful not to tangle hair). Irons with a steam feature are available, too. To avoid hair damage, don't leave hair in the curling iron more than a few seconds. Follow operating instructions carefully.

Hot Rollers: These are used just like regular rollers, but the hair is rolled dry and pretreated with specially formulated setting lotion that also protects the hair from the heat. Most hot roller units come with a selection of large, medium, and small rollers. The larger the roller, the looser the curl. Large rollers can be used to tame too-curly or frizzy hair. Like all other heated appliances, care must be taken not to overuse them and cause hair damage.

TYPES OF HAIR AIDS

Mousse: A foam product used on wet or dry hair to style and condition. Mousses come formulated for different types of hair (dry, oily, permed, etc.) and in different formulas. Alcohol-free mousses leave hair softer than those containing alcohol. Apply mousse to the hair and style by letting it dry naturally or by blowing dry.

Color Mousse: Same as above, but with color added. Colors range from wild pinks, purples, and metallics to natural-looking shades. Use the same as above for the same type of results. The color washes out when you shampoo.

Gel: Comes in solid gel or liquid gel form. Can be used on wet or dry hair. Use it to achieve the "wet" look, to slick hair back, to add volume (when applied at the roots), or to control hard-to-manage hair. Gel is not recommended for fine hair because it tends to weigh it down.

Color Gel: Same as above with color added. Colors come in the same range as color mousses. Some gels also come with glitter specks suspended in the formula. Color gels also wash out with shampoo.

Setting Lotion: A liquid formula that is applied to wet hair to add body, form curls or waves, and add more texture. Setting lotion can be applied straight from the bottle or with a mister. Comb through hair and set on rollers or blow-dry.

Setting Lotion for Heated Appliances: Spray or lotion product specially formulated to work with hot rollers and curling irons. It is sprayed on dry hair *before* the appliance is used.

Thermal Styling Lotion: Conditioning product for dry, color-treated, or fragile hair that is set with heat appliances. This product contains special ingredients to shield the hair from the heat. Apply before styling.

Hair Spray: Available in a number of formulas, from light to extremely heavy (the kind used for spiky hairdos). Hair spray keeps hair from reacting to humidity and holds a style in place. Light formulas work better in aerosol form, the heavier formulas with a pump.

COMBS AND BRUSHES

Bristle Brush: Natural or nylon bristles. Flat back, rectangular, or oval. Natural-bristle brushes with long handles work better on long hair. Brushes are used to dress and style hair. Brushing is also beneficial to the hair because it stimulates scalp circulation and helps distribute natural oils from roots to ends.

Vent Brush: Rubber or nylon prongs coming out of either a vented or raised plastic platform. Flat back. Use for brushing wet hair, detangling, and blow-drying. Can be used on wet or dry hair.

Round Brush: For use when styling with a blow dryer. The hair is rolled around it as on a roller. Comes in a number of widths. Narrower widths are for short hair and curly styles. Wider widths are for long hair or to take the curl out of very curly hair.

Wide-Tooth Comb: Comes either with or without a handle. It is used to comb wet hair and to detangle.

Styling—The Look That's Right for You

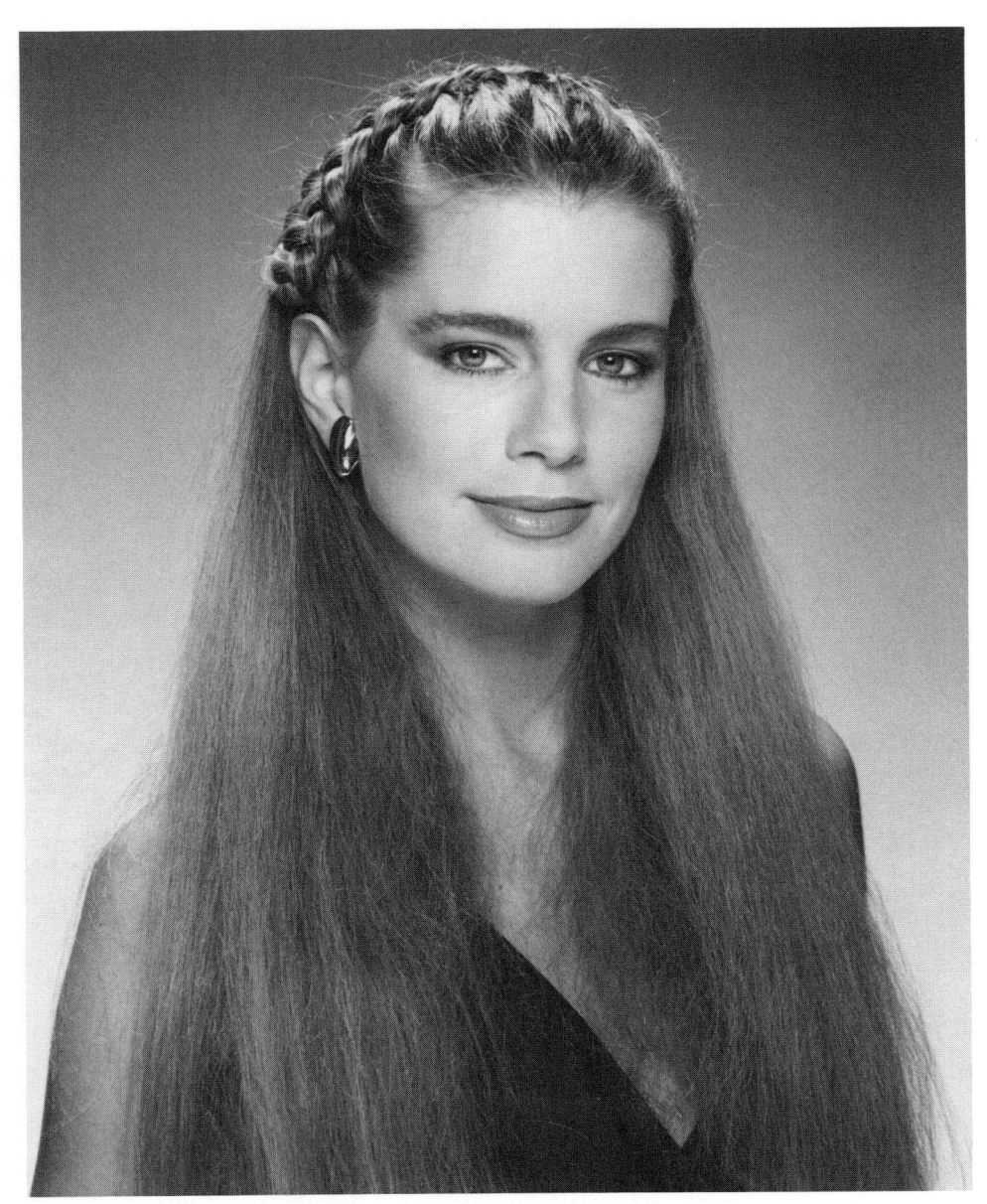

BRAIDING: Model Shelley Sterret has the perfect type of hair for braiding. I love to braid hair in many different ways, to use braids as a fashion accessory. *BRAIDED STYLE 1:* This is a great look for very long hair. Make a thin braid at each side, at ear level. Smooth the top back and cross the braids over like a headband. Arrange the rest of the hair like a veil, falling freely down the sides.

TOVAR'S CLASSIC BEAUTY

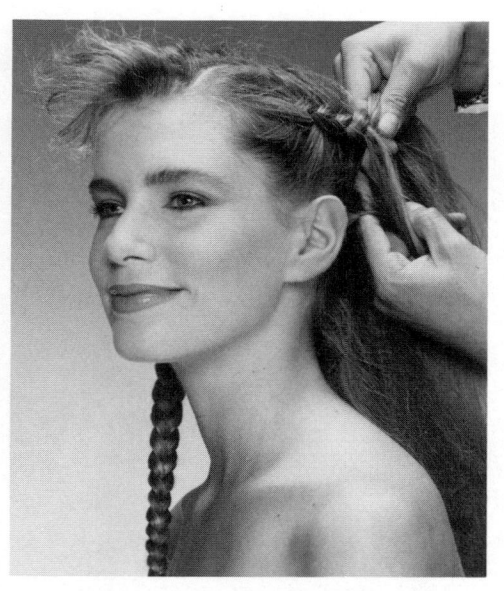

You can do an inverted french braid for a totally different look; the braid is going to pop out and look very defined. If you do a regular french braid, it is going to be a simpler look, since it lies close to the head.

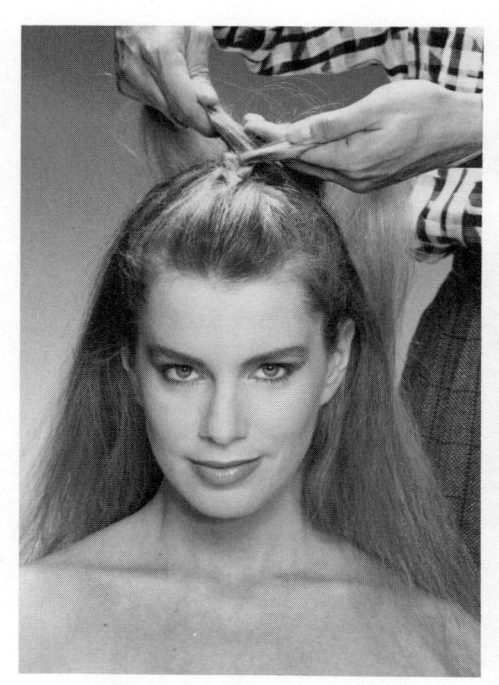

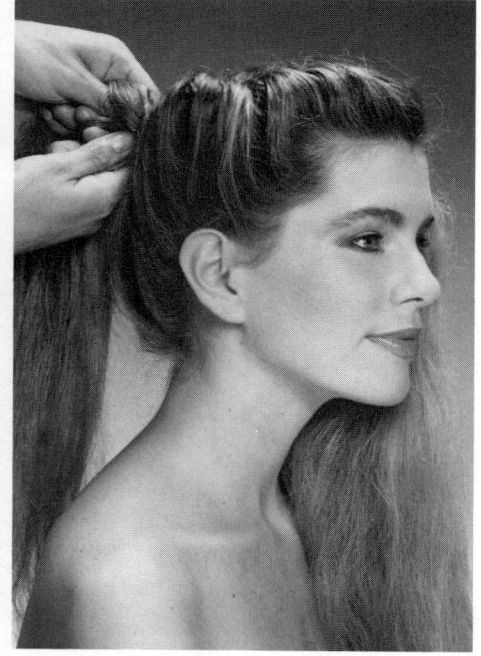

BRAIDED STYLE 2: Start the french braid with the center front section of the hair. Work the braid into one side.

Styling—The Look That's Right for You

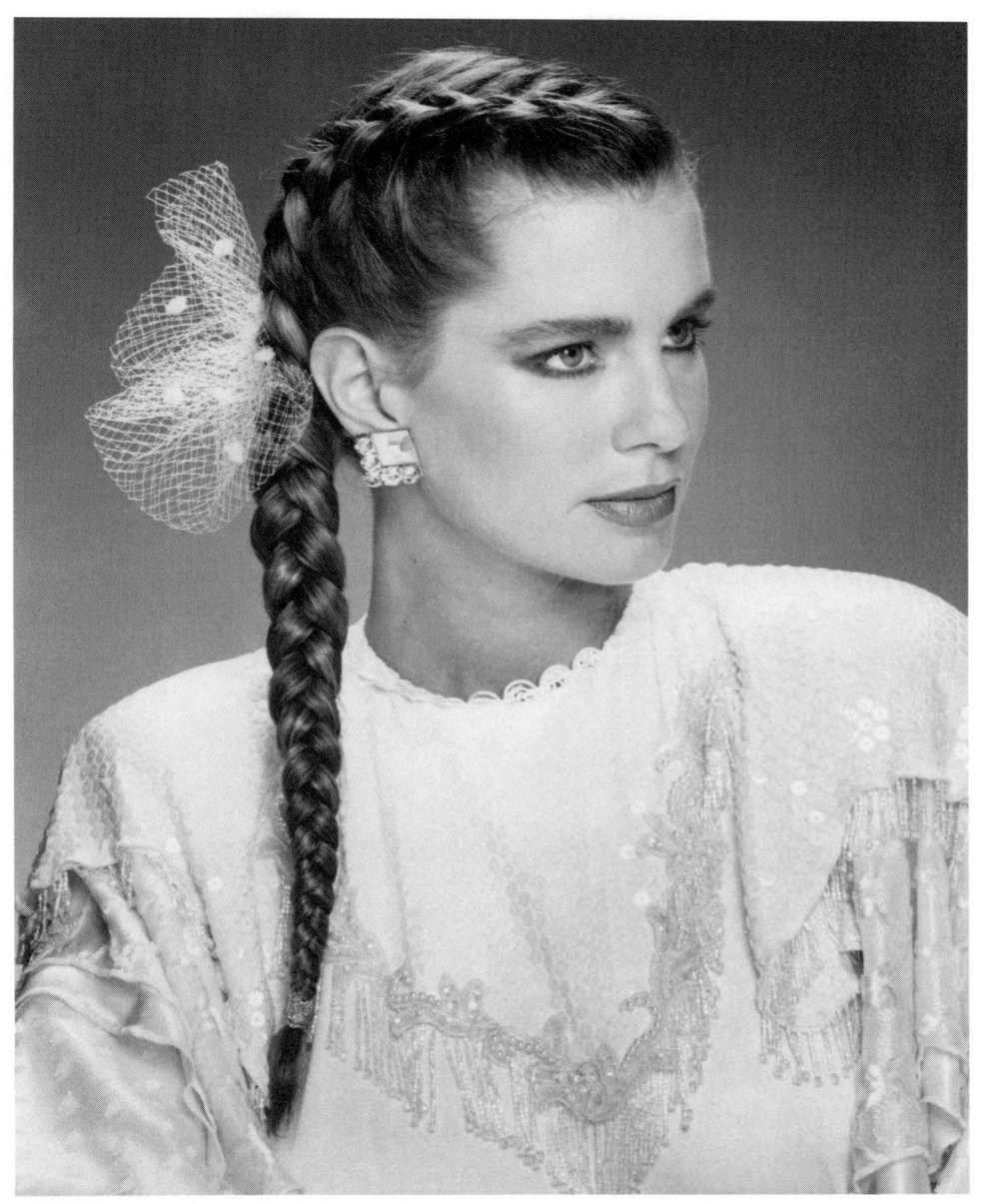

All the hair is braided over one side and accented with a net hair ornament over the ear.

Regular Comb: With teeth graduated from thin to wide, or all evenly spaced in different widths. Wide-tooth combs are used to detangle and comb wet hair, fine-tooth combs to part and groom the hair.

Rattail Comb: A fine-tooth comb with a pointed handle. The handle is used to lift, section, and separate hair for setting or styling. The comb part is used to part hair and for teasing and backcombing.

Pick: A small comb with long prongs used to lift and detangle very curly hair. It also adds volume without making hair look frizzy.

ACCESSORIES

Decorative Combs: Used to hold hair back at sides.

Rats: Synthetic mesh shapes in donut (for chignons) or sausage shapes to add as foundation to rolled hairstyles.

Ponytail Combs: Scissorlike long combs to hold hair, or round or oval combs that close around hair to hold ponytail.

Rubber Bands: Only coated rubber bands should be used on hair. Never hold wet hair with a rubber band.

STYLING TECHNIQUES

How to Blow-Dry Hair

1. Towel-dry hair to remove excess water.
2. Comb hair to follow the basic lines of the style.
3. Turn dryer on and, lifting the hair with your fingers, start drying at the root area. Be sure to keep the dryer about six inches from the hair.
4. When hair is damp-dry, apply mousse, gel, or sculpting lotion, depending on the style.
5. Start shaping the style. Turn the blower to a medium setting. Start working on the back of the head.
6. Use a round brush (for a smooth look) or your fingers (for a full, scrunched look). Whatever method you are using, work on a moderate amount of hair at a time for best results.
7. If you want to add some volume, bend down from the waist and point the dryer to the roots of the hair for a few seconds. Straighten up and finish drying with round brush or fingers.

Styling—The Look That's Right for You

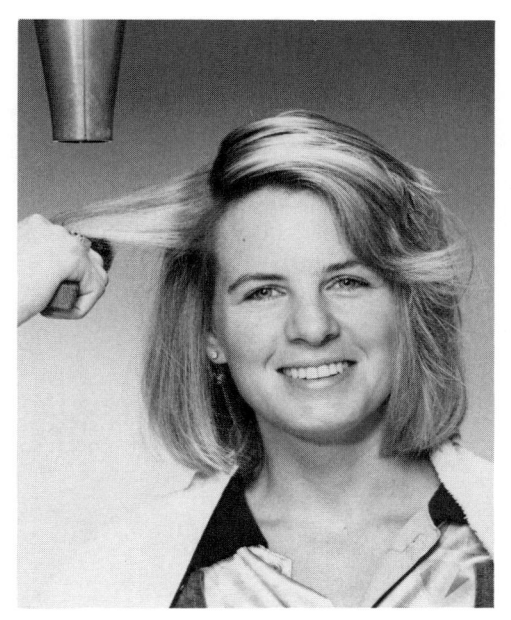

BLOW-DRYING: When finishing a smooth style such as this one, roll hair *under* and around the brush, as shown, for soft fullness that curls under. Model: Jessica Norman Pappas. Top by Marion Wagner, Los Angeles.

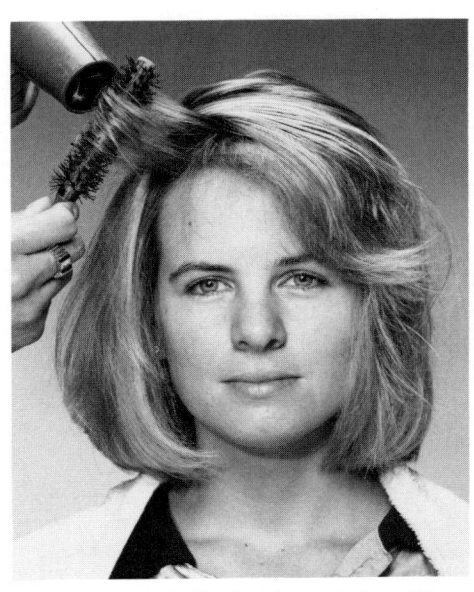

BLOW-DRYING: To finish a style with hair directed away from the face, roll it around a brush held vertically, as shown.

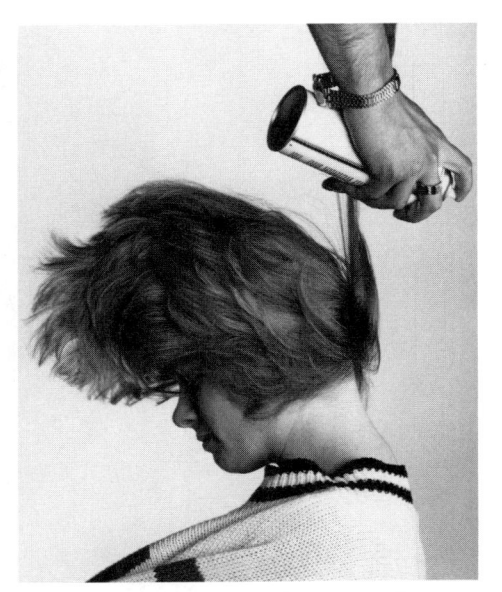

BLOW-DRYING: To add volume to any hairstyle, when hair is almost dry, bend down and blow hair from the roots to the ends.

TOVAR'S CLASSIC BEAUTY

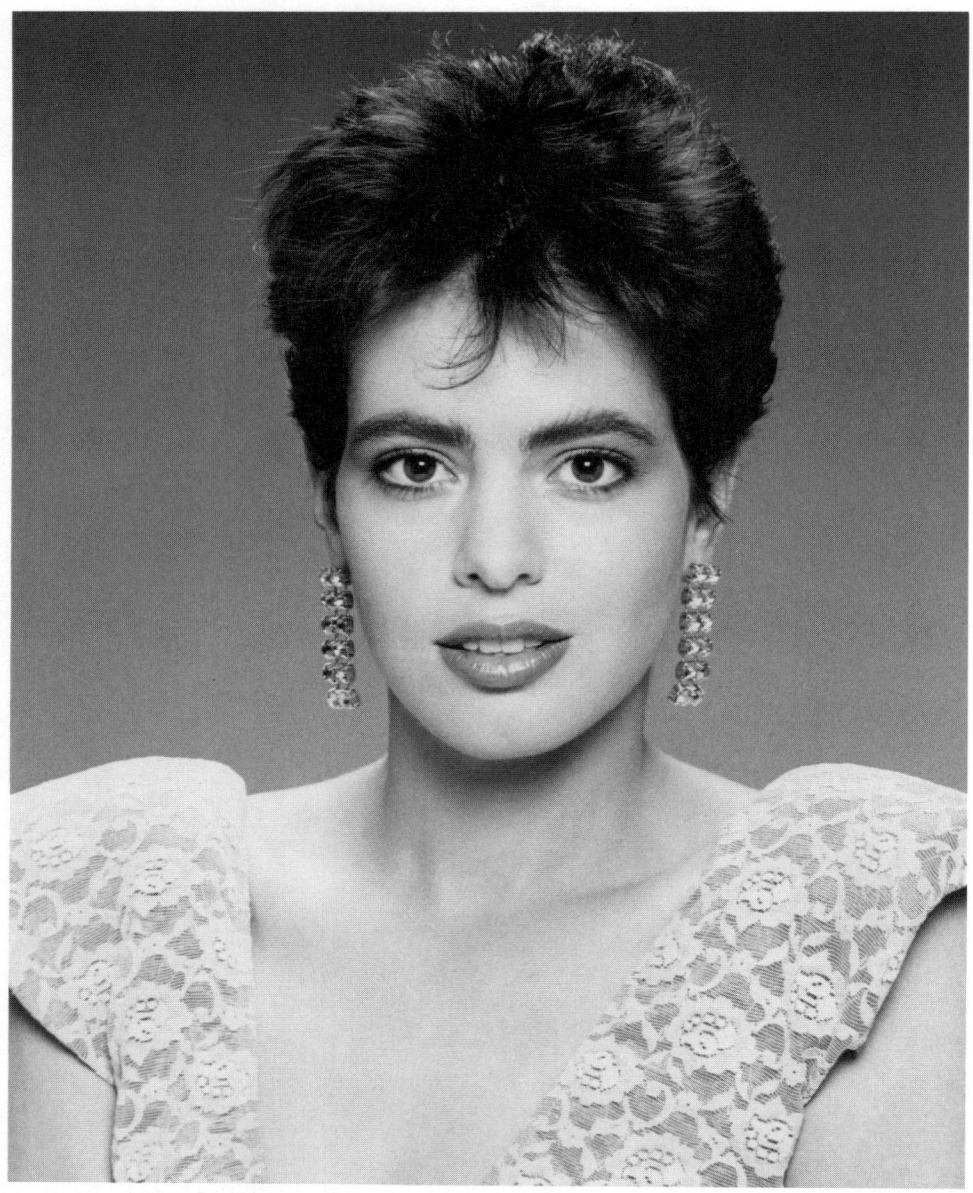

STYLE 1 FOR VERY SHORT HAIR: This model, Veronica Herrera, has thick, slightly wavy dark hair. It is cut in a very short style that requires almost no maintenance. A little blow-drying is required for fullness at the crown. A touch of mousse keeps the sides close to the head. A few strands of bangs come forward, off center over the forehead. Top and earrings by Ellene Warren, Los Angeles.

Styling—The Look That's Right for You

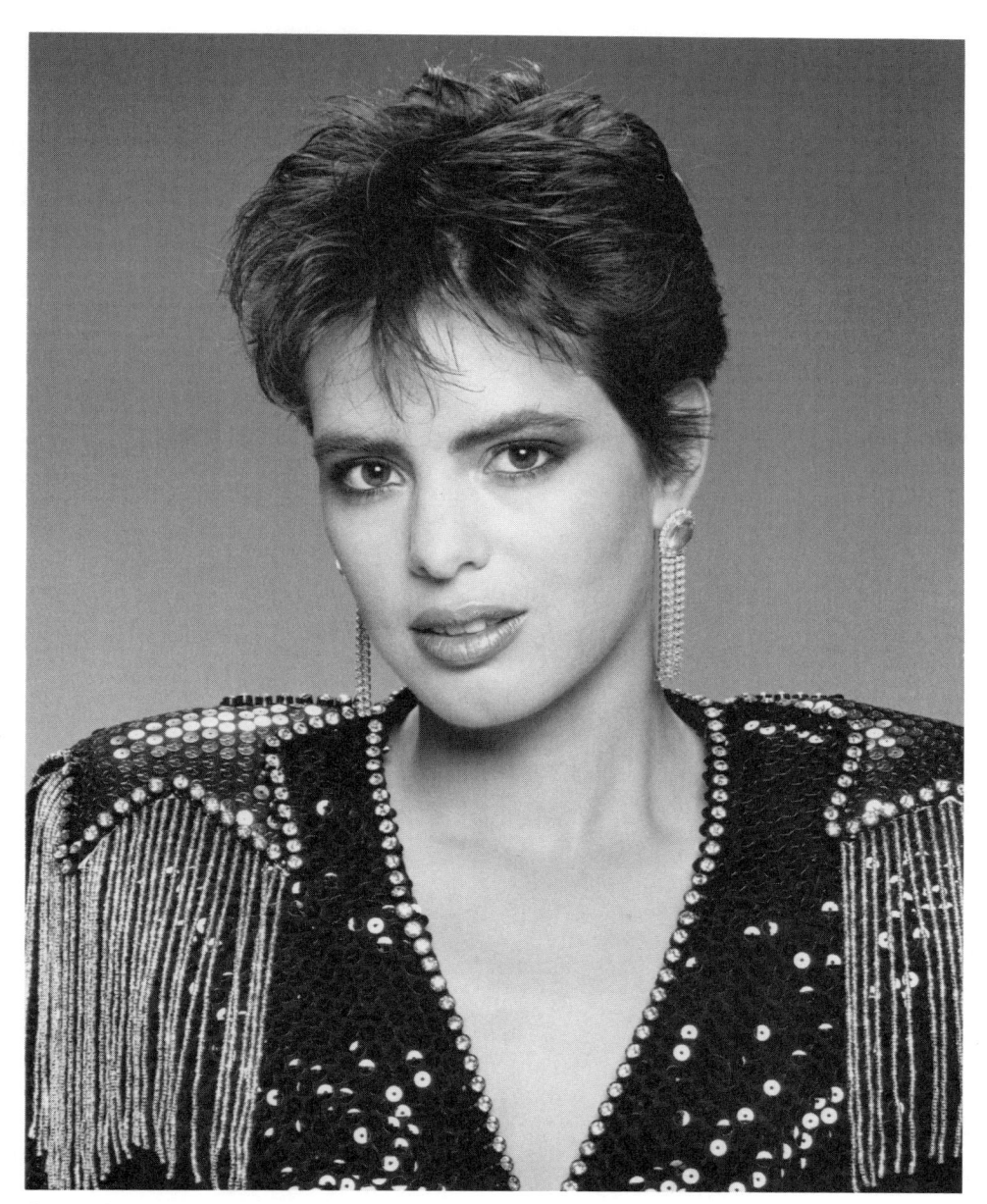

STYLE 2 FOR VERY SHORT HAIR: For a different look, add mousse to damp hair and scrunch it while using a blow dryer. Lift the hair up at the crown for volume, and bring chunky, airy, piecey bangs over the forehead.

To Finish a Short Style . . .

1. Pin top and sides out of the way.
2. Dry back, first one side from outside to center, then the other side.
3. Dry sides, toward the face or away from the face, as desired.
4. Dry top last.

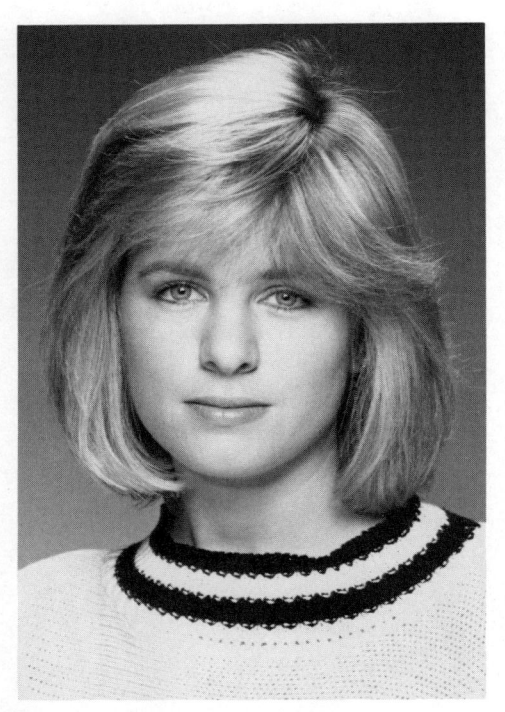

STYLE 1 FOR MEDIUM-LENGTH STRAIGHT HAIR: Jessica's smooth bob looks all one length but actually is gently layered for volume and movement. The side is parted, piecey bangs are side-swept over the forehead, and the sides curve in toward the chin.

To Finish a Medium or Long Style . . .

1. Follow basic instructions.
2. Pin crown and side hair out of the way.
3. Using a round brush (the diameter will determine whether you get a smooth or wavy look), start drying the back, rolling strands of hair around the brush.
4. Let hair cool slightly before unwinding. (This locks in the curl or bend.)
5. To style sides back, roll hair vertically and back. To style sides down, roll hair horizontally and under.

HEATHER LOCKLEAR

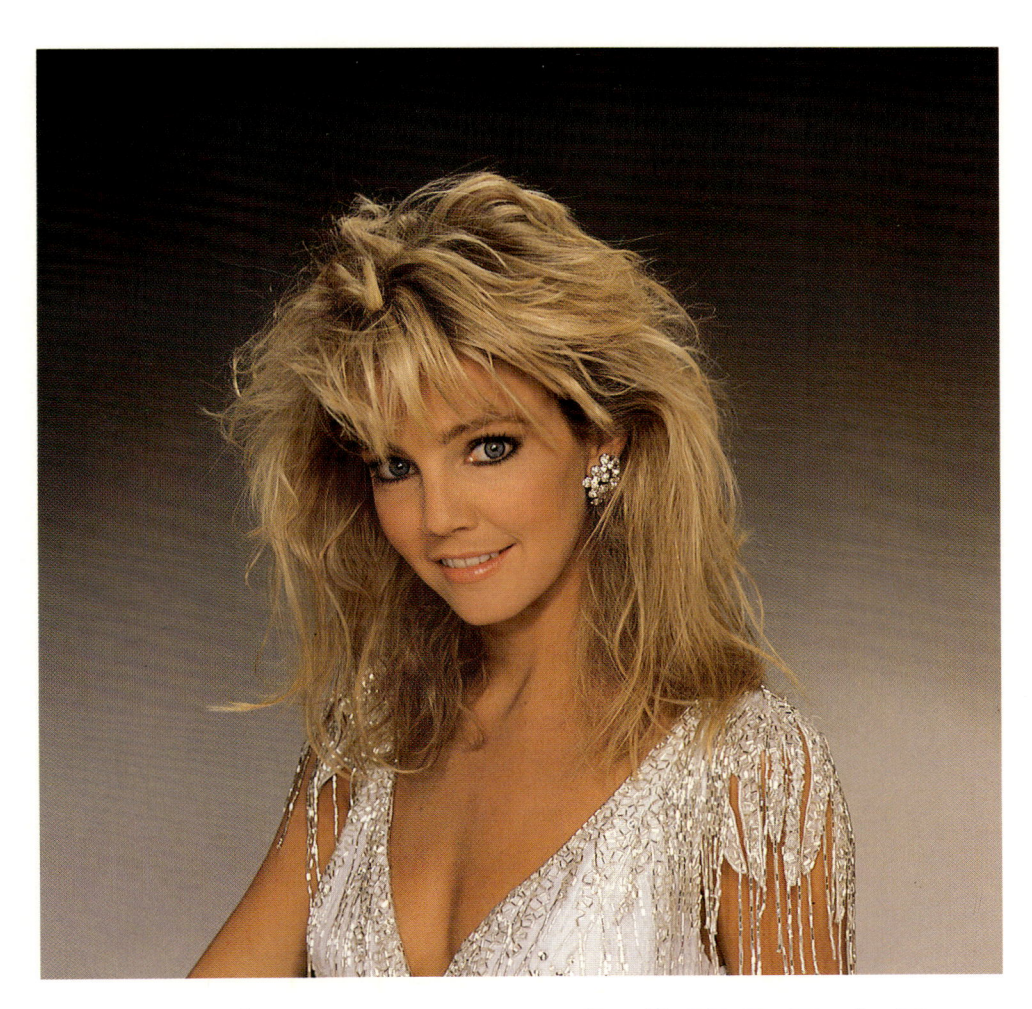

Heather Locklear, an all-American beauty, sports a new airy, softer look. The twisted pin-curl set gives her hair lots of body and volume.

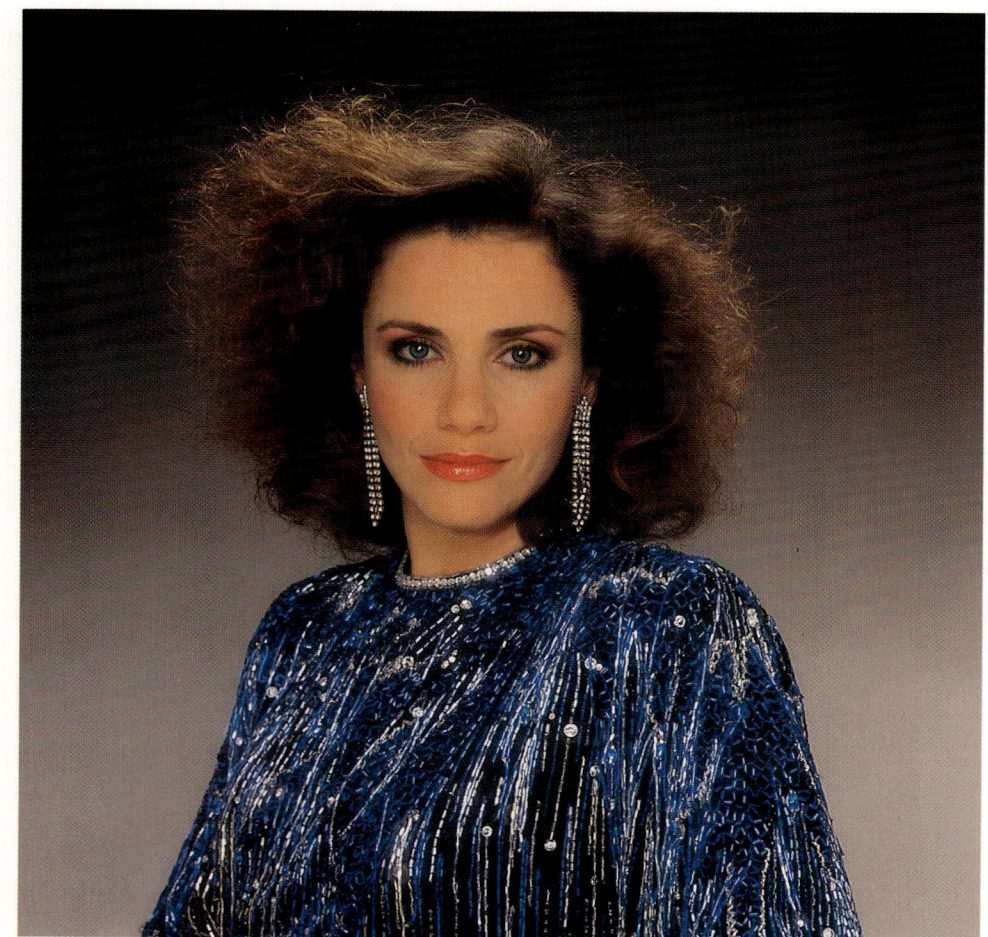

ELLEN BRY

Ellen's wonderful dark waves have been cut in moderate layers, then blown dry with a round brush to take out some of the curl for maximum volume and softness.

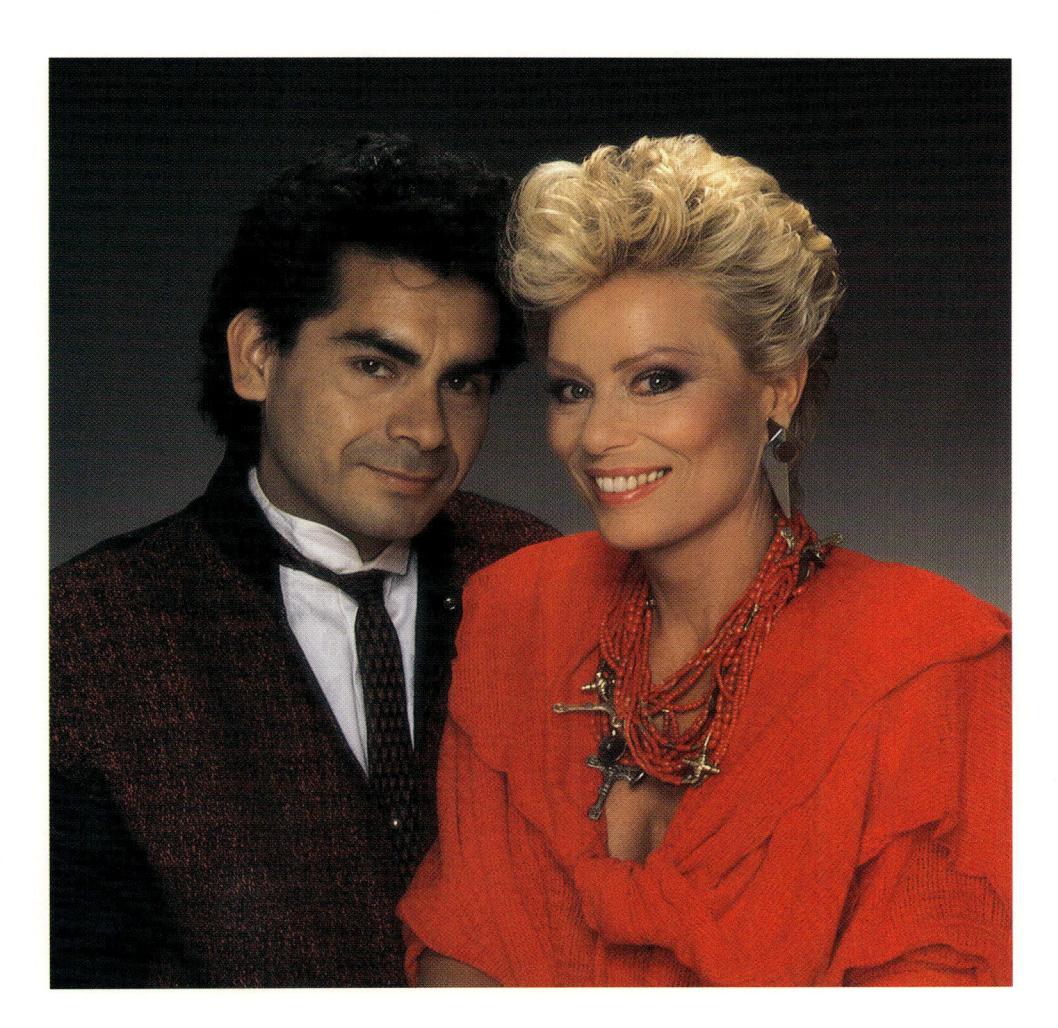

ABBY DALTON

Abby Dalton shows how youthful the right hairstyle can make you look. Abby has wonderful bone structure and can wear her hair off the face. Her hair is cut short, tapered in back, with lots of volume on top.

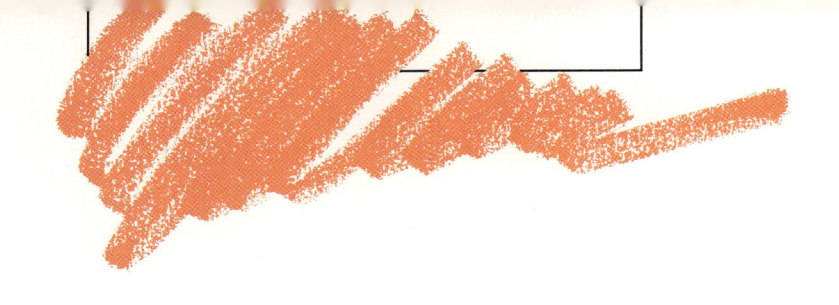

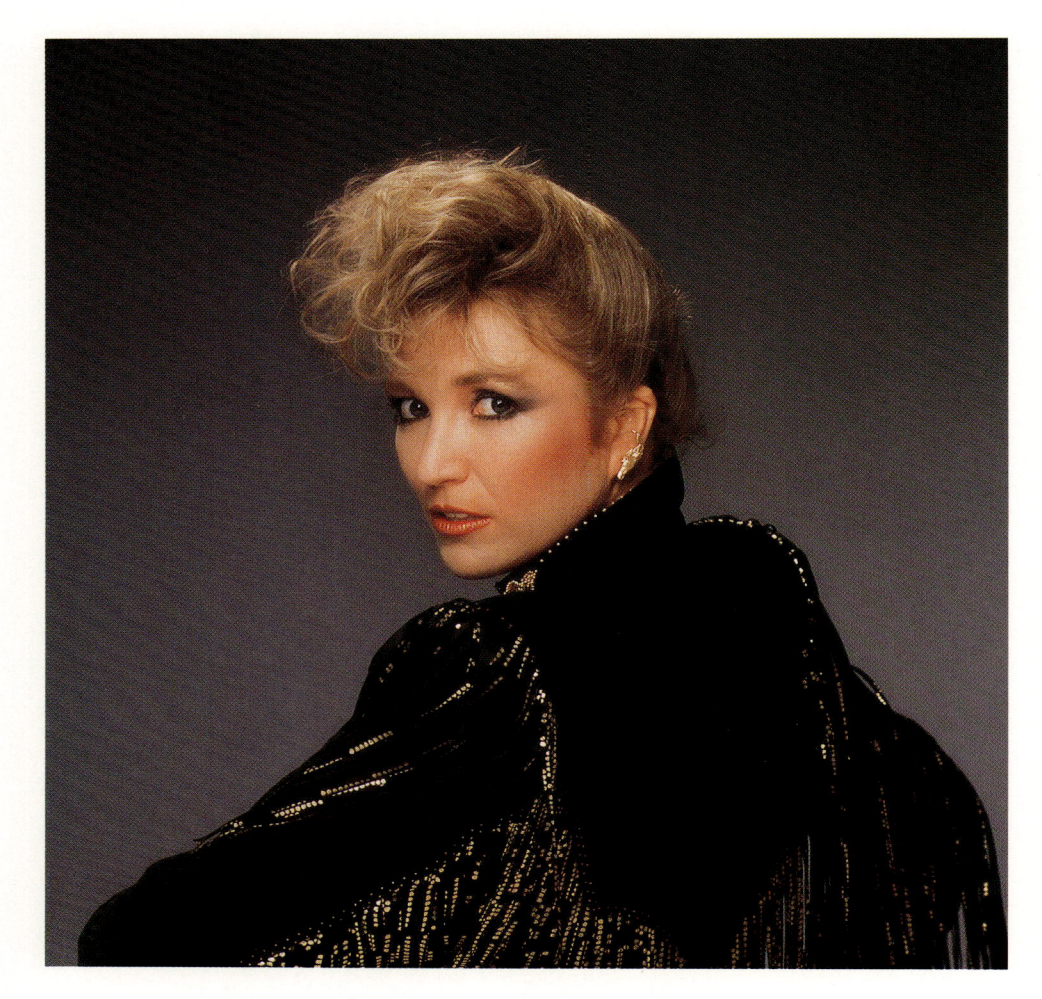

TANYA TUCKER

Tanya Tucker's fine hair is cut in short layers around the crown for height and volume. Here the longer sides and back are gathered into a French twist for a more controlled and less wild look.

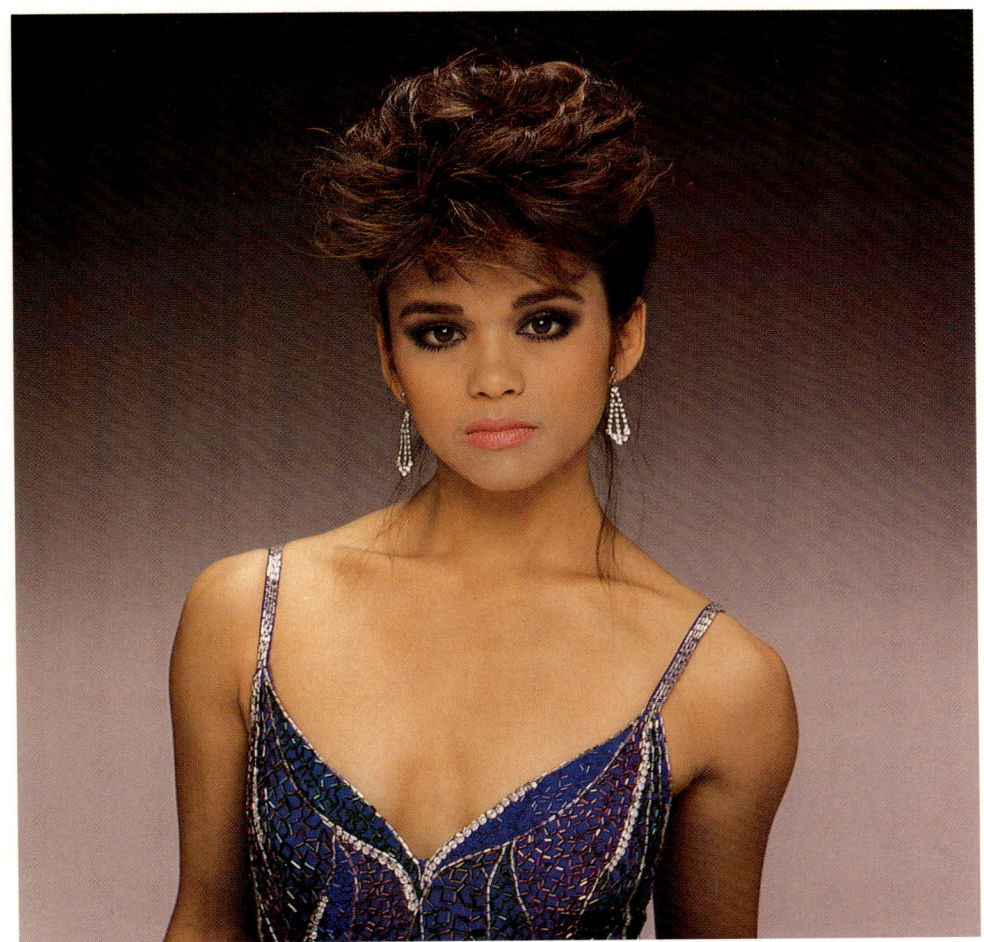

NIA PEEPLES

Nia Peeples, an exotic beauty, shows off a classic beauty style that is perfect for her petite frame. The hair is drawn into a twist in back, and the crown and bangs are swirled into soft waves that bring out her beautiful dark eyes.

CATHERINE HICKLAND

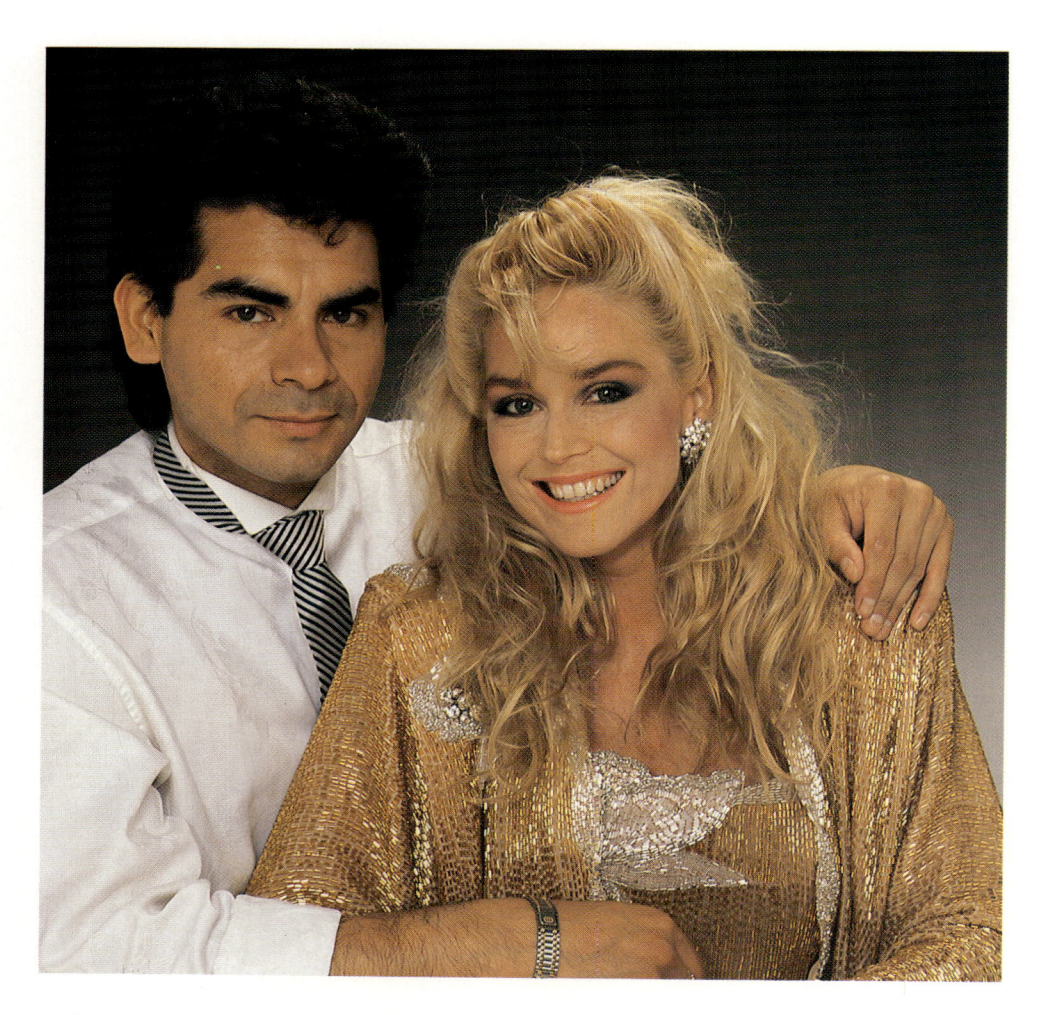

Catherine Hickland, a golden California blonde, wears her luxurious hair half up and half down. The crown is gathered into a base knot and the rest is worn down to show off the wonderful natural wave. By cutting very chunky, heavy bangs that are worn in only two strands, I've shown how to use hair as an accessory.

EMMYLOU HARRIS

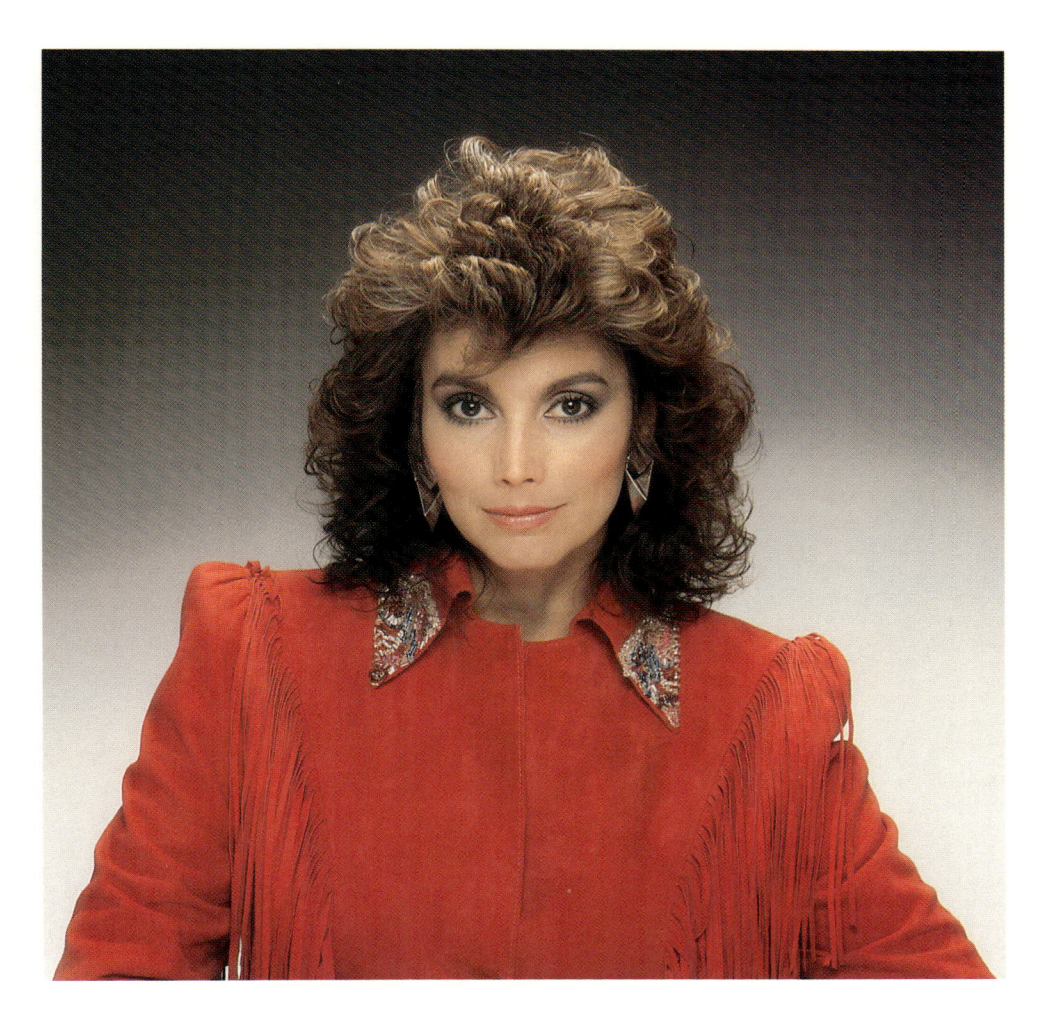

Emmylou Harris's long locks were cut to shoulder length and layered all over to give her baby-fine hair lots of movement and volume. Hot rollers and a final blow dry give her hair a soft and natural finish.

CLAIRE YARLETT

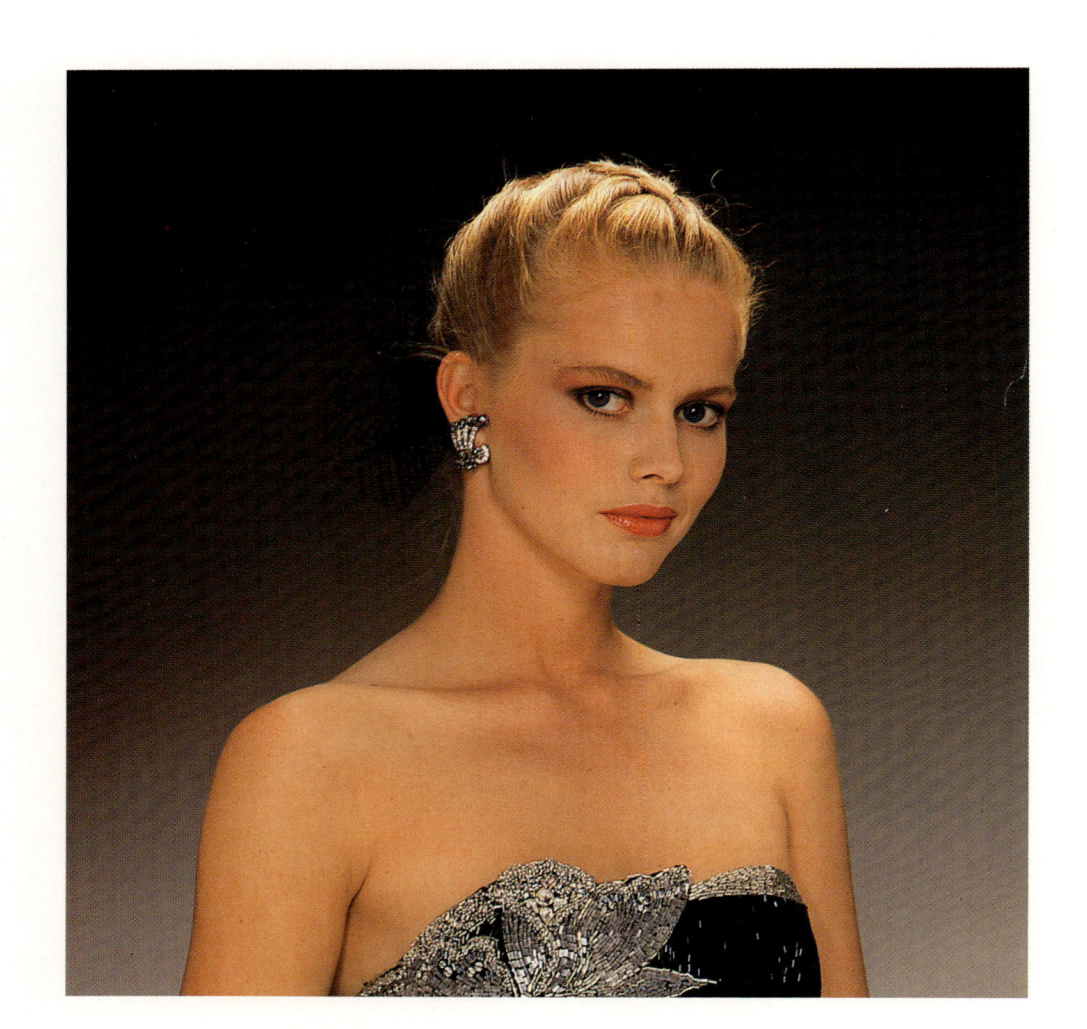

Claire Yarlett, a flawless beauty, wears her hair completely off the face. The hair is braided at the crown and arranged in a chignon in back.

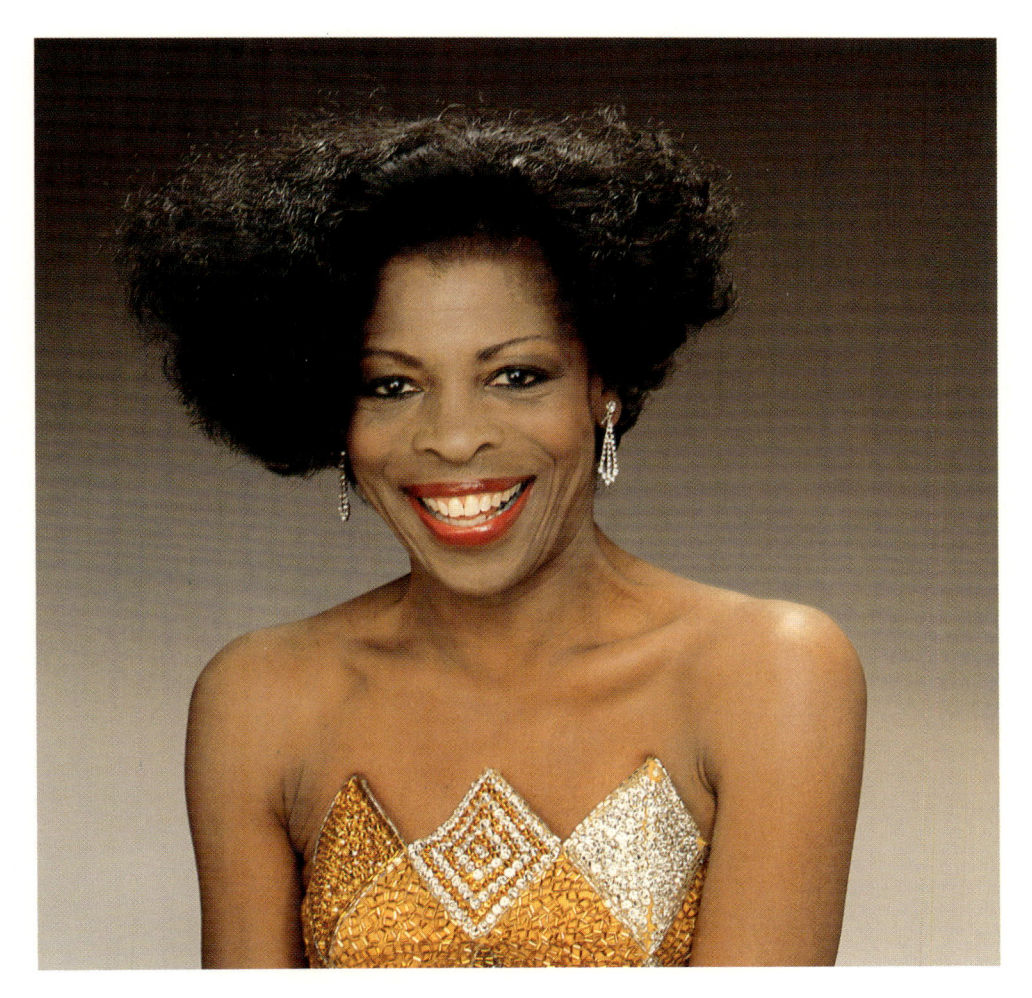

ROXIE ROKER

Roxie Roker changes her naturally curly look to a sleeker and straighter style with a wig. It's styled in a wedge bob, cut very short on top and gradually increasing in volume for fullness at the sides. Her own hair is swept over the front for a natural looking hairline.

DEBORAH MULLOWNEY

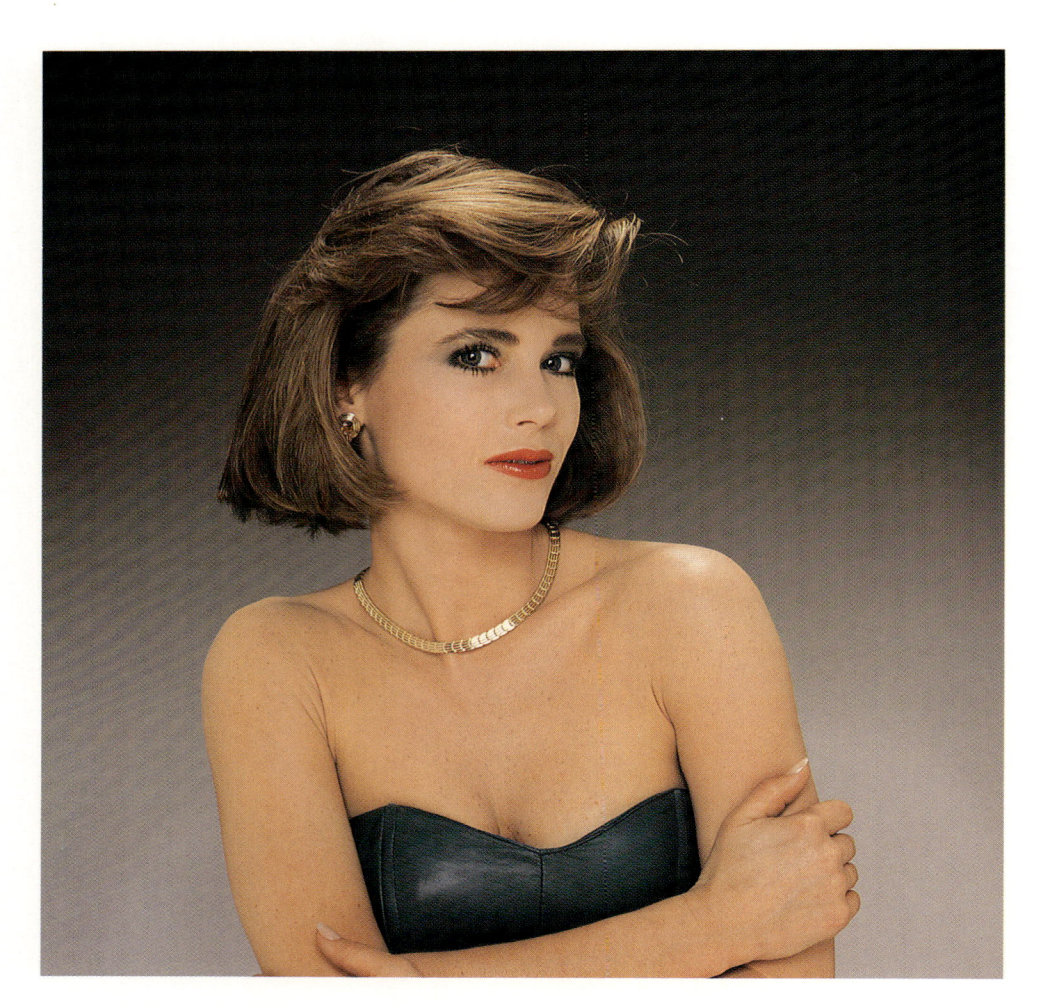

Deborah Mullowney's rich brown hair is full and thick with added golden highlights that make her hair shimmer. This versatile, chin-length, layered bob gives her the fresh clean look of a one-length cut.

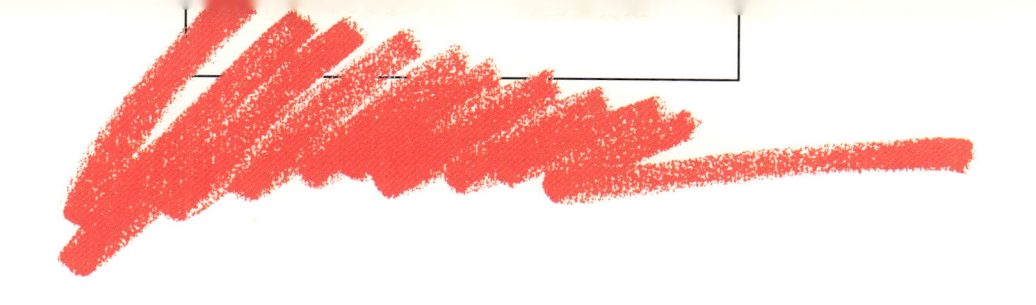

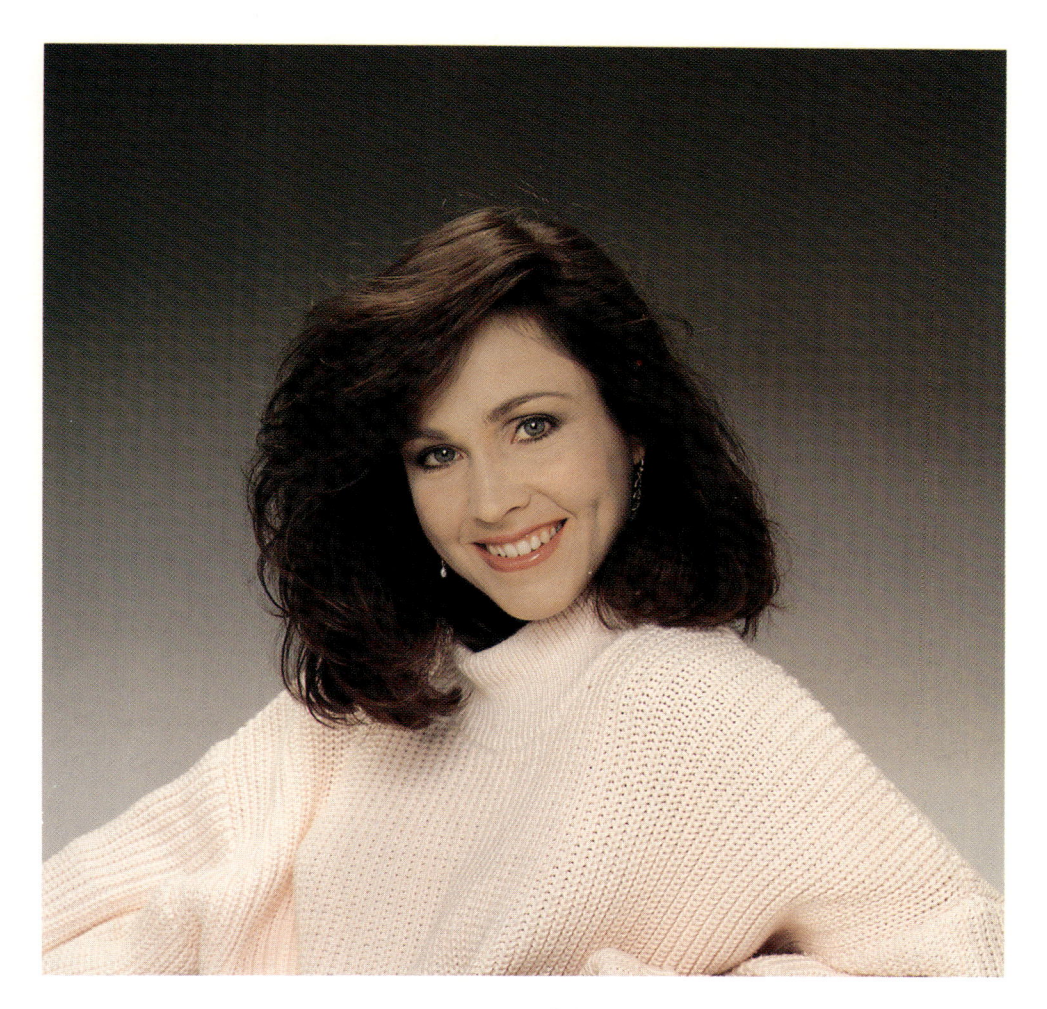

ERIN GREY

Erin Grey's thick, coffee-brown hair is best styled as naturally as possible. She's a true classic beauty. Her side-swept bangs and lots of full hair, slightly scrunched, add movement to the style.

PRISCILLA BARNES

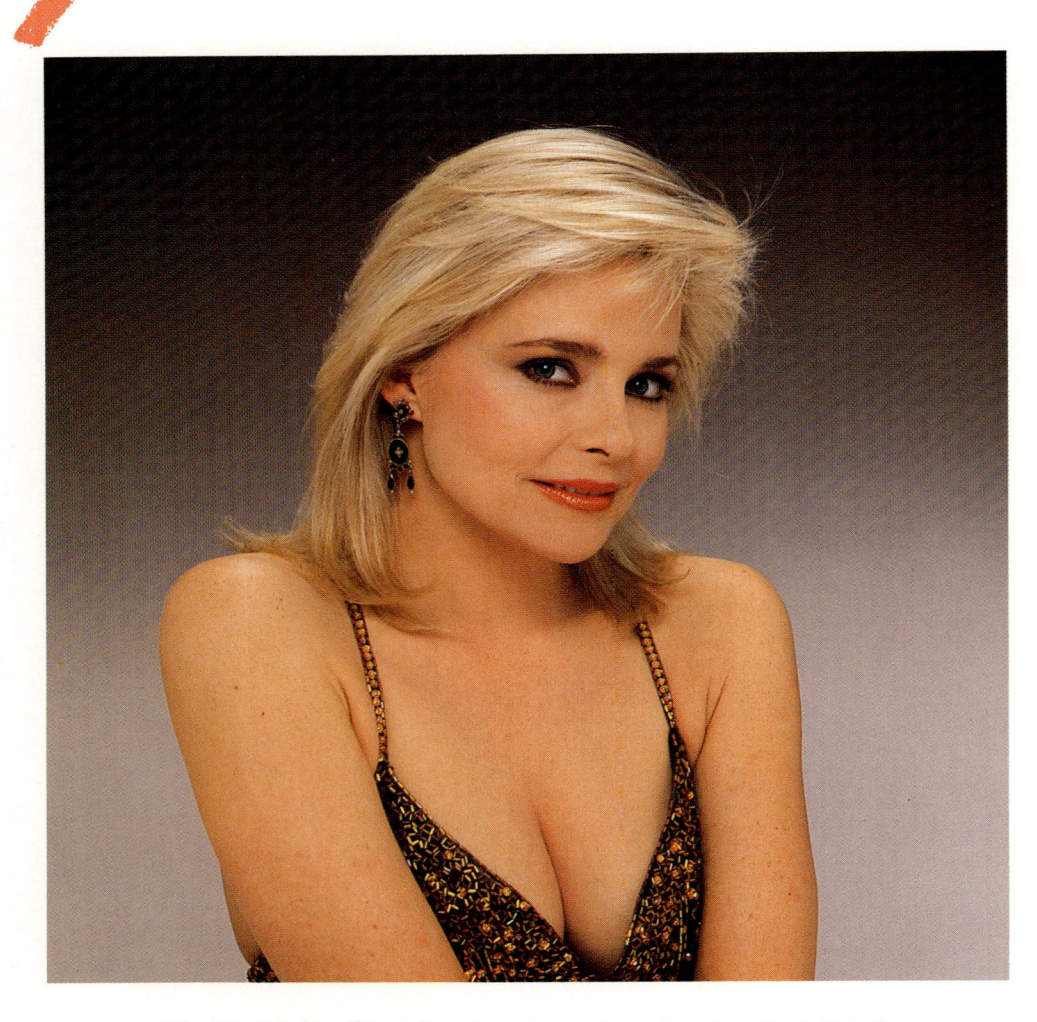

Priscilla Barnes's beautiful coloring and wonderful bone structure look best with a subtle framing. Her layered biunt-cut style shines with silvery golden highlights that have been woven into her hair.

ROSALIND CHAO

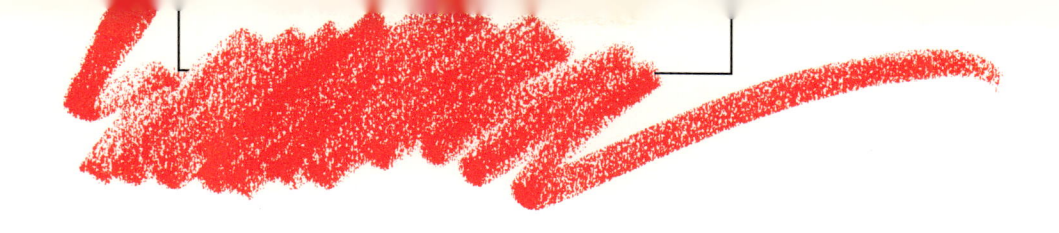

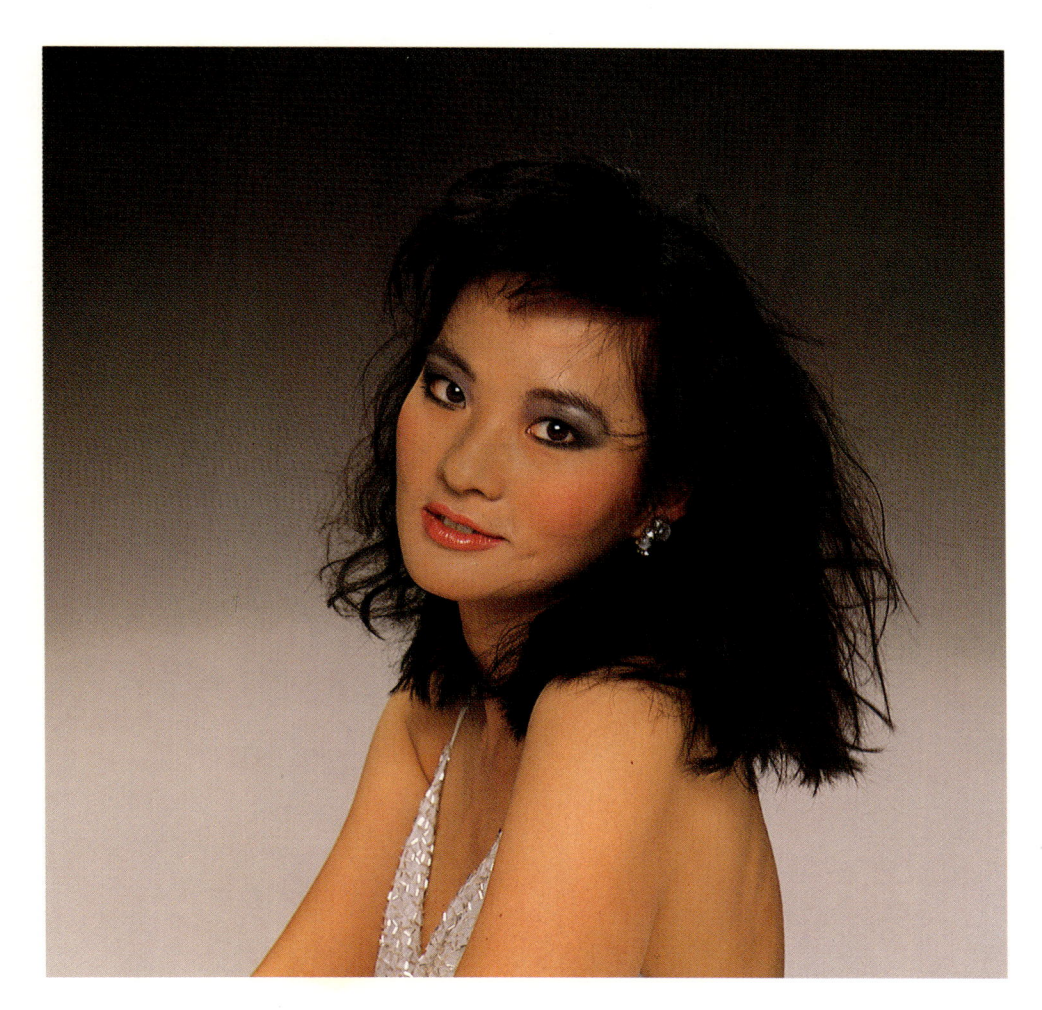

Rosalind Chao's almost blue-black hair is cut blunt with wispy bangs. For this classic beauty look, I've added mousse, scrunged the hair, and side-swept the bangs to add movement to the style.

MERETE VAN KAMP

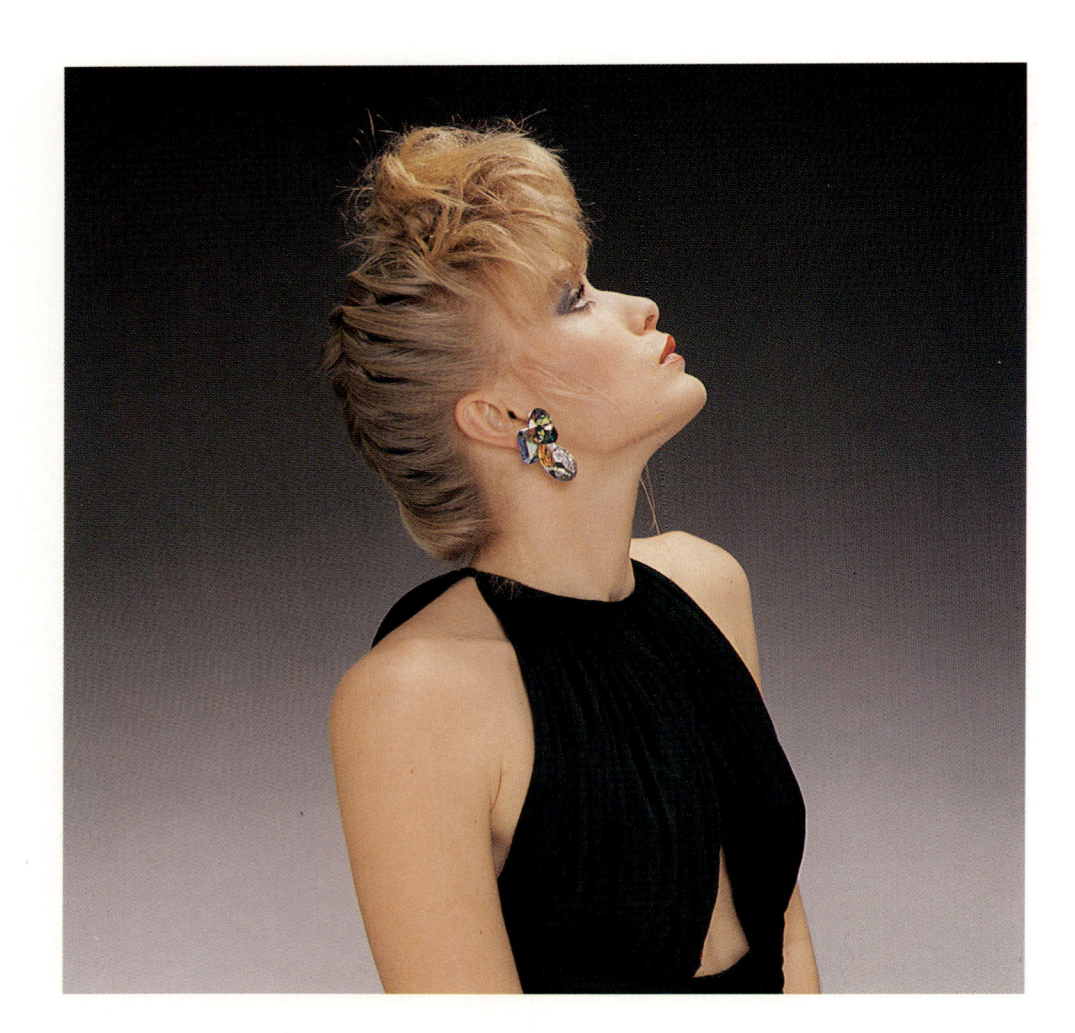

Merete Van Kamp's regal beauty look is achieved by sweeping the hair up in a French braid and curling the bangs for a full, feathery effect.

JAYNE KENNEDY OVERTON

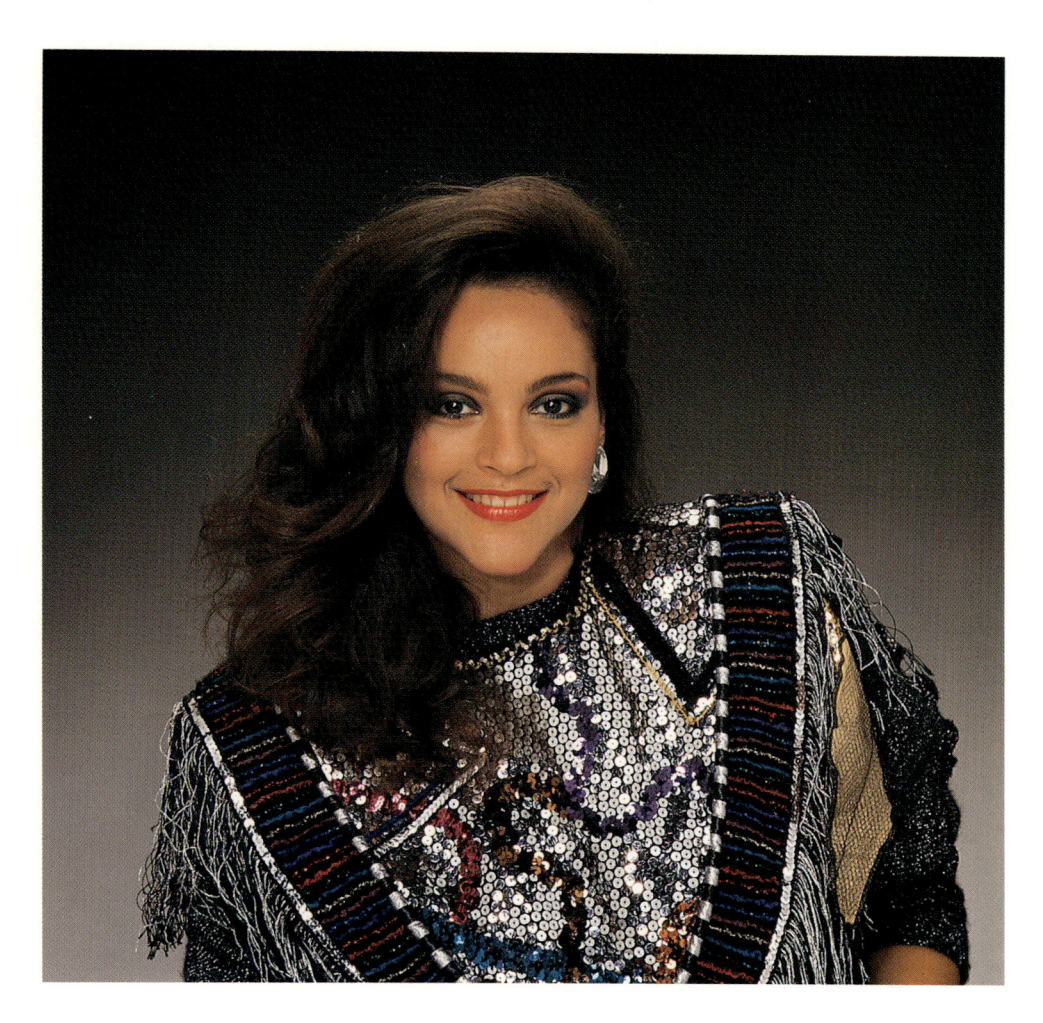

Jayne Kennedy Overton's fabulous mane is swept to one side in a loose cascade of soft waves. To avoid a bulky look and give the hair movement, I gradually layered her hair from the chin to about four inches below the shoulders.

BARBARA CARRERA

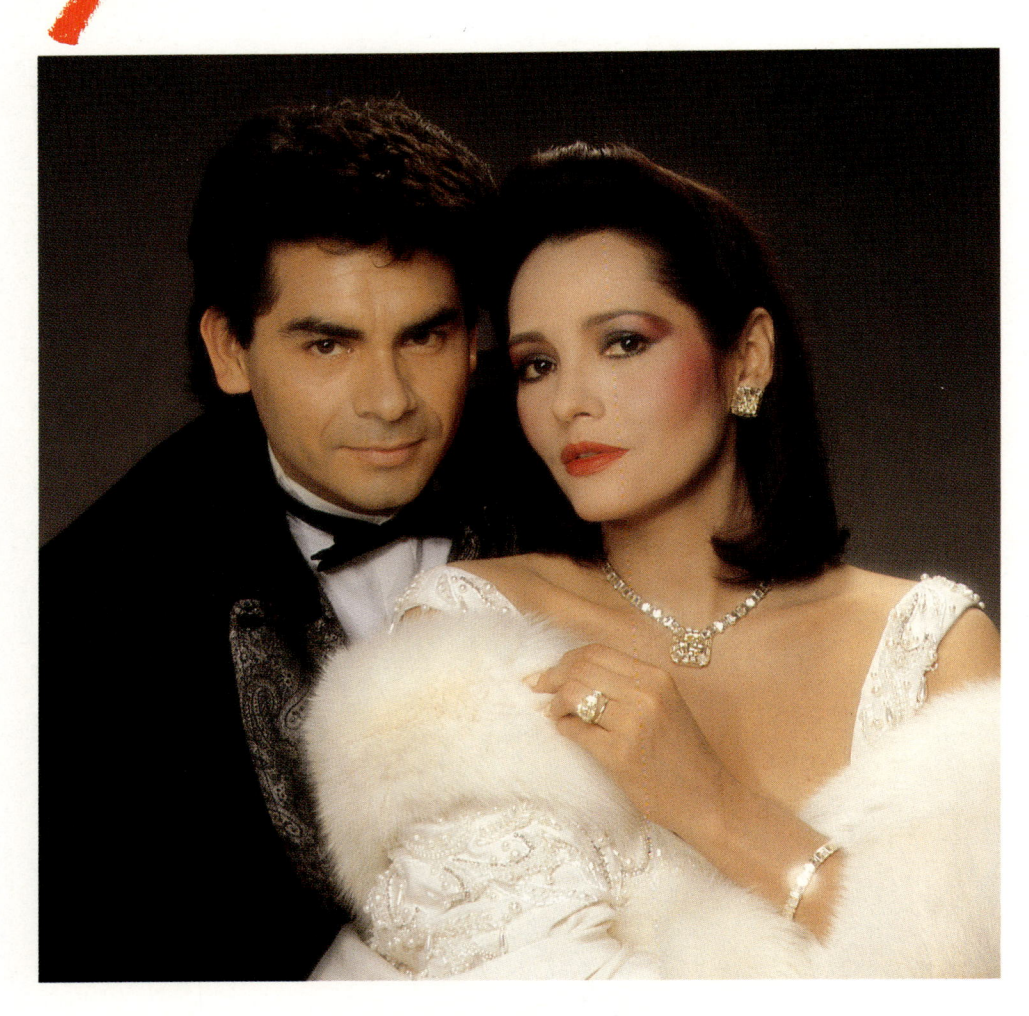

Barbara Carrera embodies the look of classic elegance. Her dark brown, abundant thin hair has been brightened to a rich berrywood red and cut to a one-length bob giving her maximum styling versatility. The smooth front roll adds height over her forehead.

Styling—The Look That's Right for You

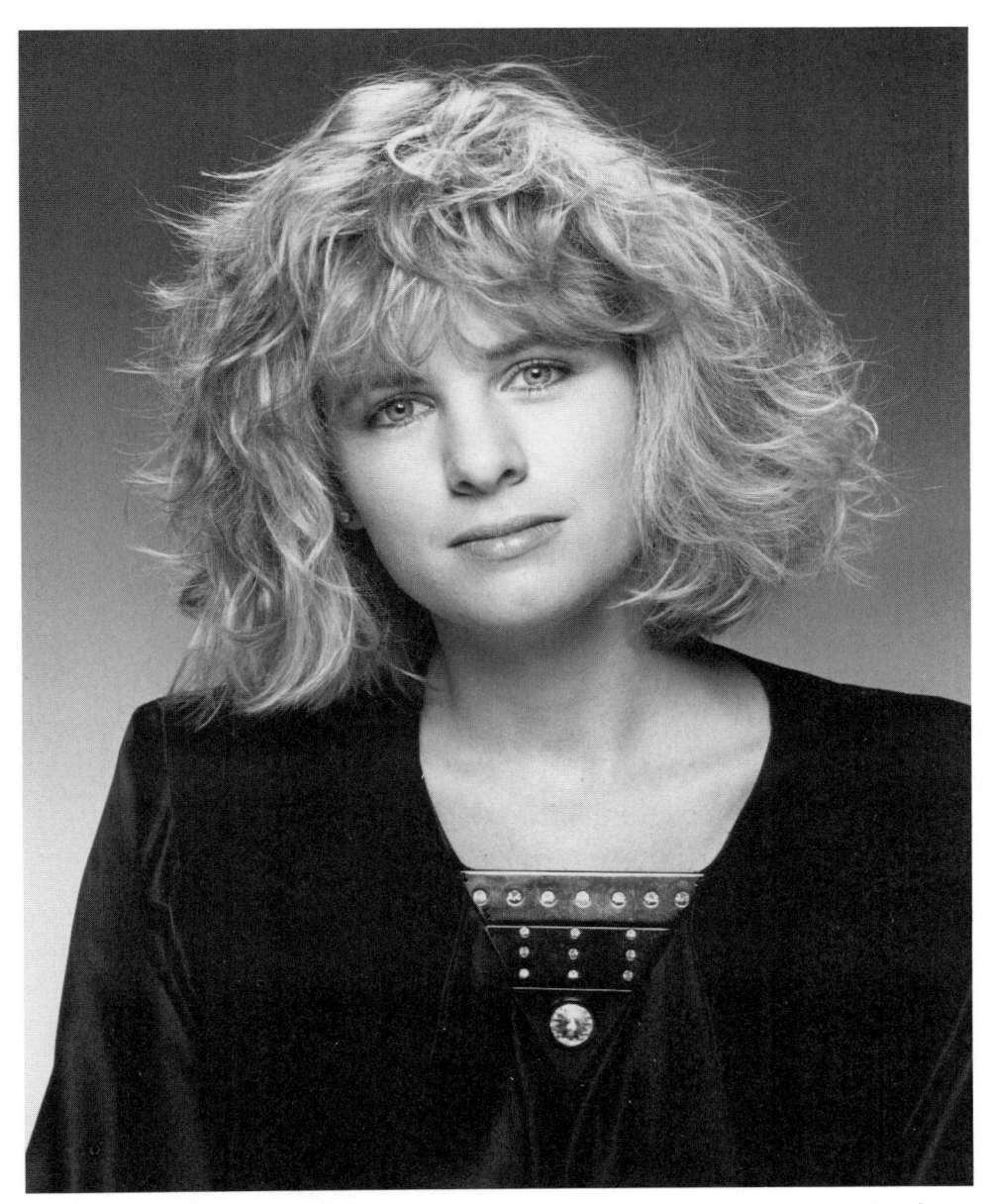

STYLE 2 FOR MEDIUM-LENGTH STRAIGHT HAIR: A full-blown style with lots of body and volume—the result of the twisted pin curl set. A little bit of scrunching adds movement as the hair is blown dry.

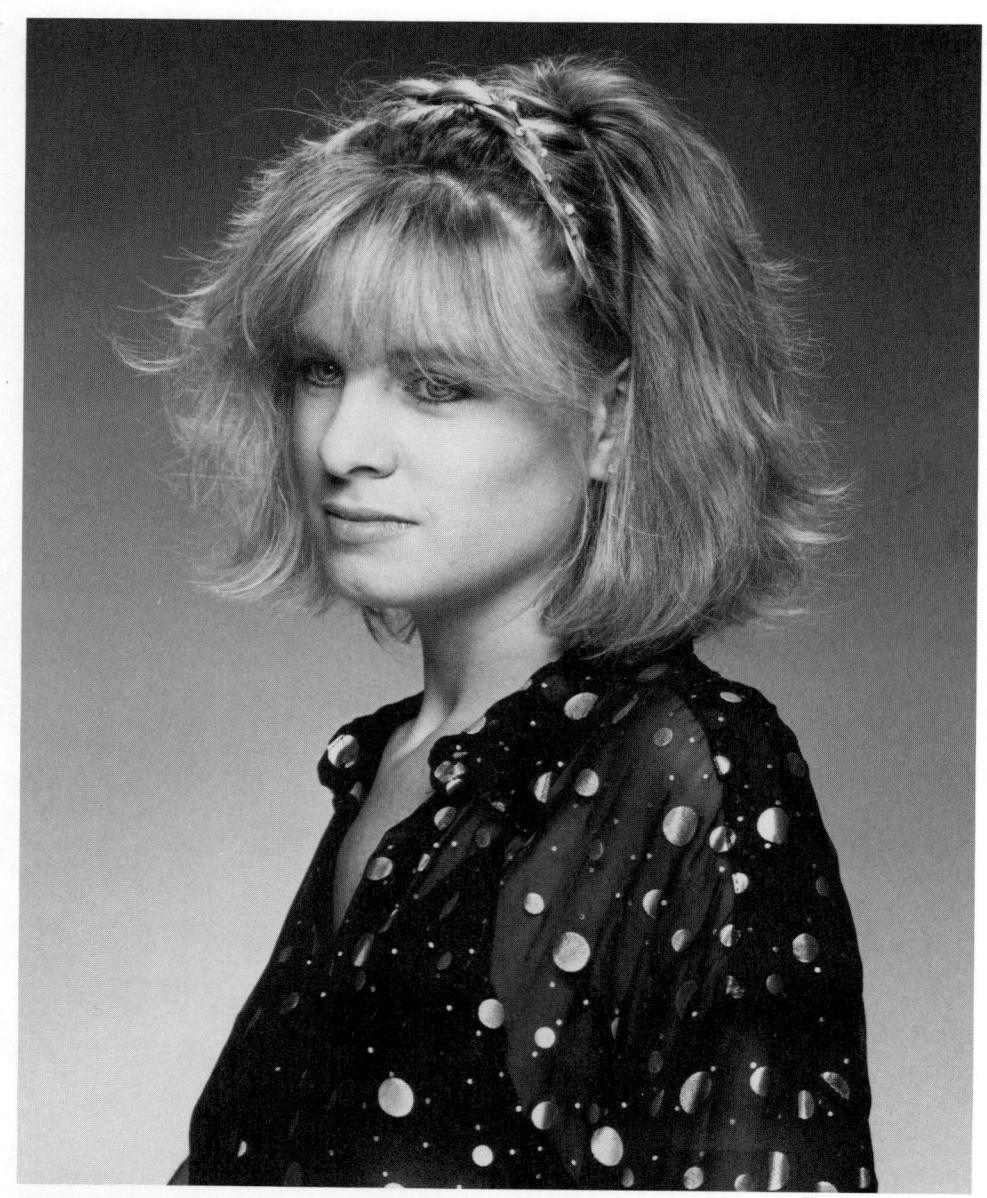

STYLE 3 FOR MEDIUM-LENGTH STRAIGHT HAIR: For a quick change of pace, make a thin braid on each side, just above the ears. Bring them up over the crown and cross them to form a natural hair headband. Airy, full bangs are brushed straight, and the rest of the hair is slightly scrunched for volume.

Styling—The Look That's Right for You

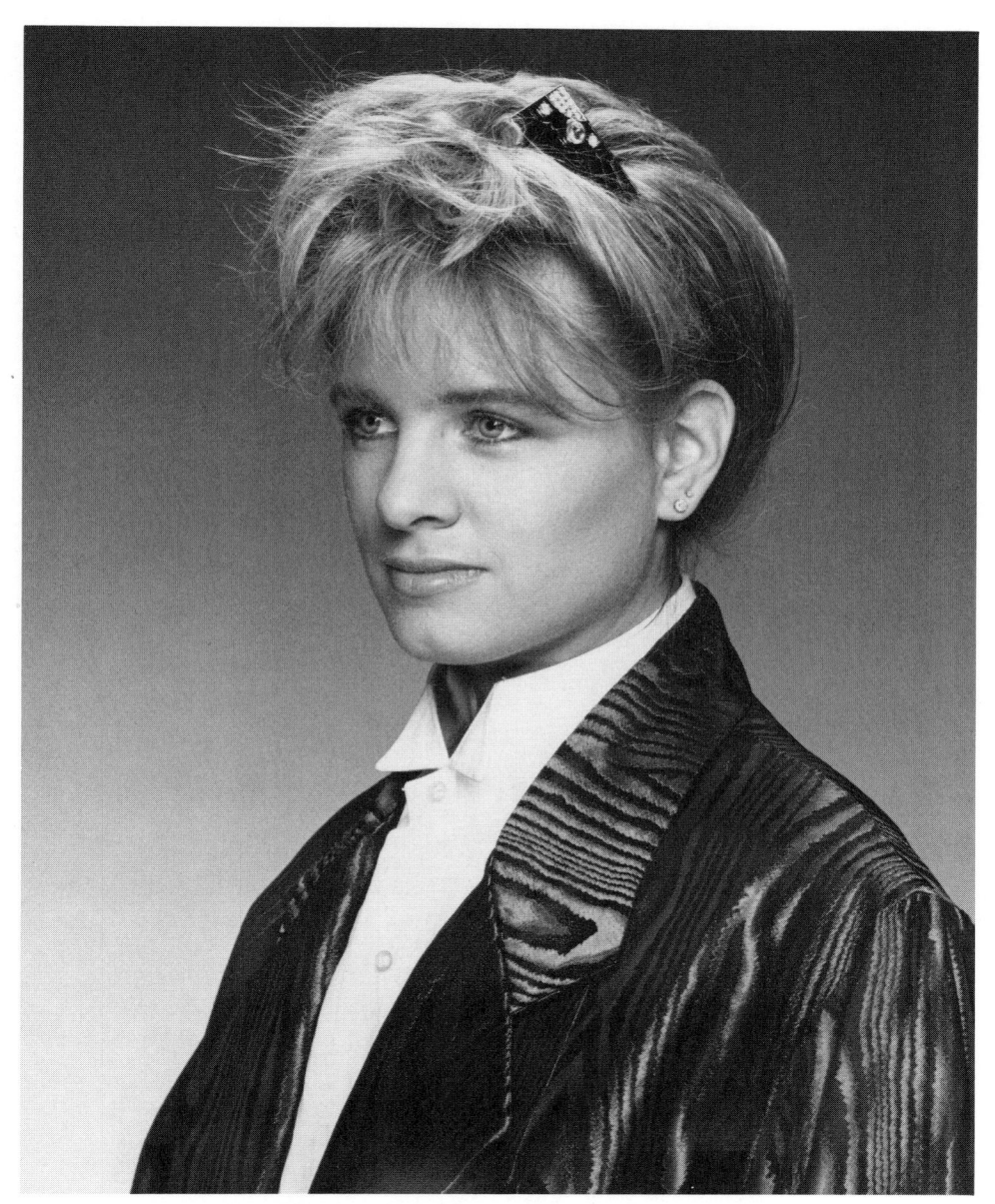

STYLE 4 FOR MEDIUM-LENGTH STRAIGHT HAIR: Up-dos can be simple and elegant, like this one. The hair is swept up and forward from the nape and pinned over the crown with a hair ornament. The front is slightly backcombed and brought over the brow in airy strands.

Twisted Pin Curl Set on Medium Hair

To add volume and fullness to medium-length hair, set the top, sides, and back in twisted pin curls.

1. Divide hair into sections—front, sides, crown, and back.
2. Lightly moisten hair with a water spritzer. Don't oversaturate. (You don't want wet hair, just slightly damp.)

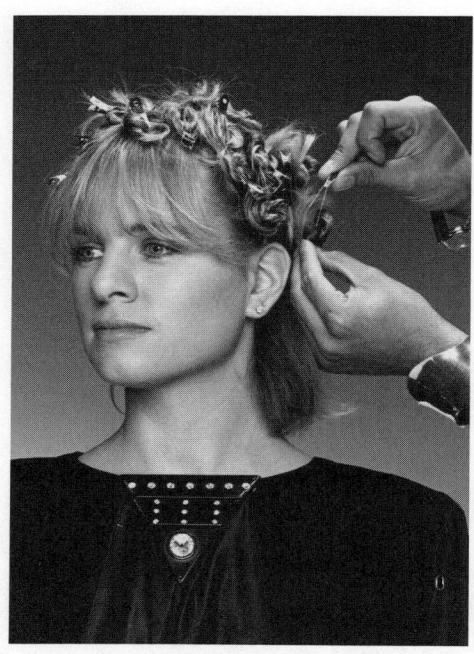

TWISTED PIN CURL SET FOR MEDIUM-LENGTH HAIR: Section the hair, and start making pin curls at the crown, then sides. This set works best on dry hair moistened with mousse. To make pin curls: section strand for pin curl (one inch wide), twist from root to end, roll into flat pin curl, and secure with a clip. For a looser curl, wind a larger strand of hair; for a tighter curl, a smaller strand.

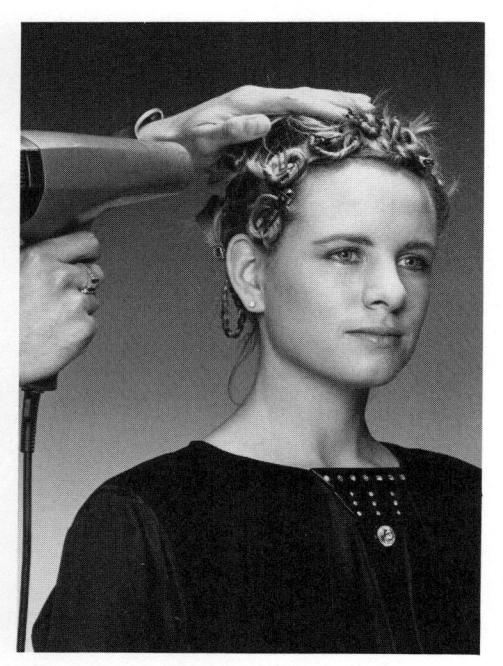

FINISHING THE PIN CURL SET: Dry hair with a blow dryer one section at a time. When hair is dry, undo pin curls, shake hair, and apply blow dryer again, using a low setting to loosen the curl a bit.

Styling—The Look That's Right for You

3. Take a small amount of mousse (about a half-dollar's size) and rub palms together to lighten thickness of mousse. Apply to hair.
4. Divide each section into strands about a half inch wide. Twist each strand from end to root. Secure in place with a pin curl clip. Finish entire head or areas that you want curled.
5. Dry with a blow dryer.
6. Remove pin curls, shake hair, and brush into place.

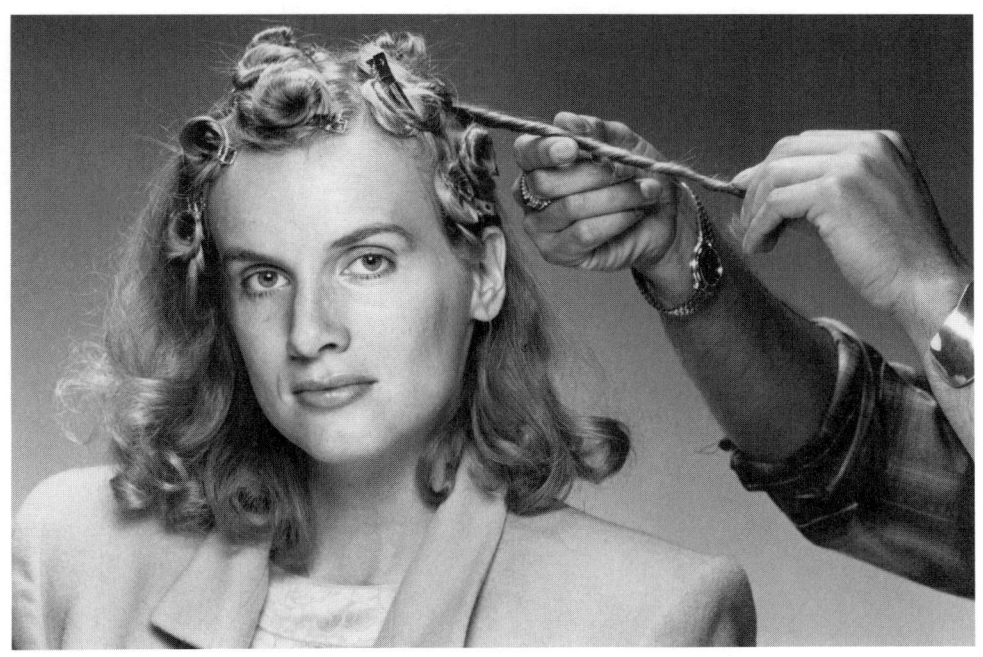

TWISTED PIN CURL SET FOR LONG HAIR: Note how model Gunilla Persson's hair is held in sections, twisted from the ends to the roots, then secured with a clip. Dress by Margi Kent, Melrose Avenue, Los Angeles.

TOVAR'S CLASSIC BEAUTY

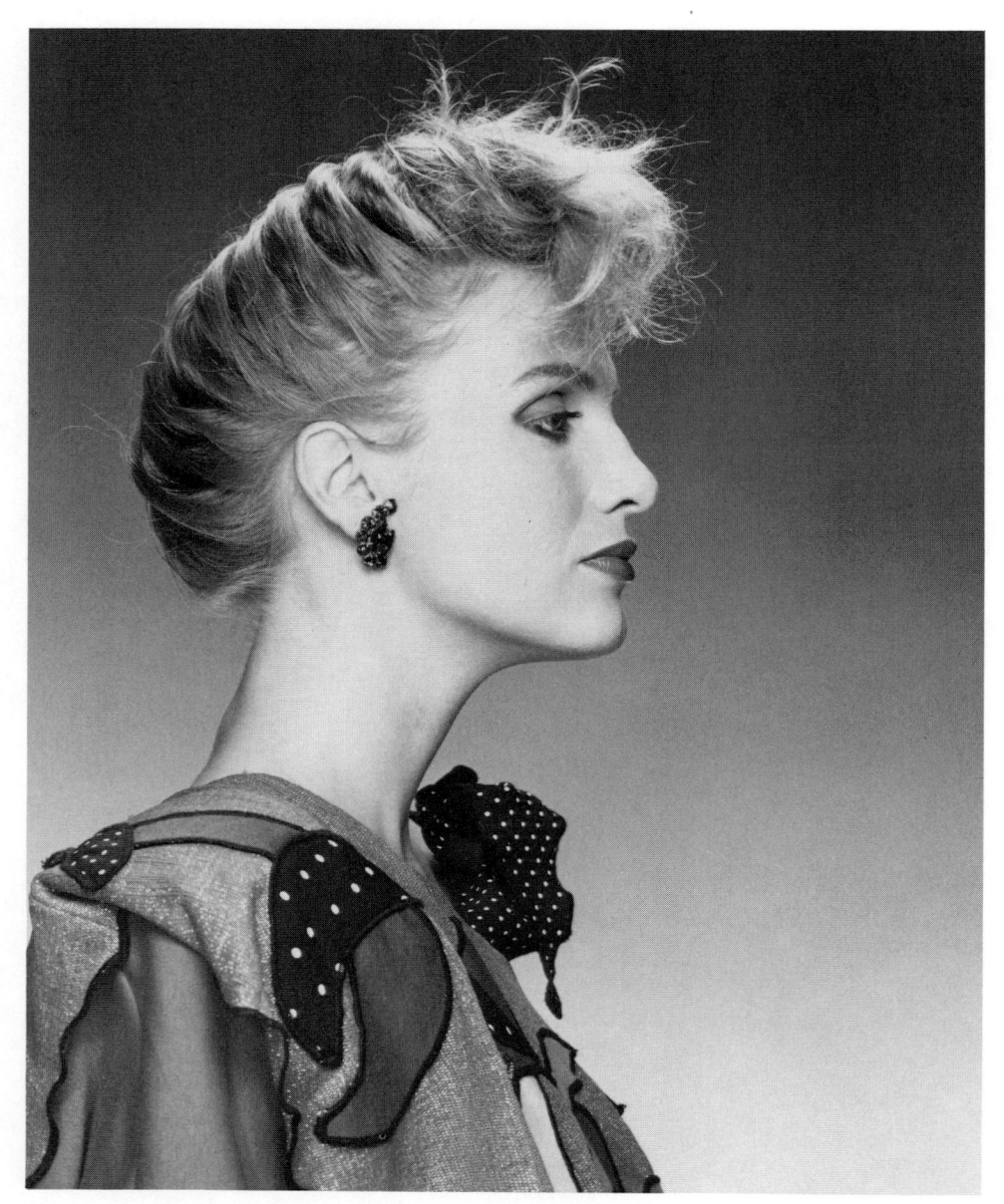

STYLE 1 FOR LAYERED SHOULDER-LENGTH HAIR: This elegant up-do is achieved with an inverted french braid begun at the nape and pinned at the crown.

Styling—The Look That's Right for You

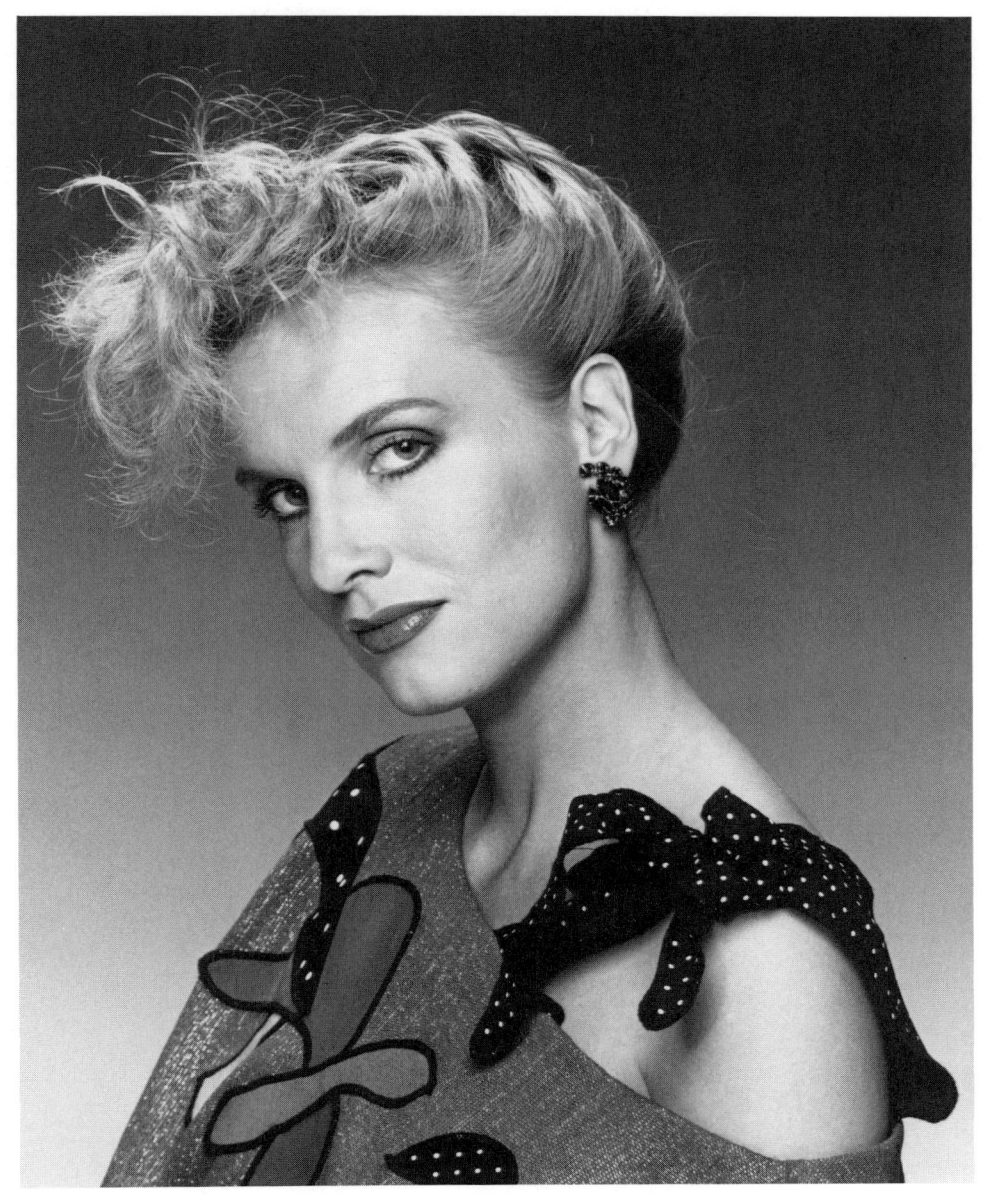

The front is scrunched and arranged falling over one side of the forehead.

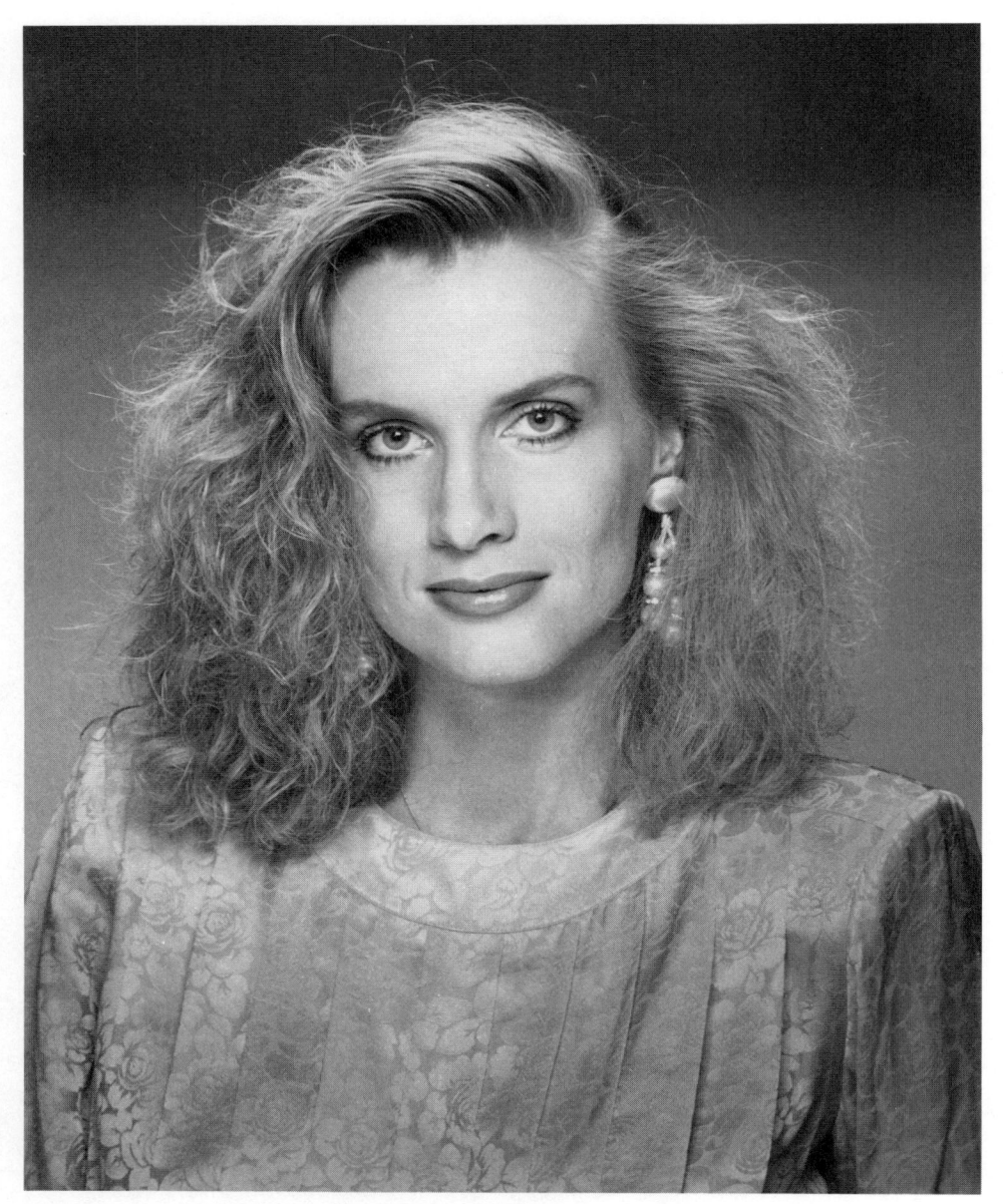

STYLE 2 FOR LAYERED SHOULDER-LENGTH HAIR: This style—sleek at the top, full-blown on the sides—is the result of the twisted pin curl set.

Styling—The Look That's Right for You

BLOW-DRYING CURLY HAIR STRAIGHT

1. Blow-dry following basic directions to step 4.
2. Using a large-diameter round brush, blow-dry as directed in steps 5 and 6. Don't squeeze hair with fingers. Keep the hair wound around the brush as tightly as possible, as shown in the photograph.

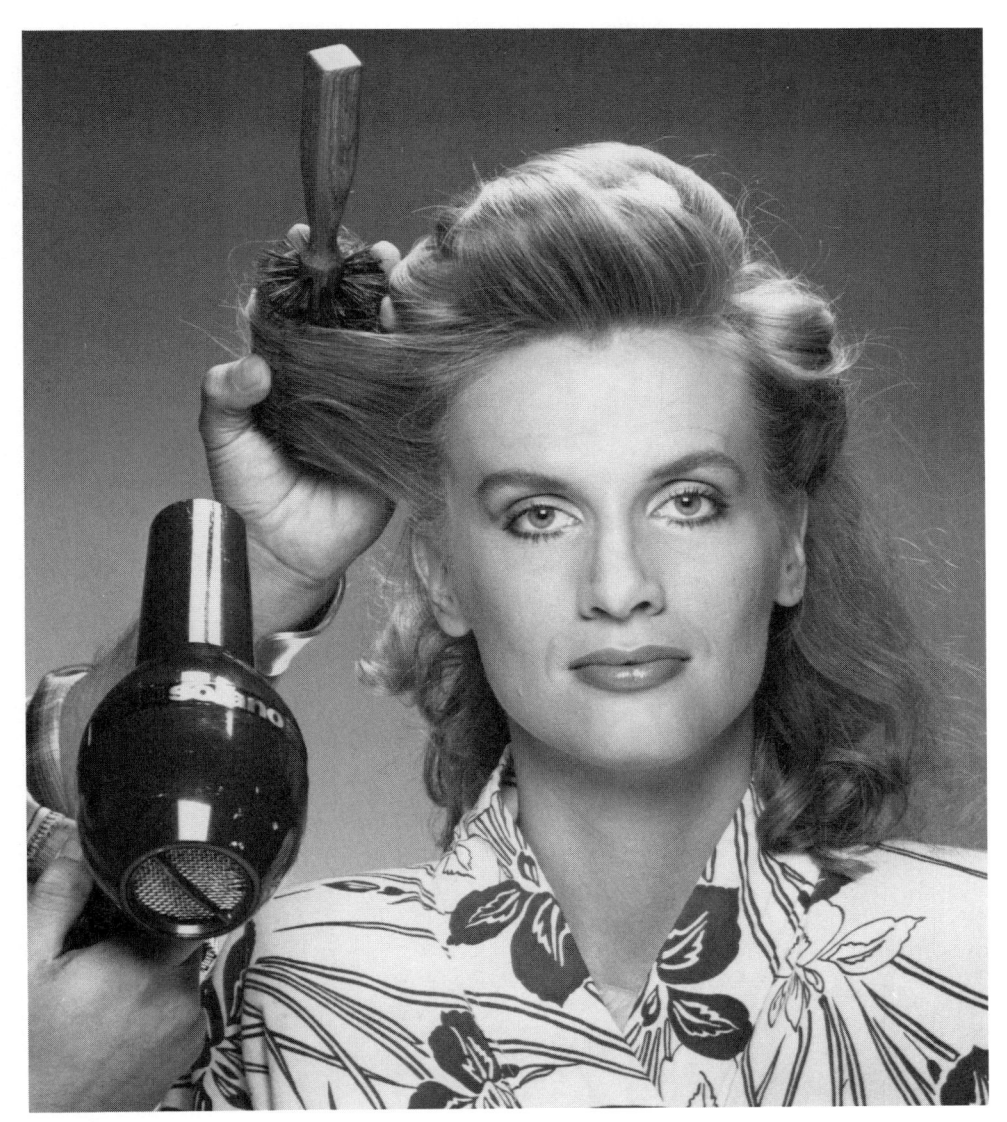

TAKING OUT THE CURL: Section the hair, pin it out of the way, and start working at the back. Use a wide round brush, wind the hair around it, and hold firmly. Use the blower on a medium setting for best results.

HOW TO USE A CURLING IRON

1. Use on *dry hair only*.
2. Open curling iron, take the strand of hair, and run it first through the hot wand from root to end. This will warm the hair and prepare it for curling.
3. Start rolling the hair around the wand from tips to root. Hold curling iron for a few seconds and release guard to let hair out.
4. Let hair cool before styling. If you style *hot* hair, the result will be frizzy, not curly or wavy.

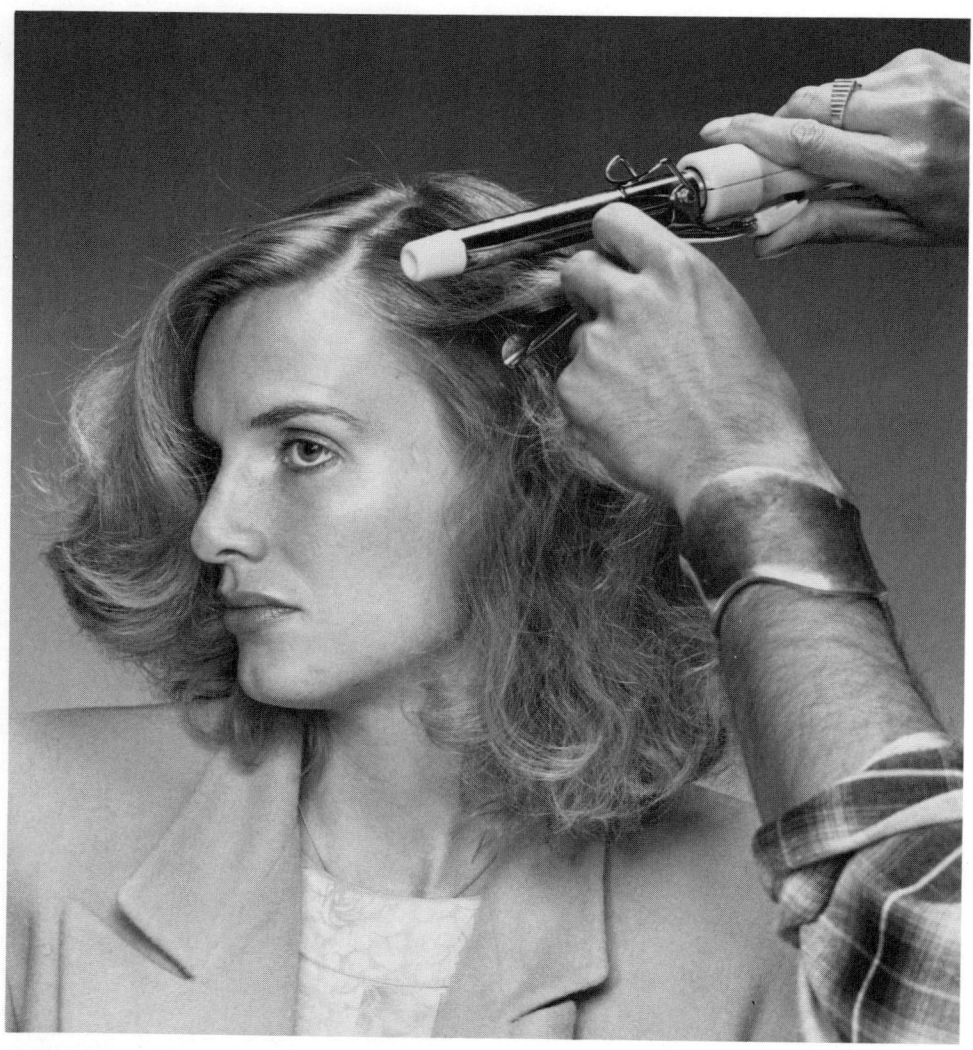

CURLING IRON: Divide hair by strands. Pass the strand to be curled through the heated iron once. Then wind around the wand. Hold for a few seconds and release. Wait for hair to cool before styling. If you have to curl a lot of hair, just hold in place with a clip to keep the curl from drooping.

Styling—The Look That's Right for You

STYLING AIDS

How to Use Mousse

One of the most common mistakes when using mousse is to use too much. Mousse abuse makes hair sticky and weighs it down.

Apply a dollop of mousse, about the size of a half-dollar, to the palms of your hands. Rub palms together to loosen mousse. Run palms through damp hair. Style hair in desired manner.

You can also apply mousse to dry hair to "set" or give direction to a style. For example, if you want to slick back the sides of your hair, add just a dab of mousse to each side and they will stay flat.

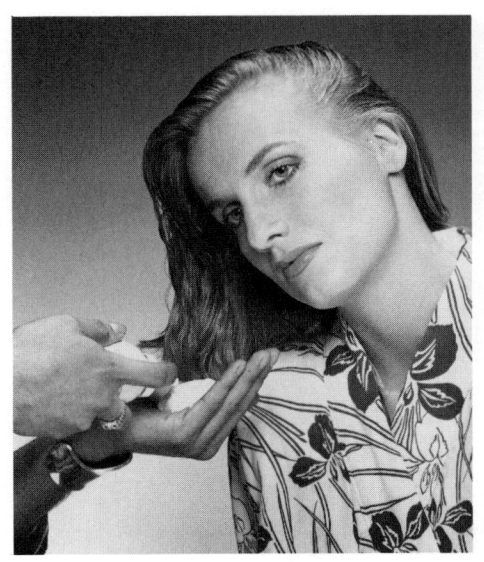

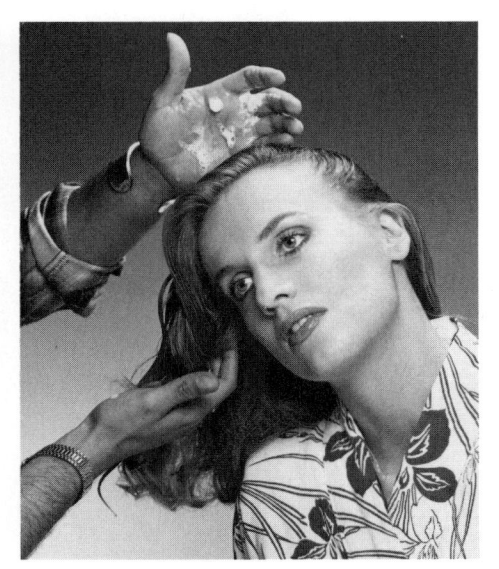

APPLYING MOUSSE: Squeeze mousse into palm of hand. Then rub palms together and apply mousse to the hair from the roots out, so that more of the product is deposited on the roots for added volume. If more mousse is deposited at the ends, the result will be flat hair.

How to Use Gel

Gel can be used to get a wet look or to add body to hair. Some curly styles require gel for finishing. Gel can be applied to wet or dry hair, depending on the look you hope to achieve.

For Wet-Looking Hair: Comb style into place. Squeeze a dot of gel (about the size of a dime) on the palm of your hands. Rub palms together to spread the gel. Run through hair. Recomb style, making sure to define waves and lines you want emphasized.

TOVAR'S CLASSIC BEAUTY

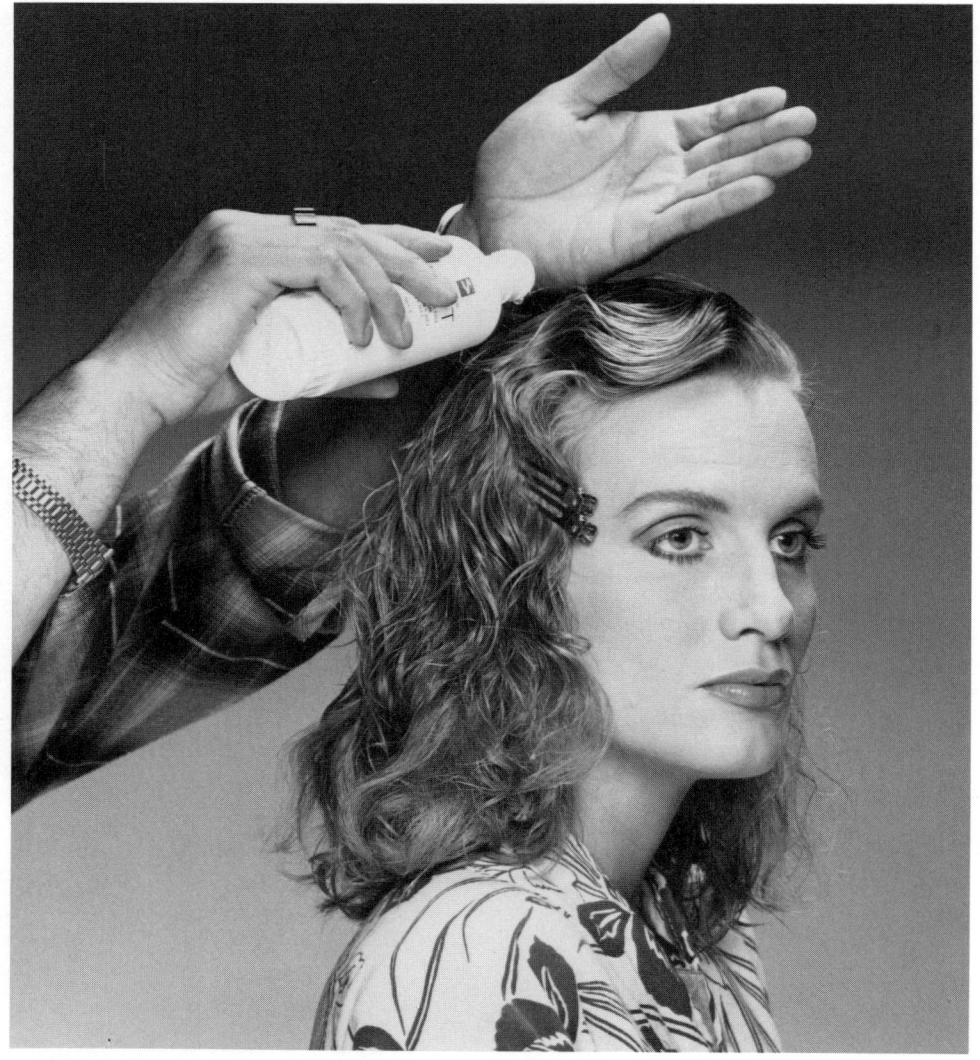

SCULPTING GEL: To sculpt waves, apply liquid gel to the palms of the hands, rub together, and run through hair. Sculpt waves with fingers.

For Body: Use same amount as above, on damp-dry hair. Apply gel *to the roots only.* Blow-dry and finish style as required.

HOW TO USE SCULPTING LOTION

Sculpting lotion is used to define waves. Comb damp hair into place. Squeeze small amount of lotion onto the palm of hands. Rub palms to spread the lotion. Apply to hair and make waves as desired. Let dry without disturbing.

Styling—The Look That's Right for You

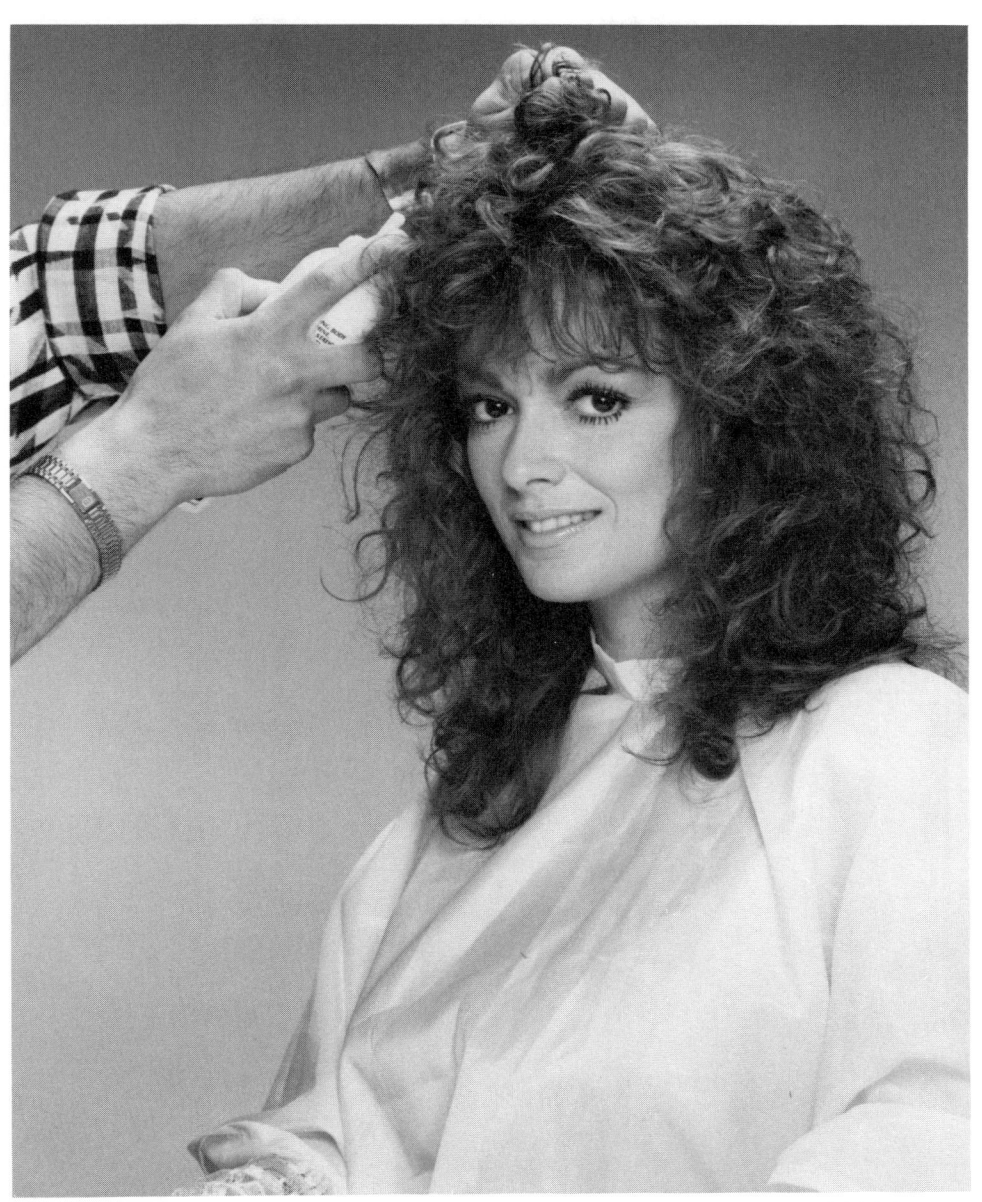

NATURALLY CURLY LONG HAIR: Sheila Aldridge, one of the singing Aldridge sisters and an actress, is one of my regular clients. Her hair is naturally curly and long, with lots of volume and kick, but because it is very heavy, it has a tendency to get flat at the crown. To avoid this, I layer it short at the crown for height; leave long, airy bangs for versatility; and layer the rest of it to end about four inches below the shoulders.

TOVAR'S CLASSIC BEAUTY

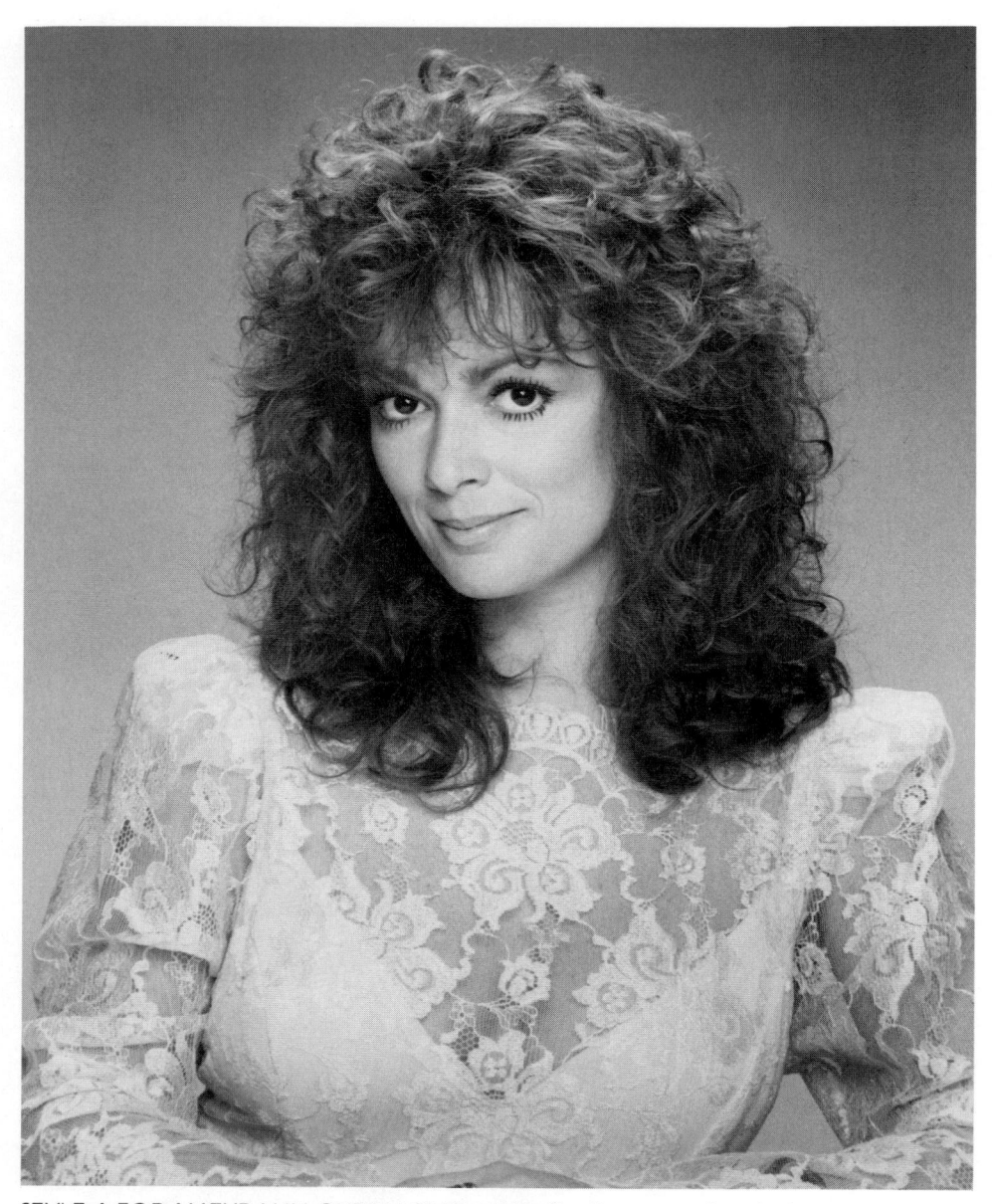

STYLE 1 FOR NATURALLY CURLY LONG HAIR: Sheila wears her hair as close to its natural state as possible, gently blow-dried and scrunched for the softly waved effect. Dress by Eletra Cassadei.

Styling—The Look That's Right for You

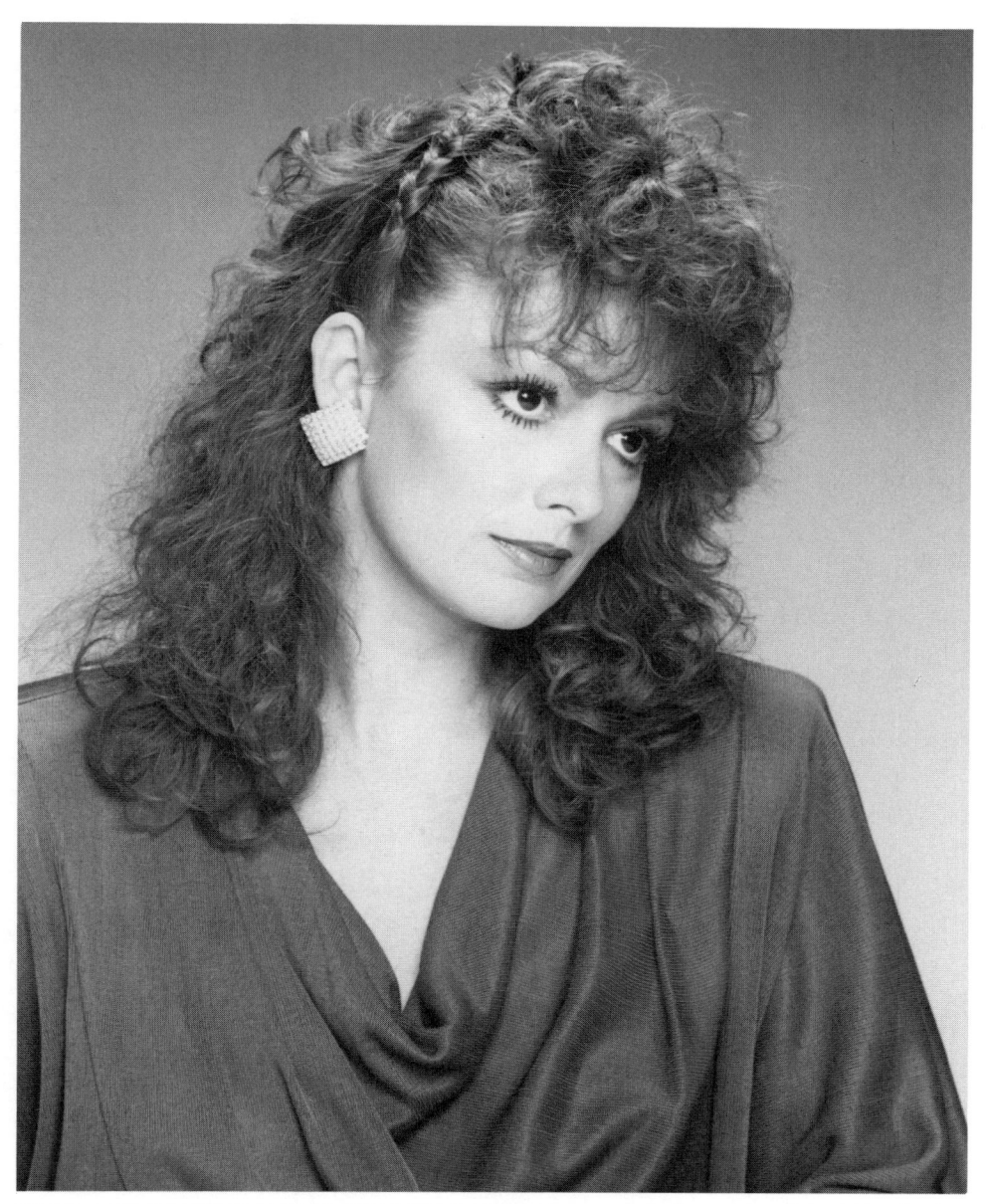

STYLE 2 FOR NATURALLY CURLY LONG HAIR: For a variation, I braided the hair on one side and left the rest down, soft and airy, cascading to just below the shoulders. Top by Margi Kent, Melrose Avenue, Los Angeles. Earrings by Bobi Leonard.

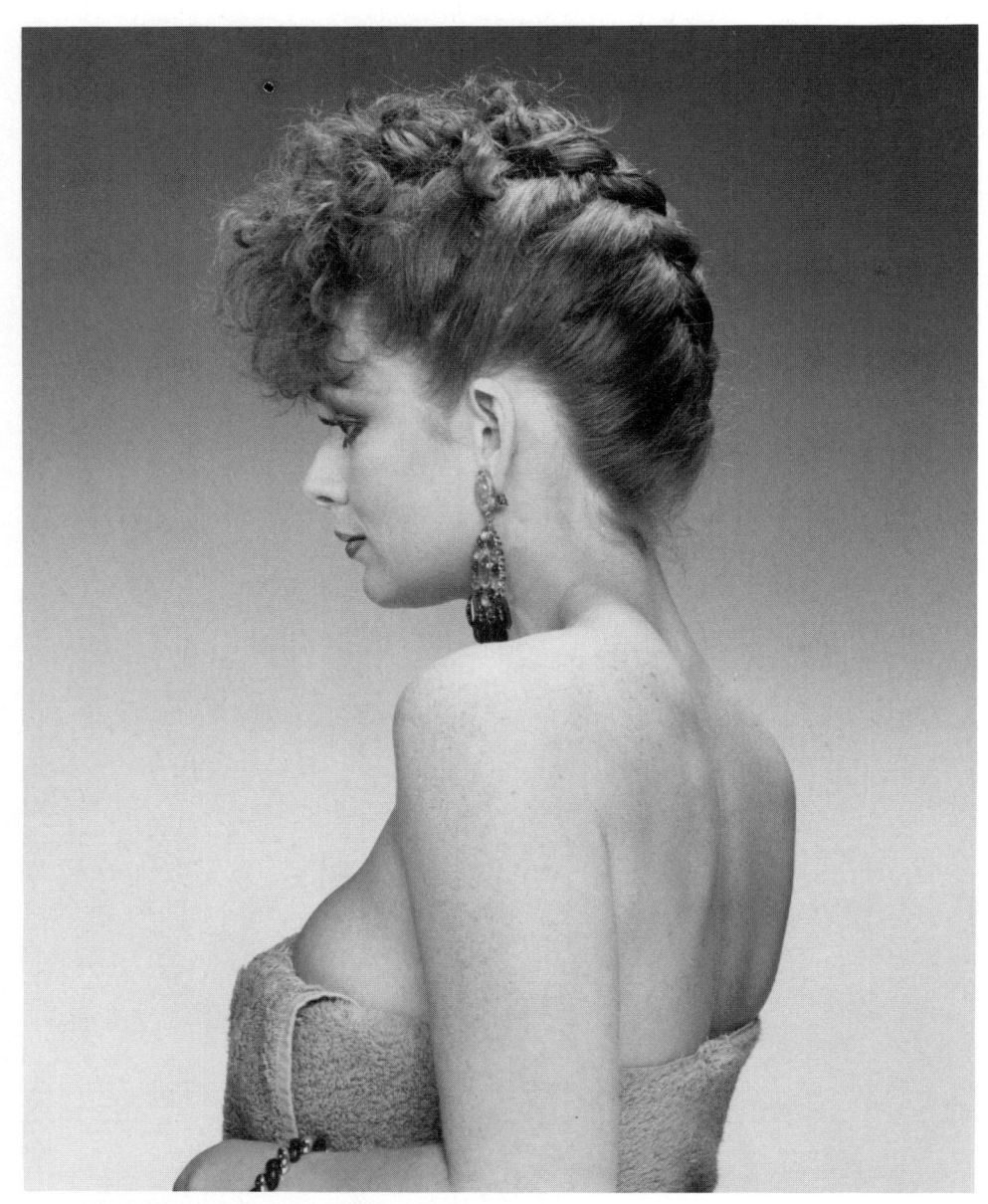

STYLE 3 FOR NATURALLY CURLY LONG HAIR: Here I put up Sheila's hair in an inverted French braid that starts at the nape and ends at the crown. The rest of the hair is very soft and sleek, except for just a fringe of very curly bangs. Very chic. Earrings by Bobi Leonard.

Styling—The Look That's Right for You

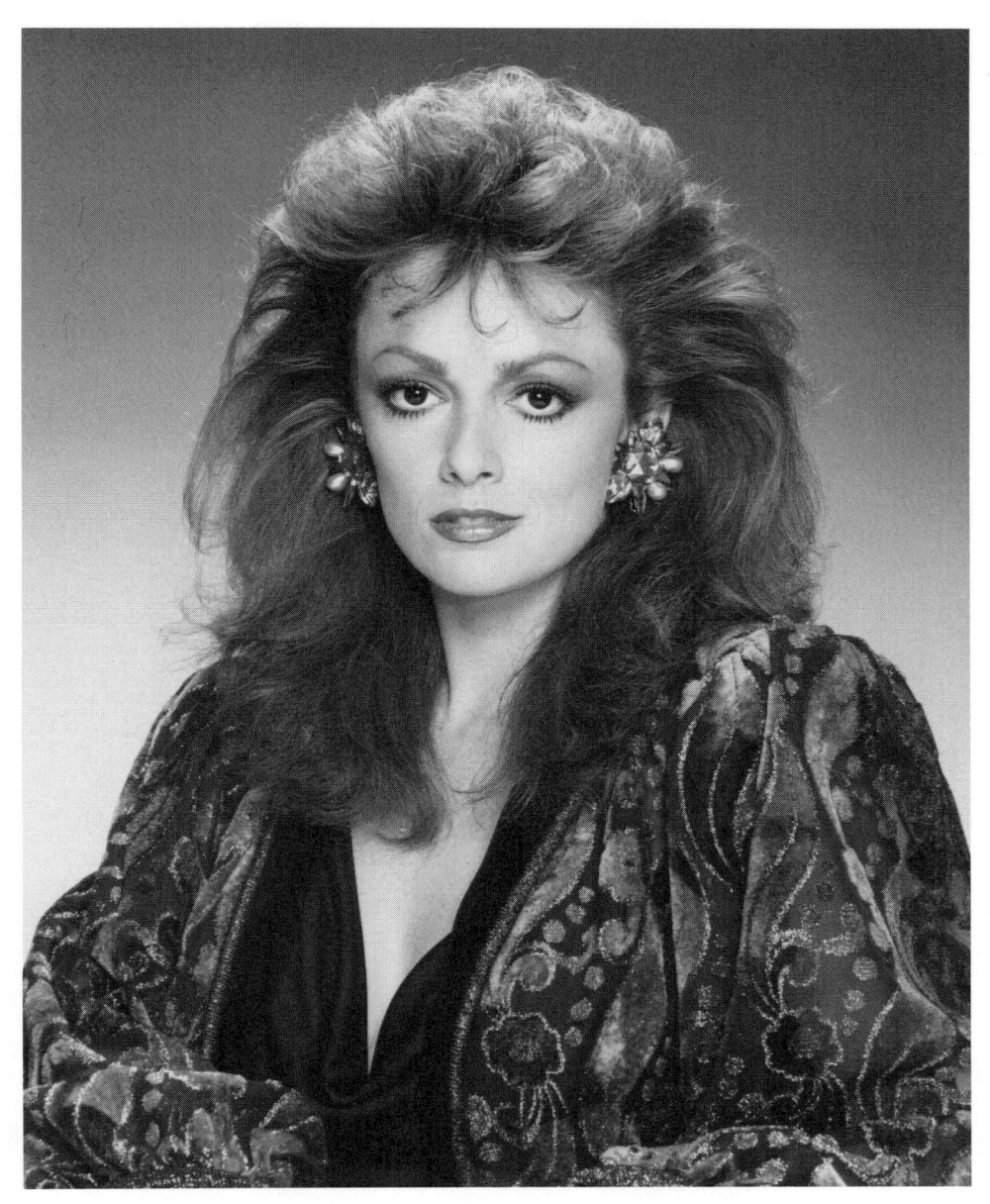

STYLE 4 FOR NATURALLY CURLY LONG HAIR: Sheila's hair is blown dry, almost straight. This look is very attractive, opens up her face, and brings out her bone structure. Bangs are swept back with just a couple of wispy tendrils over the forehead. Jacket by Margi Kent, Melrose Avenue, Los Angeles. Earrings by Bobi Leonard.

STYLING DOS AND DON'TS

Do . . .

add volume by blow-drying hair upside down with a touch of spray at the roots.

Do . . .

wear hair up for festive occasions for a change of pace and styling versatility.

Do . . .

apply mousse or gel to almost-dry hair for best results.

Do . . .

select mousses and gels for your type of hair.

Do . . .

for extra curly or permed hair, use a "leave in" conditioner (one that doesn't rinse off).

Do . . .

use end paper on ends of hair to protect it from heated rollers.

Do . . .

use combs and other hair accessories to add styling versatility to your hairdo.

Do . . .

change your style slightly, like brushing bangs to the side or slicking sides back, for a change of pace.

Styling—The Look That's Right for You

Do . . .

pay close attention when your stylist is working on you. It is the best way to learn how to handle your own hair.

Don't . . .

overkill with mousse, hair spray, or gel.

Don't . . .

ever brush wet hair with a natural- or plastic-bristle brush. Use a prong brush with very widely set prongs.

Don't . . .

use round brushes with plastic bristles. Hair gets tangled and breaks easily.

Don't . . .

use a curling iron on wet or damp hair.

Don't . . .

hold wet hair with rubber bands. Wait until hair is dry to avoid breakage.

Don't . . .

blow-dry hair with dryer fewer than six inches from the hair.

Don't . . .

blow-dry hair more than once a day.

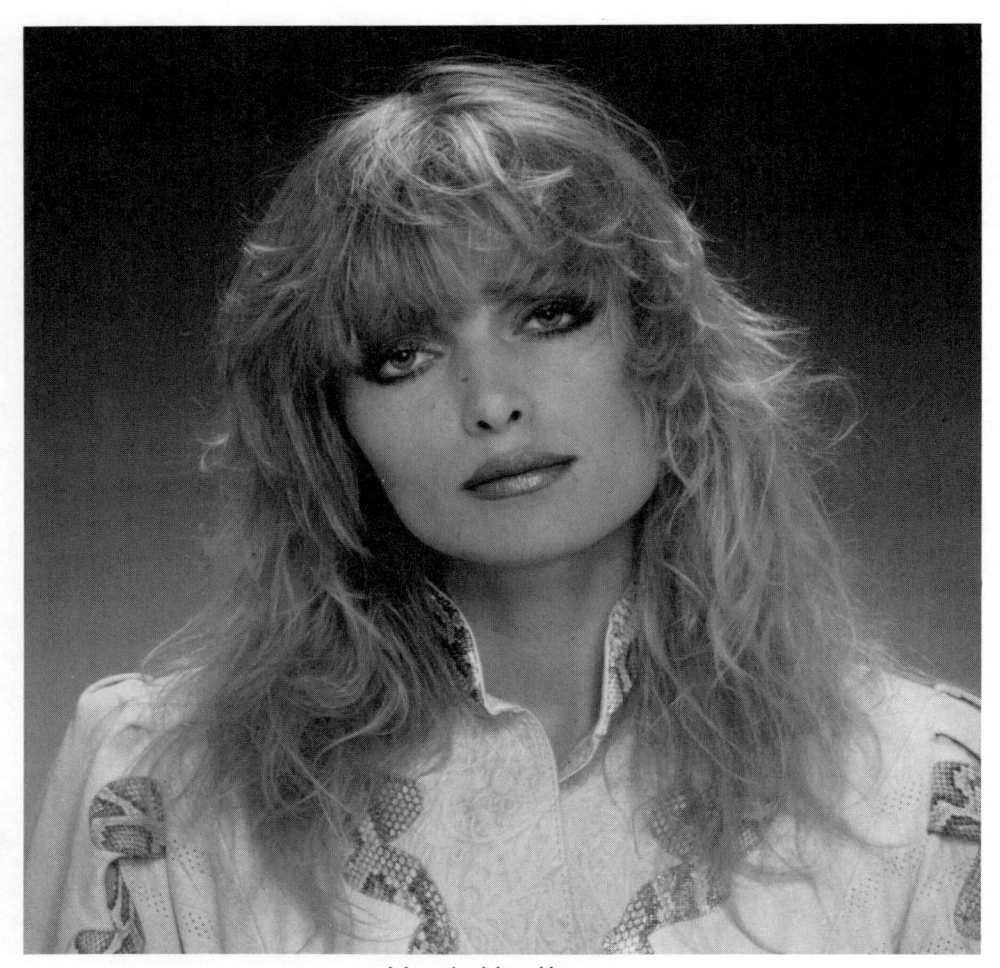

Merete Van Kamp

7
MAKEUP—DOS AND DON'TS

Makeup is like painting, and you are the canvas. But like any good artist, you want to start out with a good, clean canvas—your face. This is achieved by prepping the skin to conceal tiny imperfections, blemishes, and shadows.

I selected the makeover approach to illustrate this chapter because I feel it is the most dramatic way to illustrate what makeup can do for any face. Our three makeover models are very different beauty types. My first model, Chynna Phillips, is a professional model, very young and with the sort of classic beauty that needs very little makeup. My second model, Tamela Song, is an aspiring model, and she has a truly unusual look—a green-eyed blond who is part Chinese. My third model, Rima Uranga, shows what corrective makeup can do for a face with uneven features.

The key steps to a professional-looking makeup application are cleanse, blend, and mend. *Cleansing* refers to taking care of the skin; *blending* means that no line should ever show; *mending* refers to the corrective steps applied before the artistic part of the makeup goes on.

Makeup can totally re-create a face by reshaping it with the aid of highlighting and contouring. This combination of lights and shadows accents the positive and hides the negative.

SKINCARE ROUTINE

The basic beginning of a beautiful face is a good skincare routine. Cleansing, toning, and protecting are the first three steps to a beautiful flawless skin.

Cleansing

Use the method that most suits your skin type. Cleanse in the morning and evening—in the mornings to prep the skin for makeup application, in the evenings to remove makeup and dirt. Some types of very oily skin may need cleansing three times a day.

Toning

This step follows the cleansing step, and its purpose is to remove the last traces of cleanser, as well as to stimulate your skin. Select the type of toner that is suitable for your skin type: nonalcohol-based for dry and sensitive skin, alcohol-based for oily skin.

Protecting

There is daytime protection and evening protection. Your daytime protection should be a moisturizer with sunscreens to keep out the damaging rays of the sun that lead to wrinkles and to form a barrier against dirt and pollution that clog the pores. Your nighttime protection should be an antiwrinkle cream suitable for your skin type. The final step for total face protection is eye cream—applied morning and evening.

TOOLS

Just like a good artist, insist on the proper tools to obtain a flawless, professional finish with your makeup. Here is a list of what you will need:

Powder Brush: Large, fluffy brush used to apply loose face powder.

Blush Brush: Medium-size brush used to apply powder blush and for blending.

Makeup—Dos and Don'ts

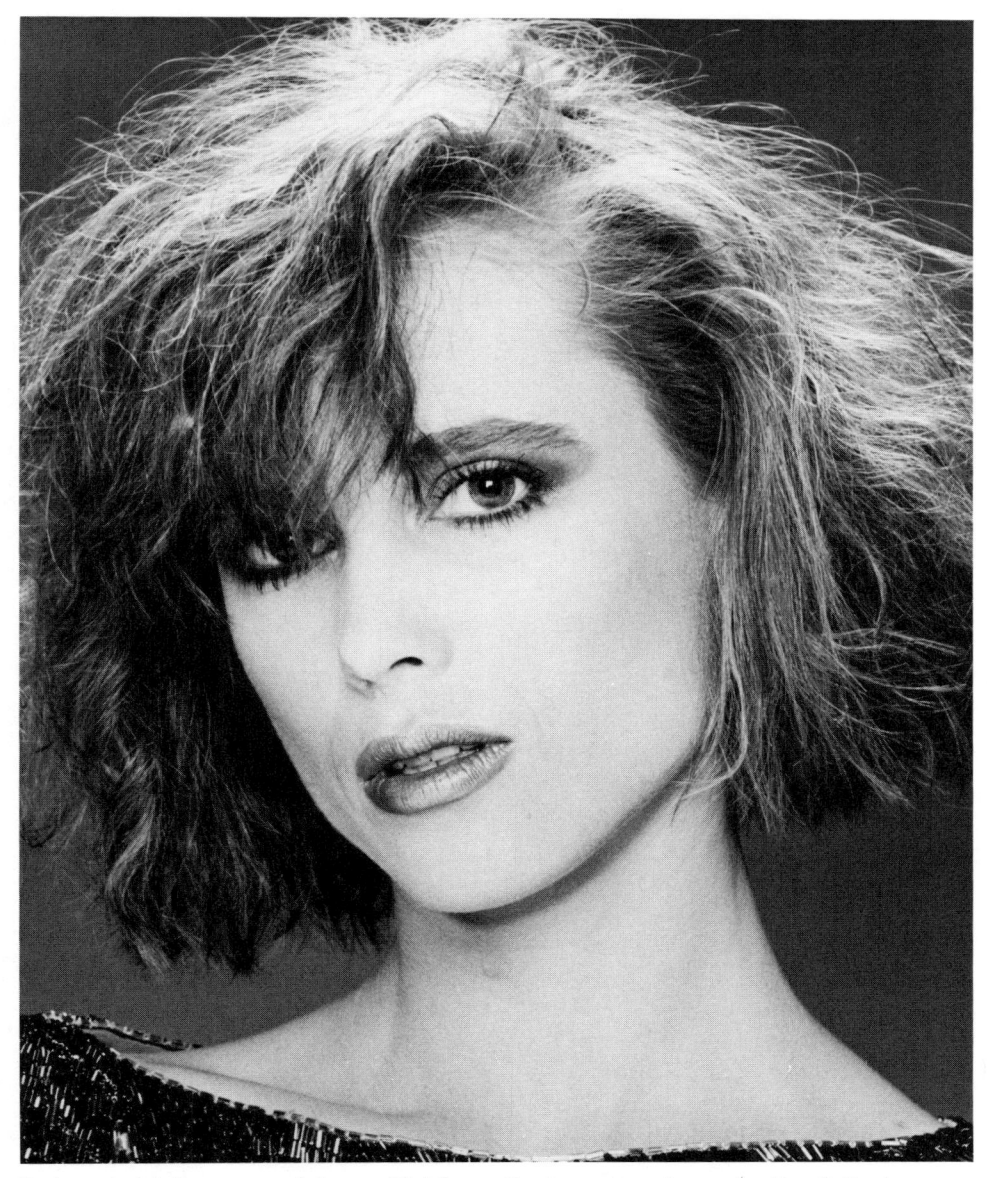

Deborah Mullowney—A beautiful face that uses makeup to the fullest advantage. Eyes are carefully lined and shadowed to bring them out, into focus. Cheeks have a gentle sweep of blush. Lips are full, moist, and ripe with glowing color.

Contour Brush: Smaller brush with blunt-cut bristles used to apply contour powder and for blending.

Sponges: I prefer synthetic sponges that can be used dry. They should be pie wedge shaped, as the corners are needed to blend makeup around the eyes and nose and the corners of the mouth. These come precut, or you can cut them yourself.

Angle Eye Brush: Small brush with bristles cut at an angle, used to apply shadow in corners of the eye and to line eyes. Also for blending.

Shadow Brush: Small brush used to apply shadow and contour to lids and to blend.

Eyebrow Brush: Shaped like a small toothbrush and used to brush brows before and after applying color. *Note:* If you have very bushy brows, a very soft bristle toothbrush might be a better bet.

Swabs: Cotton swabs are great for blending in small, hard-to-reach spaces and for softening liner.

Eyeliner Brush: Thin, small brush used to apply liquid, cake, powder, or lining with shadow.

Lipliner Brush: Thin, small brush with a longer handle used to line lips. Liner pencils can be used, too.

Lip Brush: Fuller than the lipliner brush, to be used to fill lips with color or to apply lip gloss.

Taking Care of Your Tools

Makeup tools are expensive, but with proper care they should last a long time. Wash your brushes once a week, using a mild shampoo. Fill sink with soapy, warm water and soak brushes for a few minutes. Gently rub bristles to remove all color deposits in the inner bristles. Rinse well to remove all soap. Roll brushes in a towel to remove excess water from the bristles. Let air-dry for several hours by resting them on a towel. Never dry tools near a heater or any direct source of heat, since they will be damaged. Wash shadow brushes after every application to obtain the proper shade when you change colors.

PROFESSIONAL MAKEUP APPLICATION

Here is a detailed description of all the steps necessary for a professional makeup application.

Makeup—Dos and Don'ts

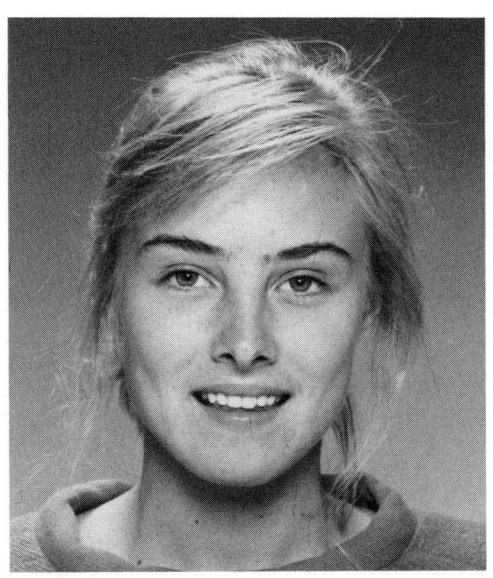

BEFORE: Chynna Phillips is a young, well-scrubbed beauty. A natural blond, she is pale and needs color to bring out her features.

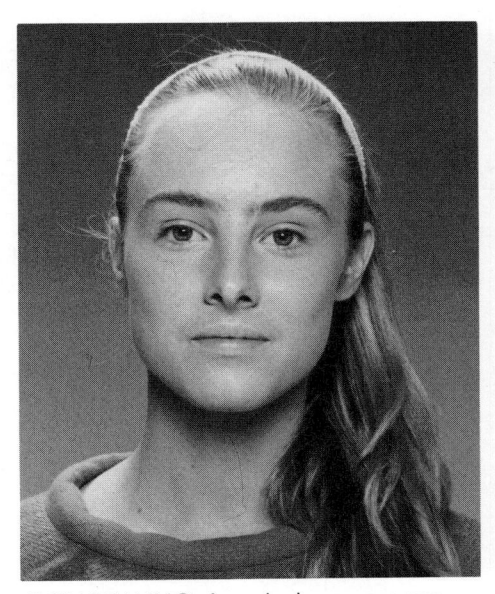

CONCEALING: A pale ivory cream (Chynna's skin is almost translucent) is used across the top of the forehead, under the eyes, around the mouth and chin. Also dotted to cover tiny blemishes where needed.

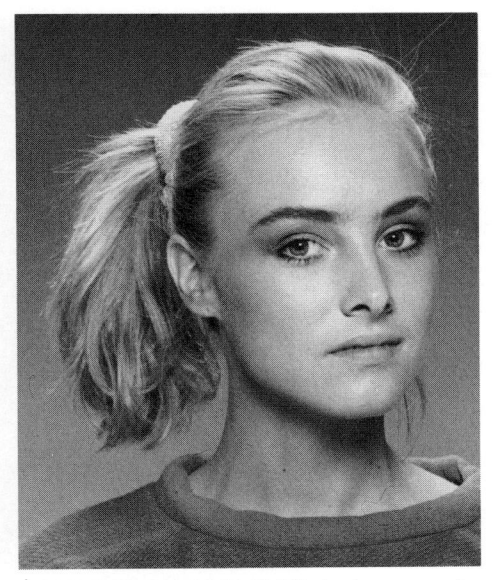

FOUNDATION AND EYES: A sheer, pale beige foundation gives a porcelain finish to the skin. To define eyes, a shell-beige shadow goes on the inner corner of the lids, golden taupe in the center, and smoky gray circles the outer corners and slightly contours the crease of the lids.

TOVAR'S CLASSIC BEAUTY

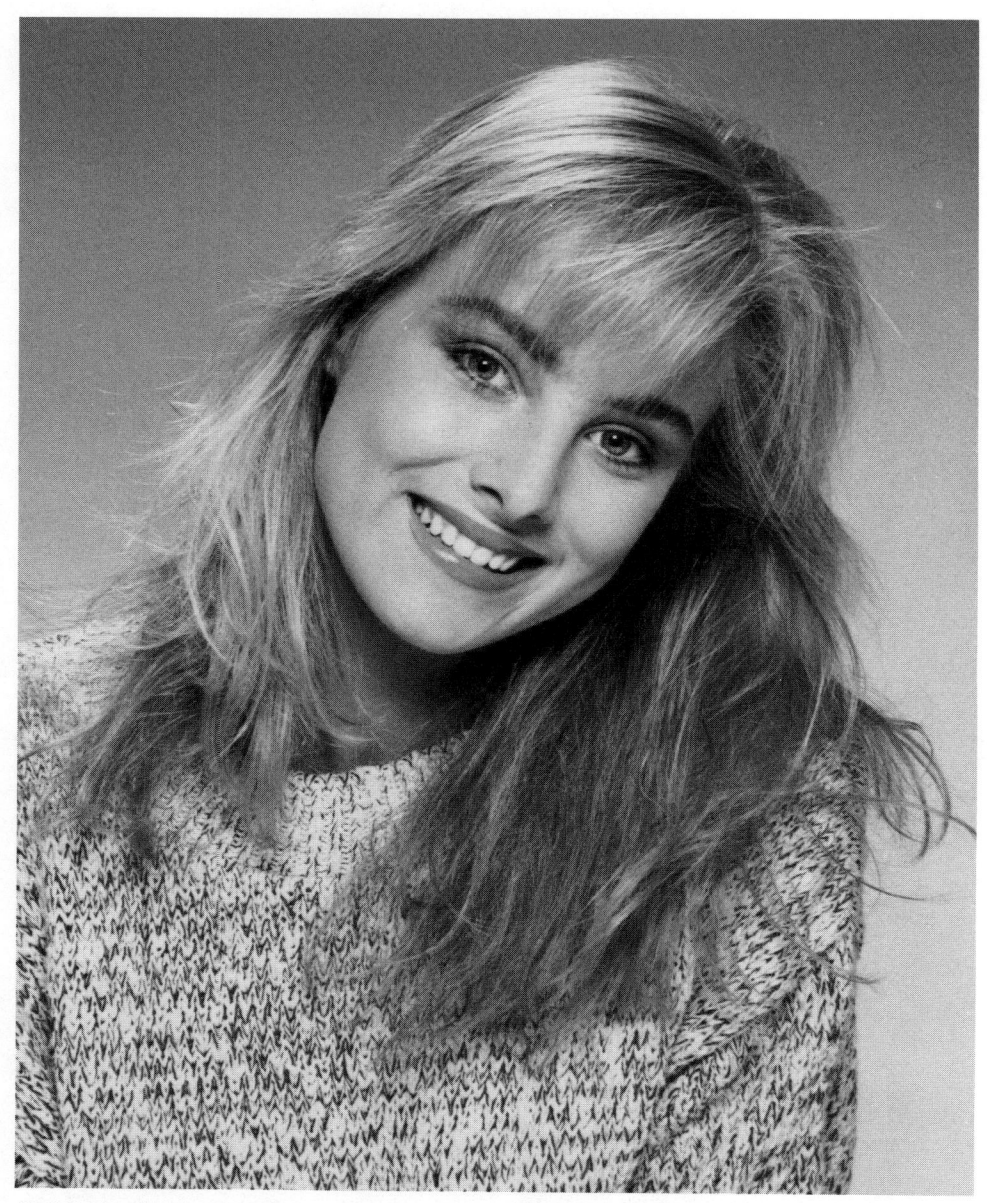

FINISHED DAYTIME LOOK: A touch of peach blusher on the cheeks and peachy pink lipstick. The hair is blown dry, scrunched at the ends, with side-swept bangs brushed over the forehead.

Concealer

This is done with a cream product known as *highlighter* or *concealer*. This cream comes in different skin tone shades, and you should select the one closest to your skin tone, but slightly darker to avoid a "fake" look.

Concealer is used to highlight around the eyes (because this area often recedes and shows dark shadows), the curved part of the forehead (around the hairline), and the chin. A concealer also can be used to cover tiny blemishes and lines. A concealer acts like an "eraser" to wipe out any shadows or flaws and bring out the features.

Once the concealer has been applied, use a dry, triangular sponge to blend the edges into the skin. If you have to cover red blotches or other areas of the skin with red undertones, select a concealer with a yellow cast to the shade. This will neutralize the red undertones.

How to Select the Right Color: The right concealer shade depends on skin undertones.. If you have a sallow complexion (yellow undertones), select a shade with a grayish tint to neutralize the yellow. If you have pale skin, an almost alabaster-white shade is right for you. If you have a ruddy complexion, stay with a medium beige. Always select a shade that is only a couple of shades lighter than your foundation shade. Avoid very white or very dark shades.

Foundation

This is the primer that readies the skin for the rest of the makeup application. Foundation comes in many forms—liquid, cream, and cake (to be applied with a damp sponge); oil-based and water-based. Water-based foundation is for oily skin and enlarged pores; oil-based foundation is for dry and normal skin. Select a shade that is close to your skin tone. I like applying makeup in "streaks"—almost like Indian war paint. Apply one streak across the forehead, one down the nose, a couple across each cheek, and one across the chin. Take a sponge and blend all the way into the hairline, under the chin, and down the neck. This is the method that I call the "fade-out." It is important that all makeup be blended to disappear and that there be no demarcation line where the makeup ends and bare skin begins.

One of the most common foundation mistakes is trying to use it to camouflage flaws. Many women feel that by applying a heavy layer of makeup they can avoid using a concealer. The result is an unattractive mask. All the covering should be done with the concealer. The foundation should be a sheer layer, which is the most effective way to enhance and make the best of the features you have.

Once you have applied your foundation, it is time to blend, blend, blend. The skin should look flawless and a little bit shiny because you have not yet added powder.

How to Select the Right Color: Your face should be a couple of shades lighter than the rest of your body. To find the spot to check for the right foundation shade, look at the underside of your wrist. This is a place that sun rarely hits directly, so it's the closest to the color of the skin on your face. Choose a warm beige shade for ruddy or sallow complexions (try to correct complexion tone with highlighter *before* applying foundation). Most pale skins look best with a cool-toned foundation. Dark skins have a lot of different pigmentation, so sometimes the best bet is to mix a couple of different colors to arrive at the most becoming shade. Test foundation colors before purchasing.

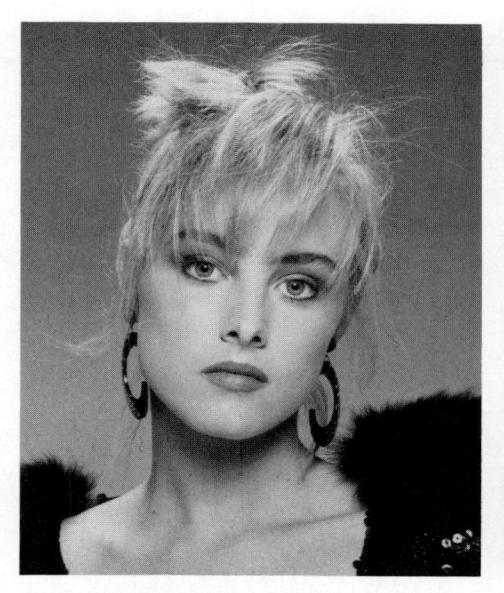

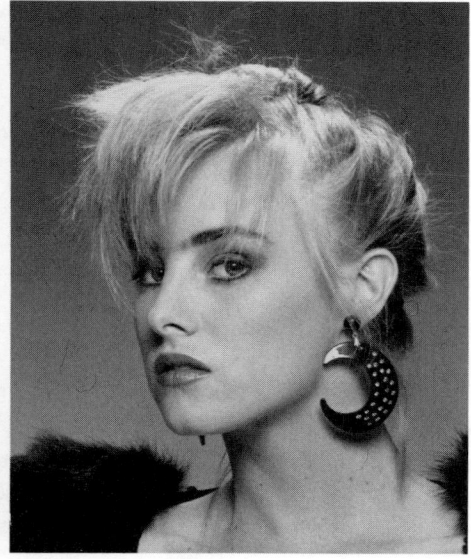

FINISHED EVENING LOOK: It starts with deeper, smoldering eyes. Glitter bronze shadow goes on the center of the eye, metallic pewter on the outer corner. A dot of gold over each pupil and under the brow bone. Two coats of lush, black mascara. Golden-bronze blusher and a golden-red lipstick give the finishing touches to the burnished, glittering look.

Eyes:

They have been called "the mirrors of the soul" and they are perhaps the most obvious feature on a face. Start at the outer corner of the eye and apply the darkest-color shadow (this will be from the color family you have selected). Apply the medium shade right in the center of the eye, over the pupil. Apply the lightest shade on the inner corner of the eye, running the color up to the bone under the brow. After you have applied the three colors, take a clean shadow

Makeup—Dos and Don'ts

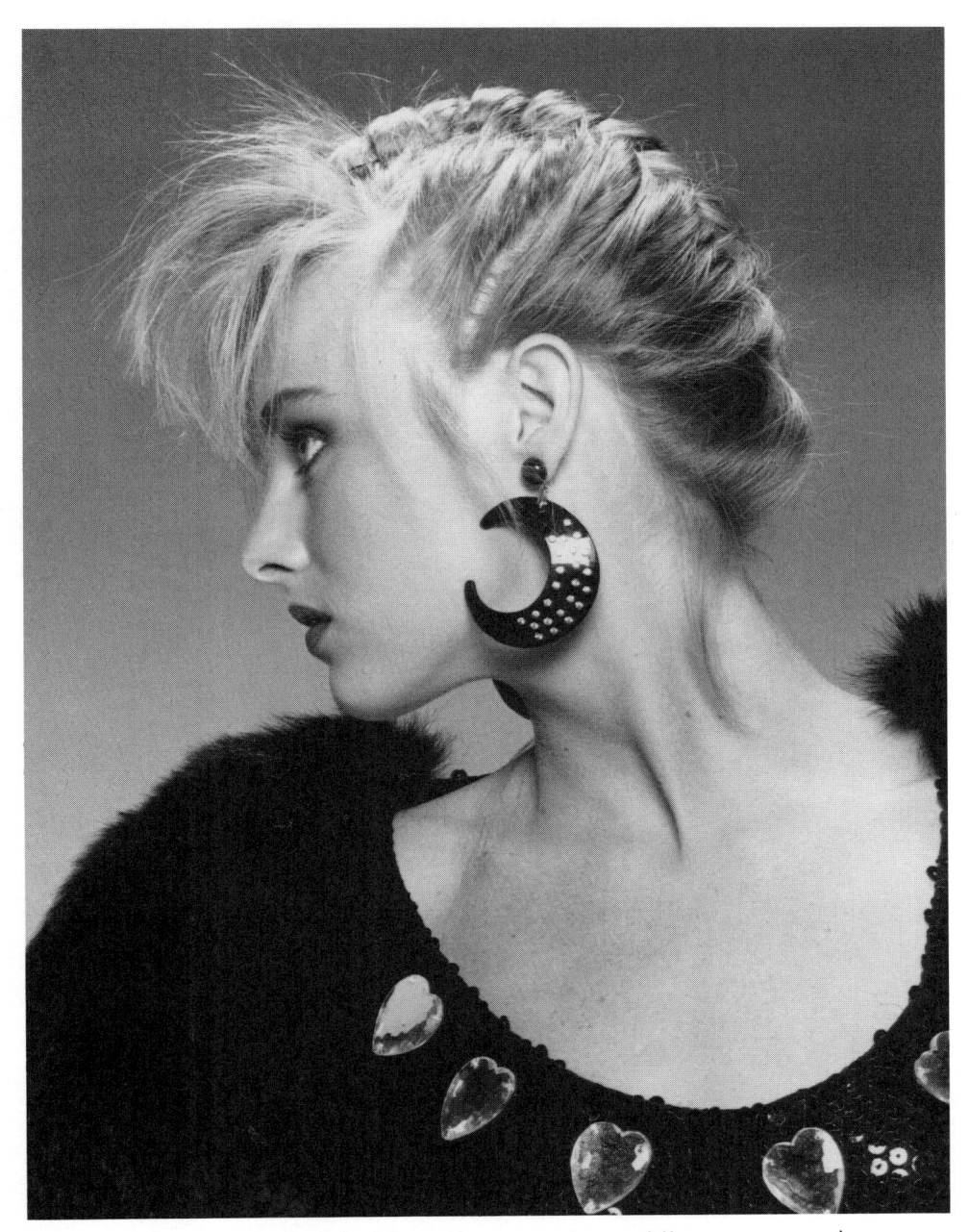

The hair is pulled up, braided from the nape toward the crown, and arranged in spiky strands on the top and forehead. Top by Ellene Warren, Los Angeles.

TOVAR'S CLASSIC BEAUTY

brush and blend the edges of each color into the next one so there is no definition of where one color begins and the other ends.

Line eyes with pencil, drawing a line as close to the bed of the lashes as possible, from corner to corner of the eye and on both upper and lower lids. After you have drawn the line, take a clean brush or cotton swab and run gently over the pencil line to soften it. Again, I would like to add that the key factor in a successful makeup application is blending. When in doubt, blend, blend, blend.

The next step is to apply the mascara. First I prep the lashes by curling them with an eyelash curler. Mascara should be applied from the bed of the lashes upward. Make sure that you don't use too much mascara; it tends to make the lashes clump together. To avoid this, wipe the mascara brush lightly with a tissue to remove the excess

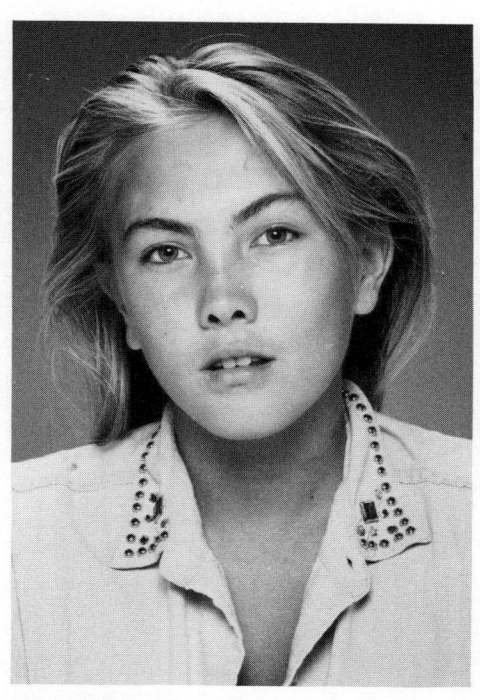

BEFORE: Tamela Song has a childlike, pretty face with unusual features. Her face still shows some "baby fat."

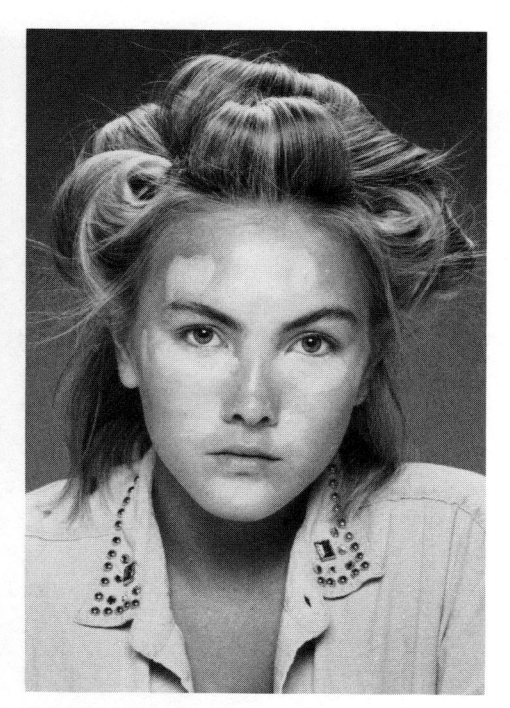

CONTOURING: At the corners of the forehead and around the cheekbones to conceal her "baby fat."

that collects when it is stored in the container. Next I separate the lashes with a tiny comb, apply a second coat, and repeat the comb step. Mascara should be applied to the lower lashes in the same way. Nothing brings out those eyes more than a thick fringe of lashes. For years, women have achieved a lot by batting their eyelashes, so make sure yours are in good shape.

Brows should follow the natural line. I like to emphasize them with brown or taupe shadow—pencil makes a harsh and obvious line. The only time I use a pencil is when lashes are too sparse or uneven; then the pencil line creates a new line. Before applying color to brows, brush them, apply color, and brush them again to soften the color. If you are using pencil, apply it with very short light strokes, almost as if you were painting hairs on.

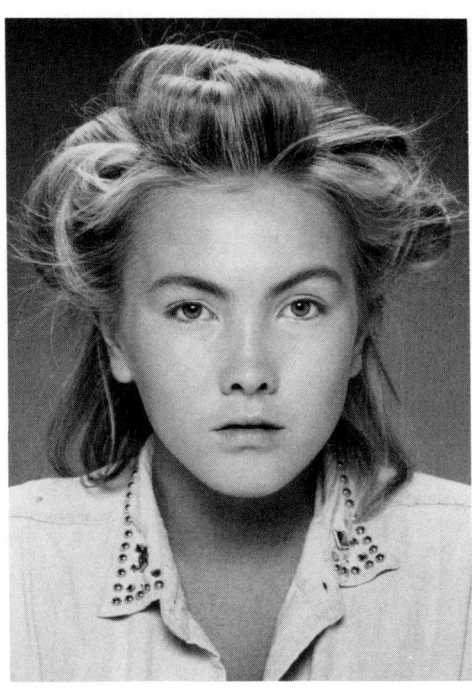

FOUNDATION: Next is a medium beige foundation to provide the canvas where makeup will be applied.

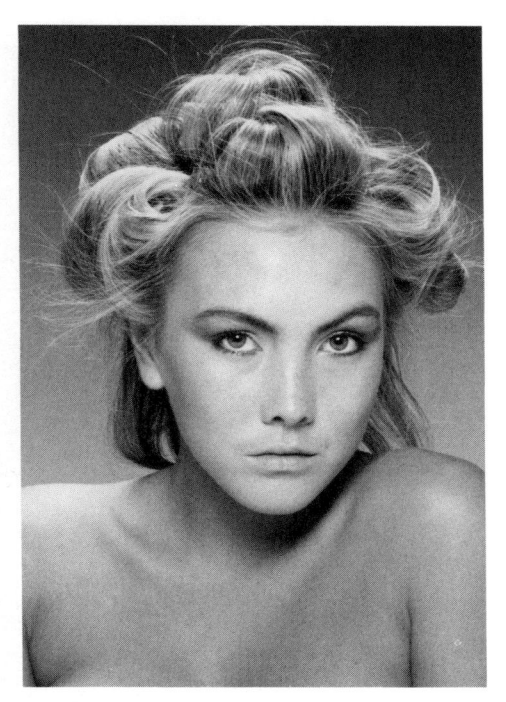

EYES: Modifed "cat eyes" to emphasize Tamela's Oriental ancestry. Shell-beige shadow goes on the inner corners of the eye, medium gray over the center, and deeper gray on the outer corners, slanting upward.

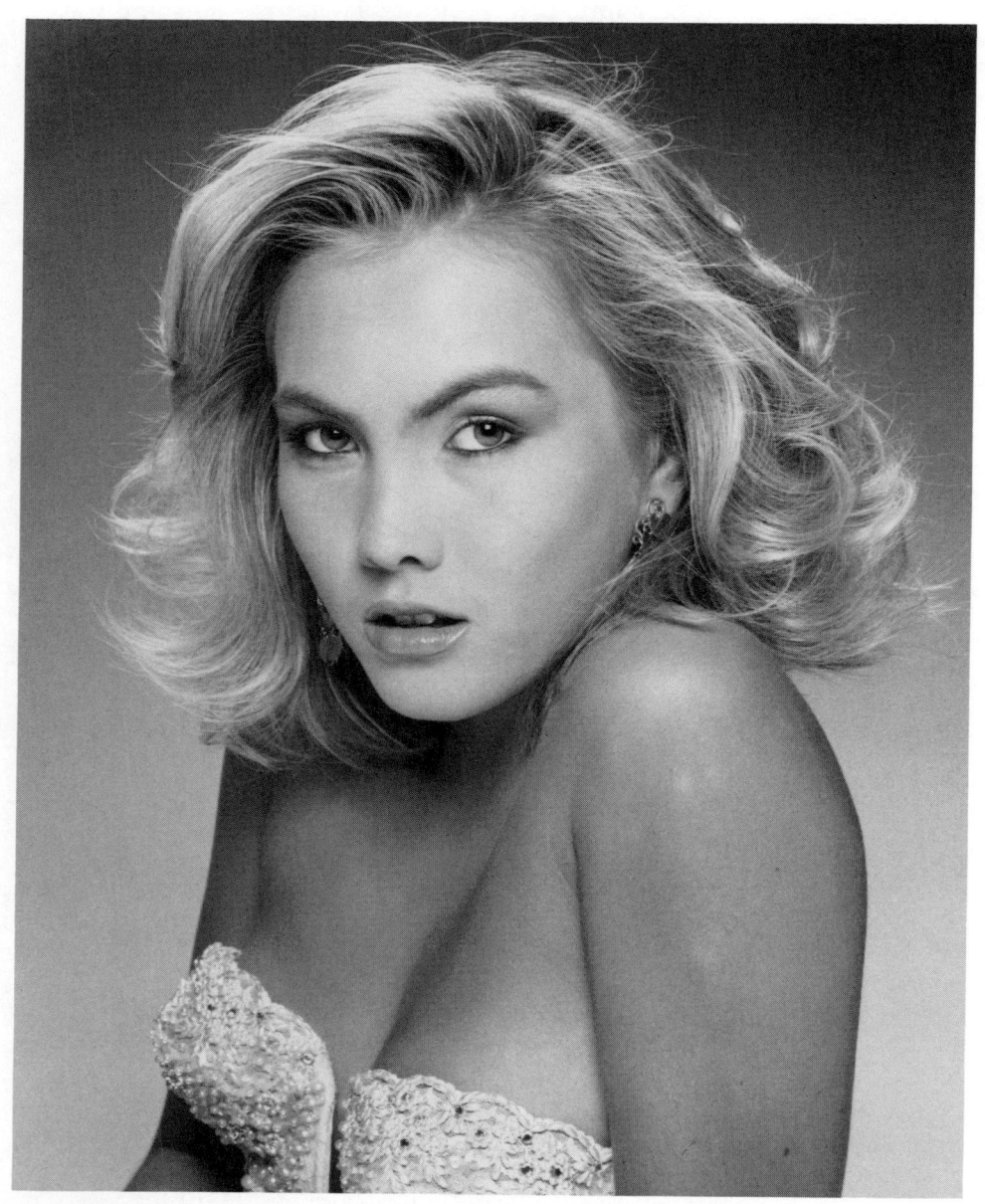

FINISHED DAYTIME LOOK: Rosy pink blusher adds a soft glow to the cheeks, and pale pink lipstick colors the lips. Tamela's hair is brushed smooth and wavy from a side part. Fashions by Ellene Warren, Los Angeles.

Makeup—Dos and Don'ts

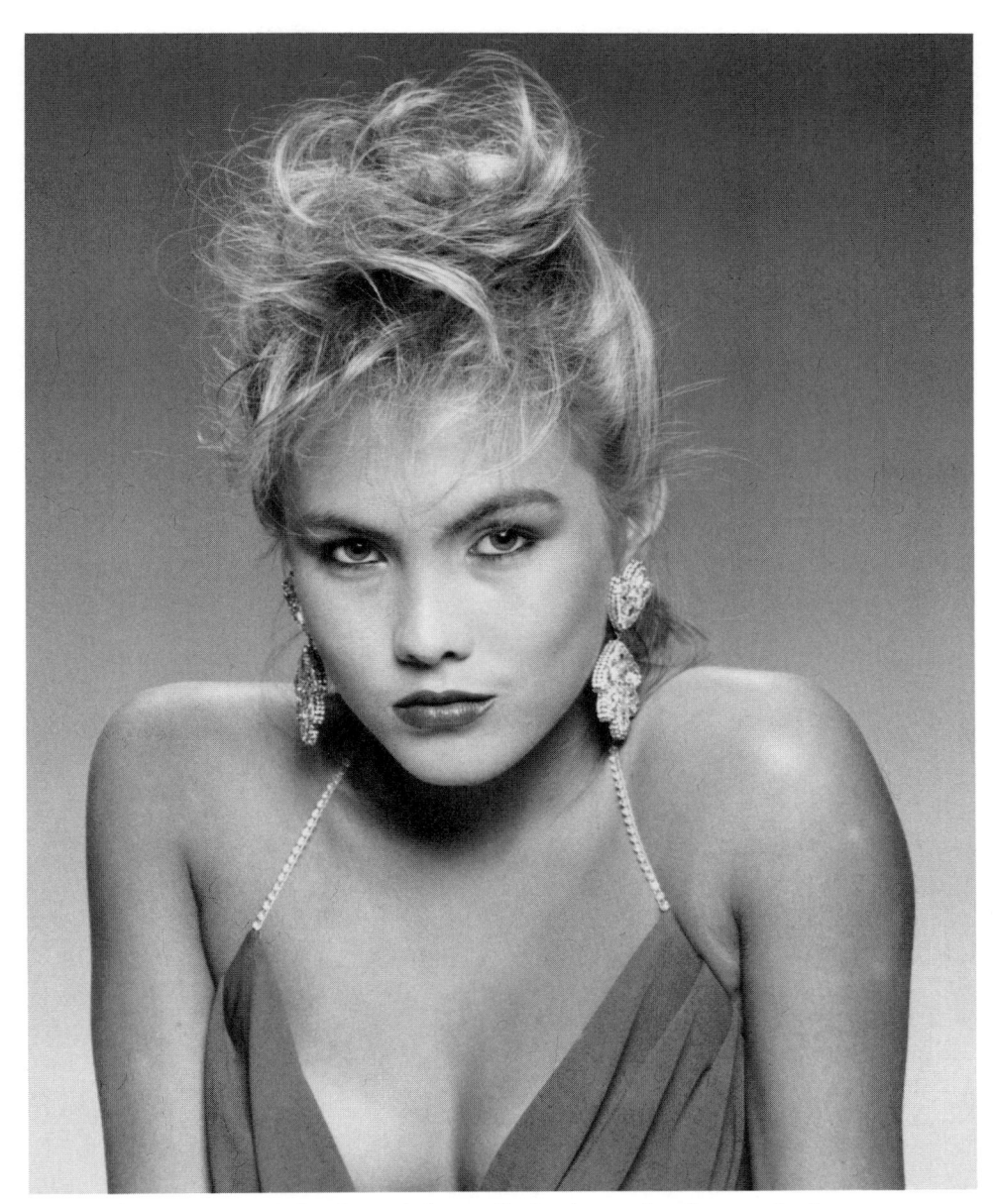

FINISHED EVENING LOOK: Tamela's exotic looks make the perfect background for a dramatic evening makeup. Eyes are touched with turquoise shadow on the center of the lid to make her green eyes look deeper and lined with black pencil on the inner rim of the lashes. Burnished bronze blusher and ruby-red lipstick add to the dramatic color effect. Her hair is wrapped into a french twist in the back and brought forward into a riotous froth of waves over the crown and forehead. Fashions by Ellene Warren, Los Angeles.

TOVAR'S CLASSIC BEAUTY

Contouring

This is a very individual step, depending on the shape of the face. I find that most faces fall into four categories: round, oval (the ideal shape), oblong (long and narrow), and heart-shaped (or triangular). Each area of the face should be contoured differently. The purpose of contouring is to achieve the look of the perfect oval face.

In contouring a round face, the purpose is to break the circular effect by adding angles. So the corners of the forehead, under the chin, and under the cheekbones are contoured to create a feeling of sharpness.

The opposite is done with a square or oblong face. Instead of sharpening the angles, the contouring will be applied to soften the angular corners of the face. Draw contouring across the sharp corners in a round, almost half-moon effect.

For the heart-shaped or triangular face, you will contour around the forehead and cheeks and soften the pointed chin. To soften the chin, start applying the heaviest concentration of contourer at the jawline, fading out toward the center.

Whatever contouring method you need to follow, be sure to blend all the contouring until no edges show.

Lips

It is best to try to follow the natural lipline as much as possible. If your lipline needs correction, it is best to draw the new lipline in with pencil or brush before applying lipstick. Whether you have to correct your lipline or work with yours, you will get a neater lipstick application by lining the lips first.

Draw a line from the bow to each corner of the lips, then on the bottom from one corner to create a half circle ending at the opposite corner. The shade of liner selected should *match*, not contrast with, your lipstick.

Then apply lipstick, making sure the color covers the line. Highlight the center of the lower lip with a tiny dot of clear or colored gloss to match your lipstick.

Makeup—Dos and Don'ts

Powder

Loose powder is used to "set" the makeup and take the shine off the skin. Dust powder all over the face using a large brush. Repowder during the day as necessary to keep the shine off.

Blusher

Add color to the cheeks last. Select a light shade. Nothing looks more dated than red "apple cheeks" or the brown streaks look. A pretty pink or peach is a more becoming shade. Apply blusher with a brush. After picking up color with the brush, blow slightly to remove excess color. Blend blusher very well with a brush to make edges "melt" into the surface.

Evening Makeup

Follow the same basic steps, but you can be a little more creative when it comes to color, selecting stronger, more daring shades. Also, glitter and frosted colors are effective for evenings.

Eye makeup can be more intense for evenings, too. You can use heavier liner: a good technique is to line the inner rim of the lids with a black or blue pencil, which makes the whites look whiter. This trick makes eyes stand out and be emphasized. Be careful not to apply the liner very heavily, or the look will be very hard instead of dramatic.

Blusher should be darker, with a touch of glitter if you like. Powder that contains little specks of glitter provides a sparkling finishing touch to your evening makeup.

Follow the same contouring guidelines as for day. The only thing I add for evenings that I won't use for day makeup is contouring the nose. The effect is too obvious in daylight, but it works after dark. See instructions earlier in this chapter for ways to contour.

TOVAR'S CLASSIC BEAUTY
CORRECTIVE MAKEUP

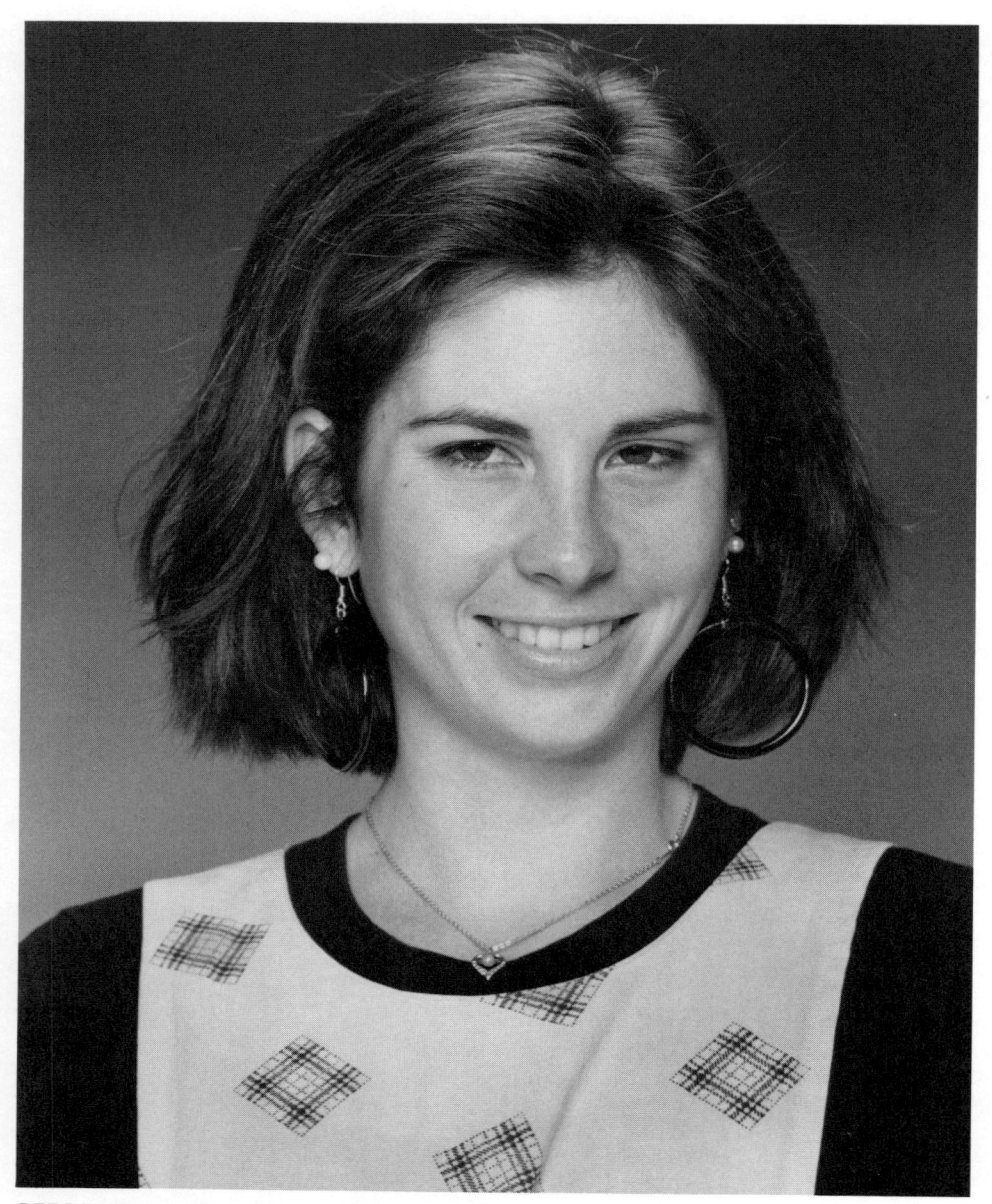

BEFORE: Rima Urana has deep-set eyes, a wide nose, and a wide jawline. I chose her as my model for the corrective makeup section because she had the type of facial structure to which I could apply many of the corrective makeup techniques.

Makeup—Dos and Don'ts

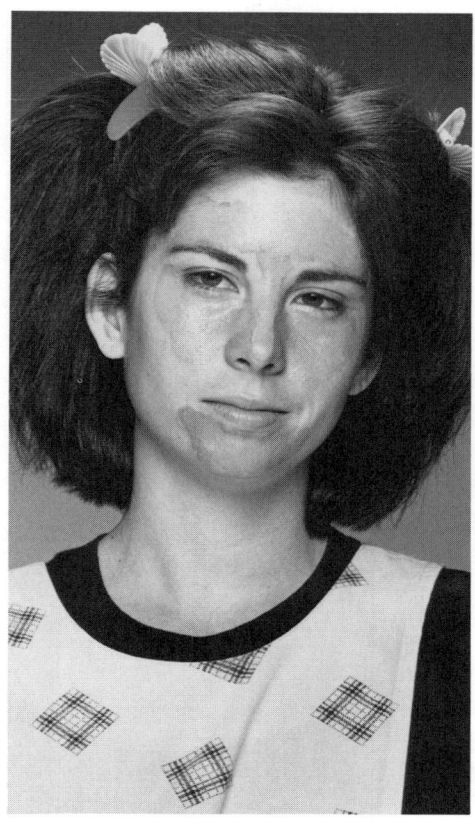

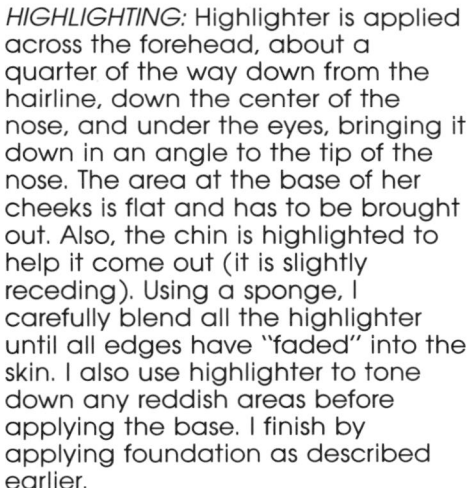

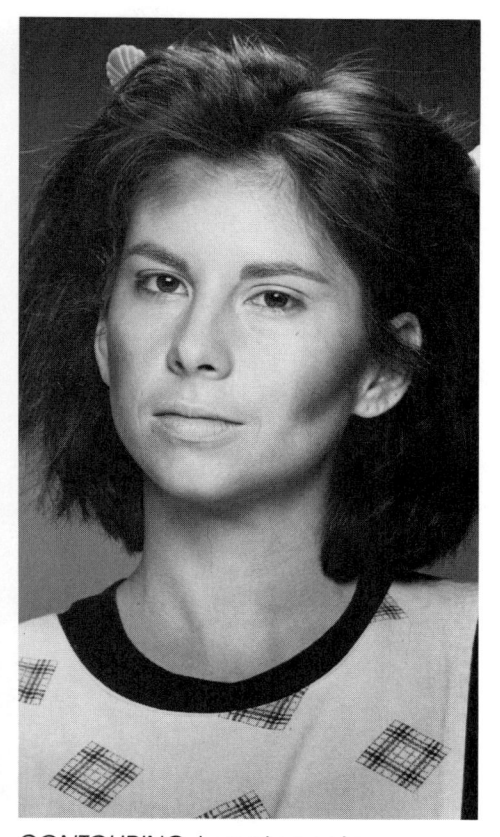

HIGHLIGHTING: Highlighter is applied across the forehead, about a quarter of the way down from the hairline, down the center of the nose, and under the eyes, bringing it down in an angle to the tip of the nose. The area at the base of her cheeks is flat and has to be brought out. Also, the chin is highlighted to help it come out (it is slightly receding). Using a sponge, I carefully blend all the highlighter until all edges have "faded" into the skin. I also use highlighter to tone down any reddish areas before applying the base. I finish by applying foundation as described earlier.

CONTOURING: I apply contour powder under the cheekbones, at the jawline, and on the chin, applying some under the chin to give more depth to the area and make the neck appear longer. Then I blend in all the contour with a sponge. To contour the nose, I draw a line down from between the brows to the tip of the nose and draw another line on each side of the nose and one across the tip. Then I blend very well with a sponge to "fade" contour lines into the skin.

TOVAR'S CLASSIC BEAUTY

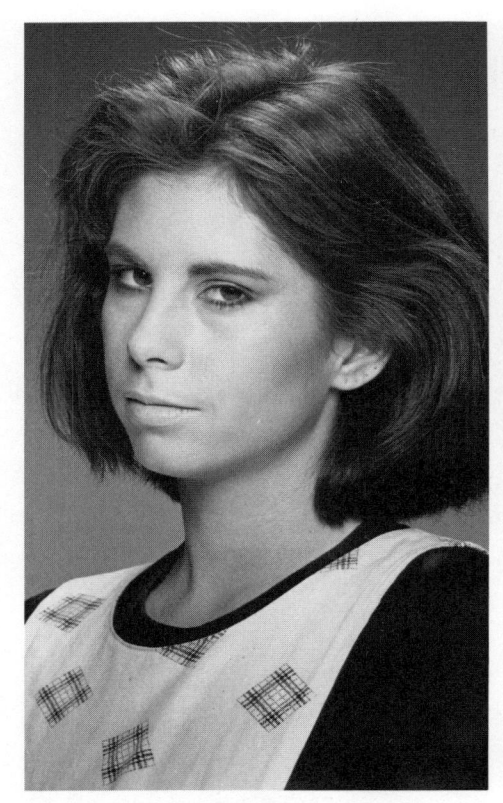

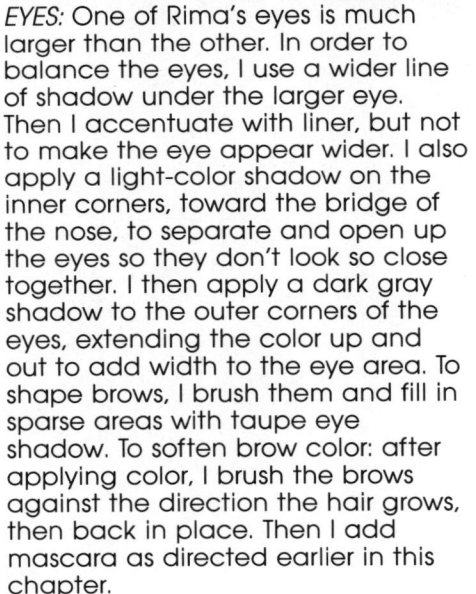

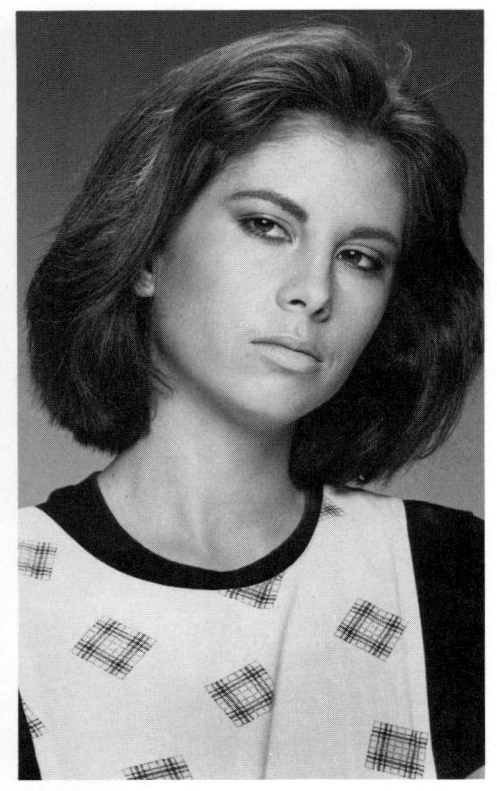

EYES: One of Rima's eyes is much larger than the other. In order to balance the eyes, I use a wider line of shadow under the larger eye. Then I accentuate with liner, but not to make the eye appear wider. I also apply a light-color shadow on the inner corners, toward the bridge of the nose, to separate and open up the eyes so they don't look so close together. I then apply a dark gray shadow to the outer corners of the eyes, extending the color up and out to add width to the eye area. To shape brows, I brush them and fill in sparse areas with taupe eye shadow. To soften brow color: after applying color, I brush the brows against the direction the hair grows, then back in place. Then I add mascara as directed earlier in this chapter.

LIPS: I follow Rima's natural lipline to just before the corners. Rima's lip corners tend to fade away, so I draw a firm line connecting them. Because her lips are rather flat, I fill them in using three different shades of lipstick; this gives them some depth. I use the darkest color at the center of the lips to make this area come out.

Makeup—Dos and Don'ts

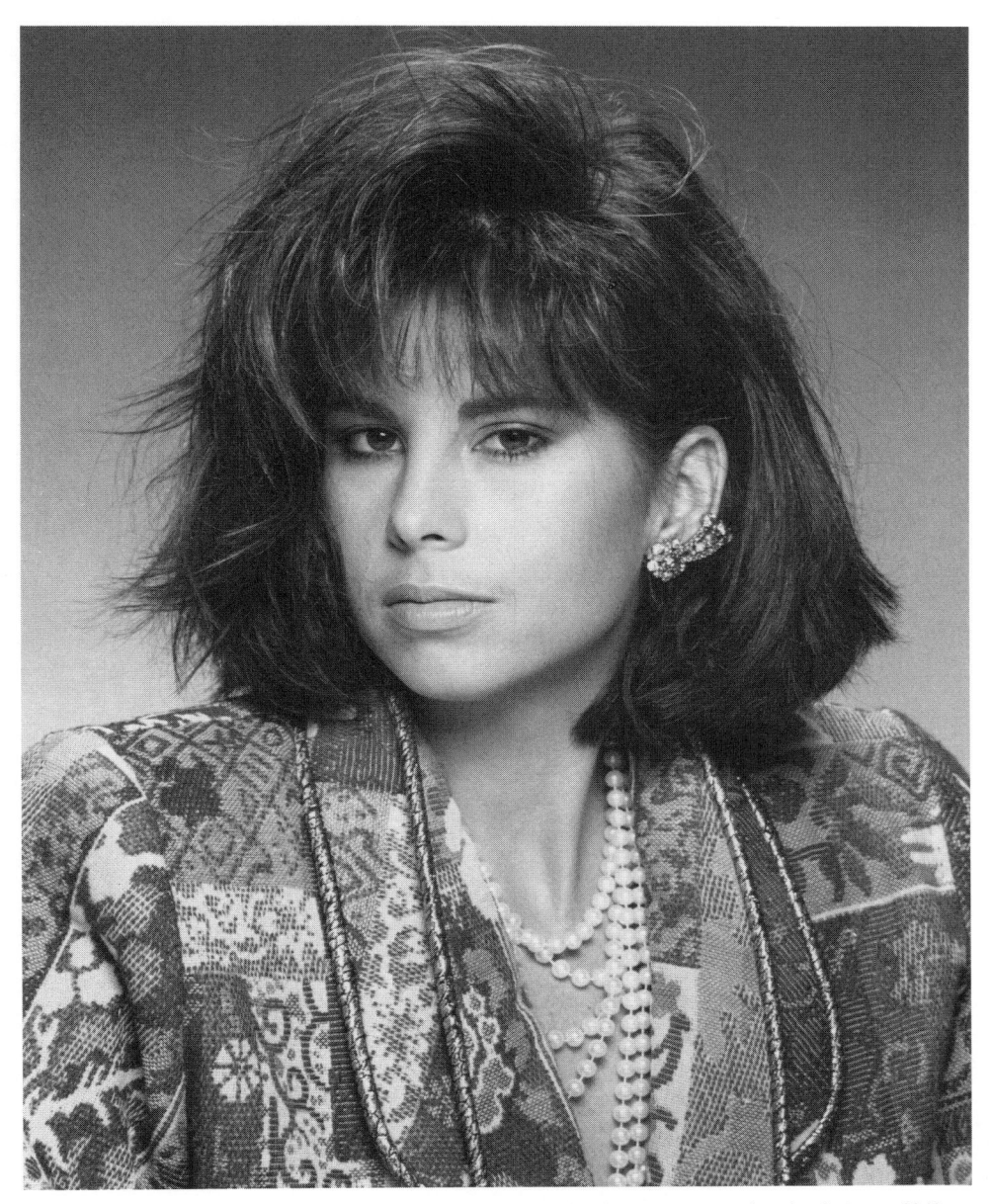

FINISHING: I finish the face with a sheer "veil" of loose powder to take off the shine. Her hair too is styled to accentuate the positive and minimize the negative. Bangs accentuate the eyes; the asymetrical lines—one side forward, the other back—balance the uneven features; and fullness and height at the crown balance the nose and chin. Outfit by Margi Kent, Melrose Avenue, Los Angeles.

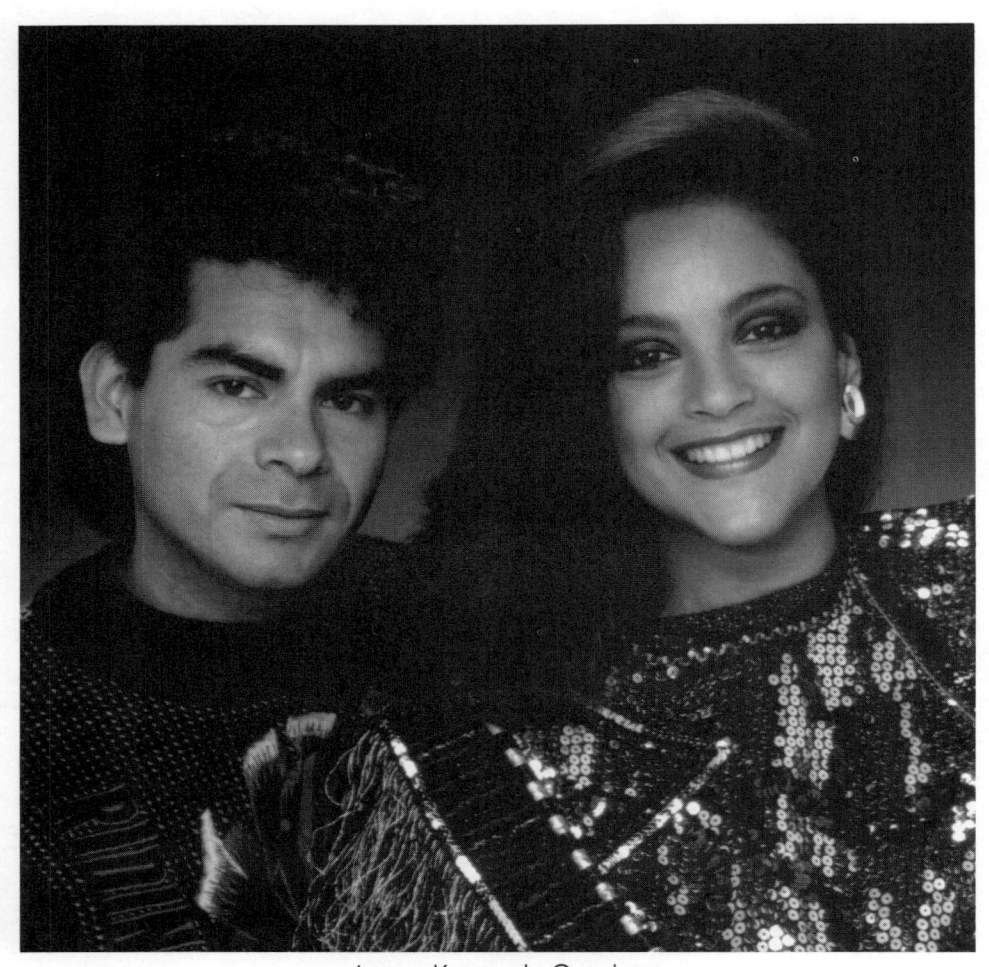

Jayne Kennedy Overton

8
CLASSIC BEAUTIES AND THEIR STYLES

BARBARA CARRERA

Barbara, the all-time classic beauty, has the type of good looks and screen personality that shout out STAR!

A former model, Barbara is famous for her scheming-temptress screen roles—Fatima Blush, the hired assassin in the Bond film *Never Say Never Again*; and most recently, Angelica Nero, the international villainess who gives J. R. a run for his money in "Dallas."

Barbara's dark brown, abundant thin hair is worn in an elegant one-length bob to the shoulders. Barbara wore her hair much longer until she became my client. I created her new look just before she started appearing in "Dallas." Her hair was cut four inches shorter to its present length. I also added some wispy bangs for versatility. Barbara can add the bangs to her hairstyle or brush them back and blend them into the crown hair. I also suggested a very subtle hair color change. Her natural dark brown was changed to a rich berrywood red, a shade that brings out hot burgundy undertones in the hair.

Barbara was recently named one of the 10 Most Beautiful Women in Hollywood by *Los Angeles* magazine and was featured on the cover of its special "Hollywood Beauty" issue.

TOVAR'S CLASSIC BEAUTY

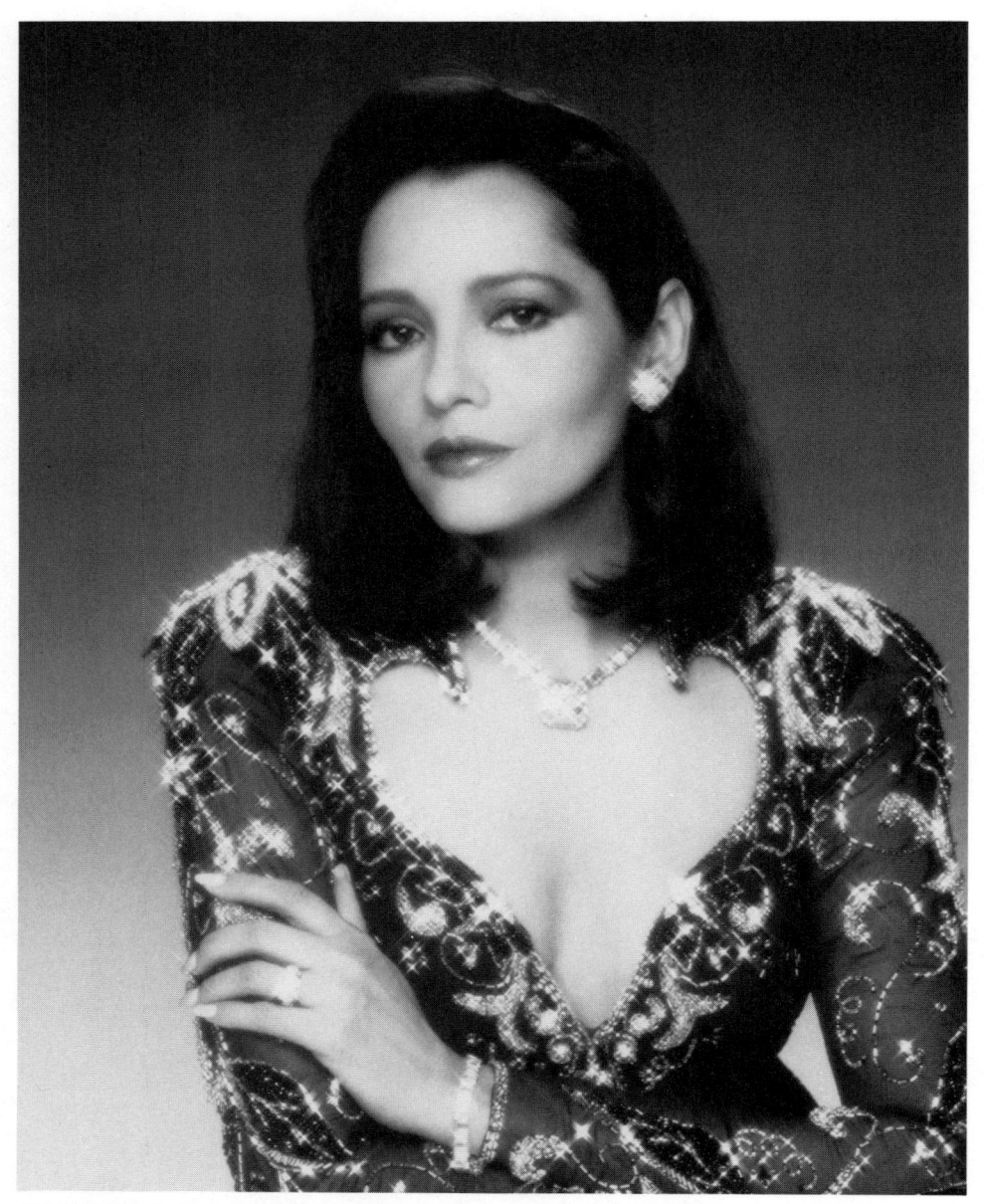

STYLE 1: Barbara's classic look—smooth, sleek, side-parted, and gently folded under at the ends, showing off those wonderful burgundy highlights. The black gown with ornate silver beading by Jeran Designs, Los Angeles. Diamond jewelry by Nova Stylings, Inc.

Classic Beauties and Their Styles

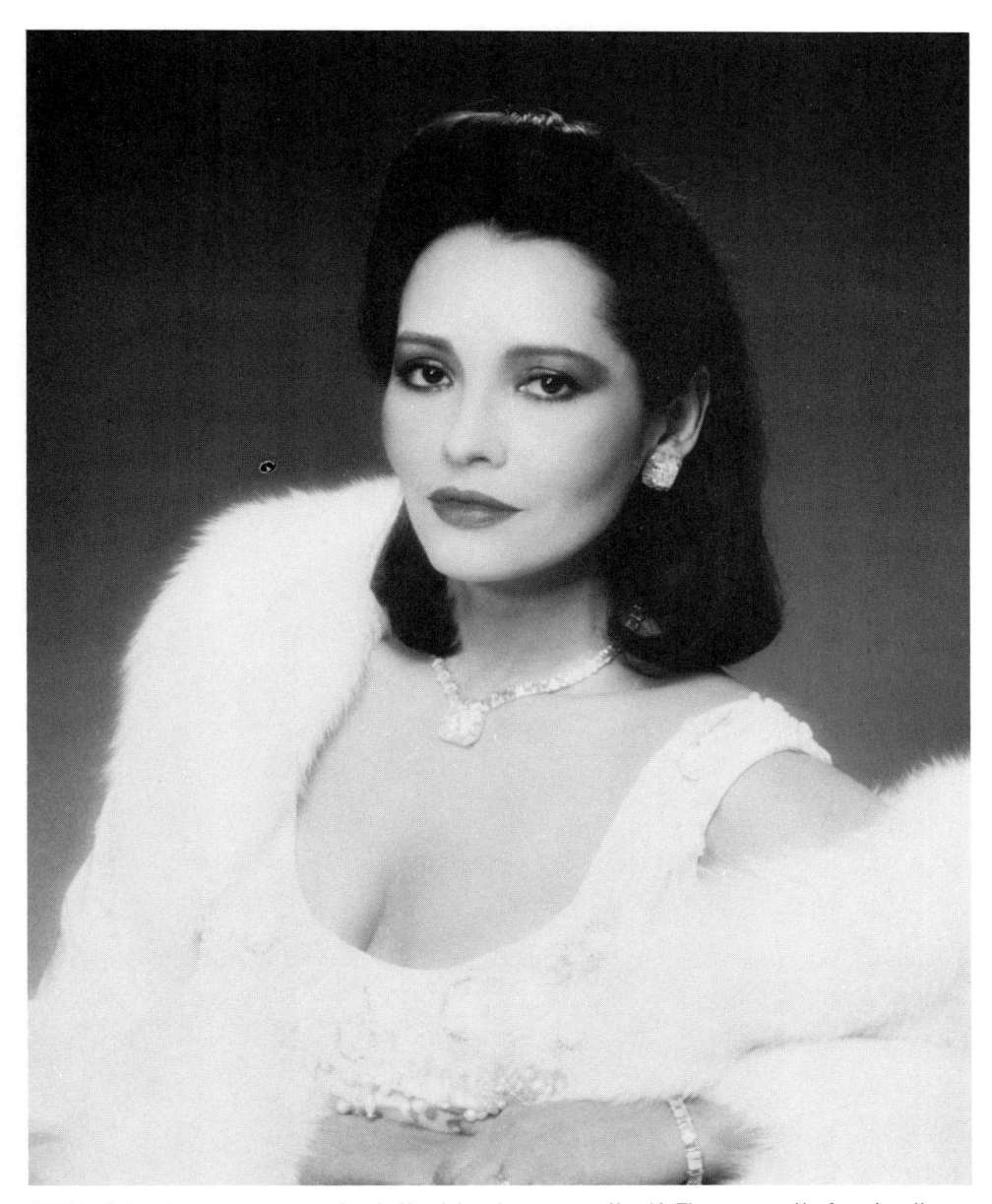

STYLE 2: Barbara wears a look that is elegance itself. The smooth front roll (her own hair rolled around a "rat" foundation) adds height over the forehead. The rest of the hair is just brushed smooth and sleek. The white gown with fur-trimmed jacket by Ruven Panis, Los Angeles. Diamond jewely by Nova Stylings, Inc.

TOVAR'S CLASSIC BEAUTY

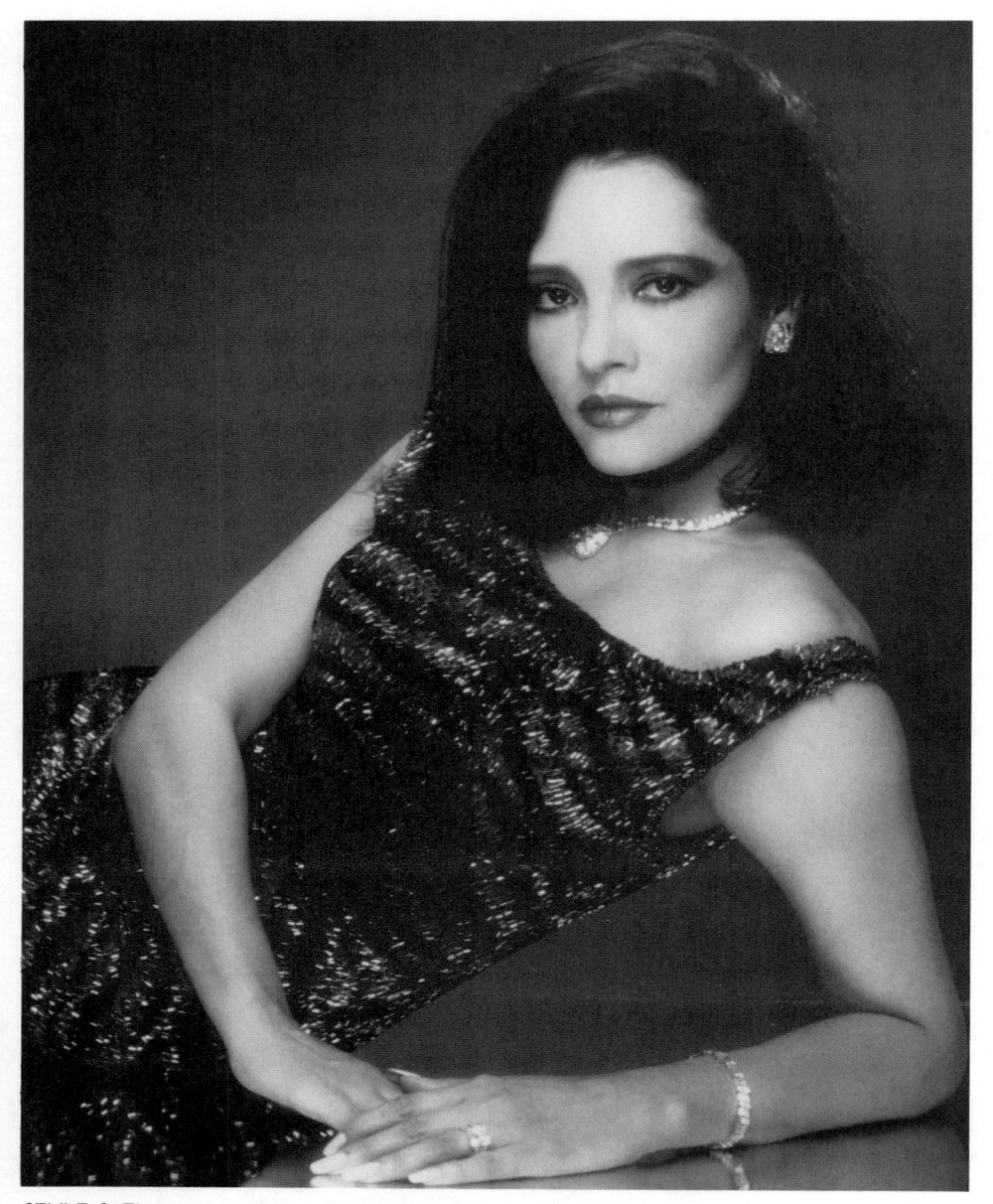

STYLE 3: Elegance doesn't have to mean every hair in place. Here Barbara's bob is brushed loose for a windblown effect to go with her wild evening costume. Tiger-striped beaded gown by Jeran Designs, Los Angeles. Diamond jewelry by Nova Stylings, Inc.

Classic Beauties and Their Styles

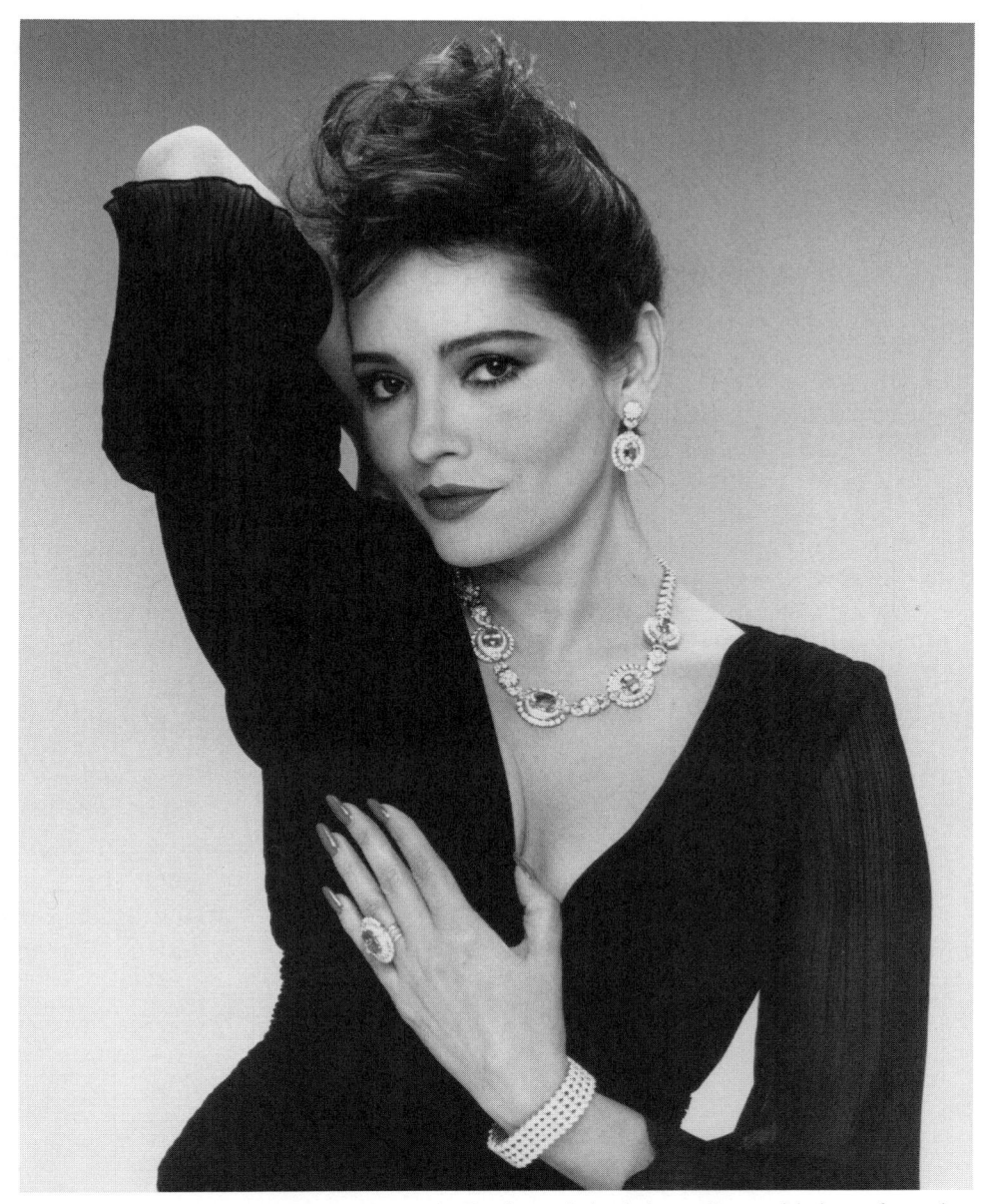

STYLE 4: For this classic beauty look, Barbara's hair is gathered into a french twist in back, brought up to the crown, and backcombed to give it some height. Light, wispy bangs touch the forehead. I put some gel on the sides to make them very sleek, to emphasize the volume at the crown. Crystal pleated chiffon gown by Jill Richards. Jewelry by Layken, et Cie., Los Angeles.

LINDA THOMPSON JENNER

A sandy blond with a bubbly personality, Linda has been my client for some time. She is one of those ladies who know how to work with their hair. She can do it herself as well as I can.

Linda is a multitalented lady, a native of Memphis, Tennessee, the birthplace of the blues and home of much of the country music we enjoy today. She writes poetry and lyrics for songs recorded by Kenny Rogers and others. Linda also acts and has coanchored a number of NBC "Sports World" shows and specials with her husband Bruce.

Linda and Bruce are sports and fitness fanatics and have their own exercise video. Linda's hairstyle has to be tailored to her active lifestyle. Her hair is very fine and difficult to work with, and she doesn't like body perms. Although I don't promote roller sets because I don't like the "doey" look, Linda is one of my clients for whom I set hair on hot rollers. She needs that volume and body. Another volume trick is to brush the hair forward when the rollers are removed.

I cut Linda's hair in a bob with long layers and some wispy bangs. Linda wears her hair long enough to be able to put it up when she wants to. Linda looks very good wearing her hair up; her fine bone structure and long neck really come into focus when the hair is drawn to the top or back of the head.

Classic Beauties and Their Styles

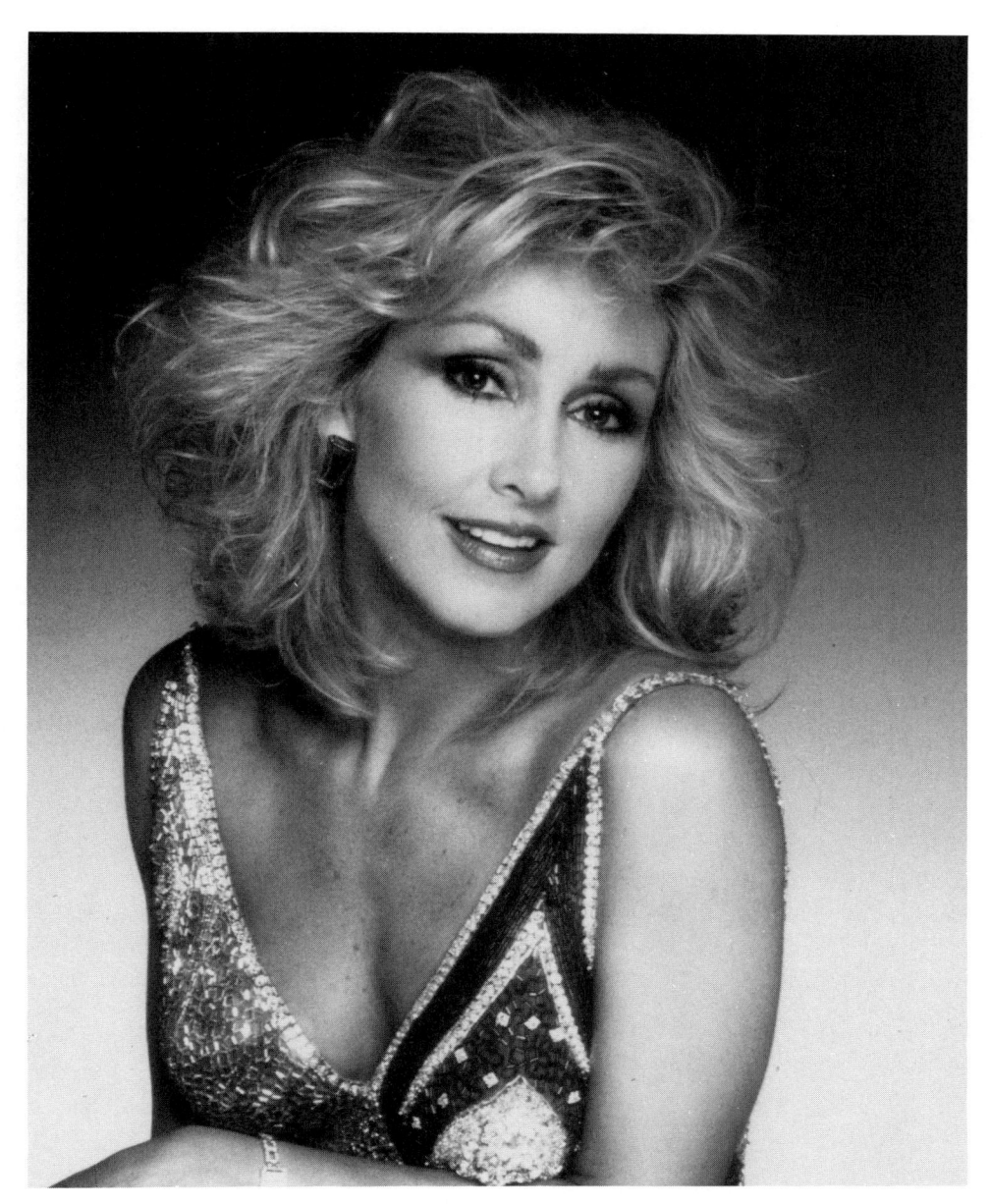

STYLE 1: A soft feathery, windblown style. Side-parted and swept over the crown and back from the sides. Because of layering, the hair can be tousled for an almost wild, very voluminous look. Silver and blue beaded dress by Jeran, Los Angeles.

TOVAR'S CLASSIC BEAUTY

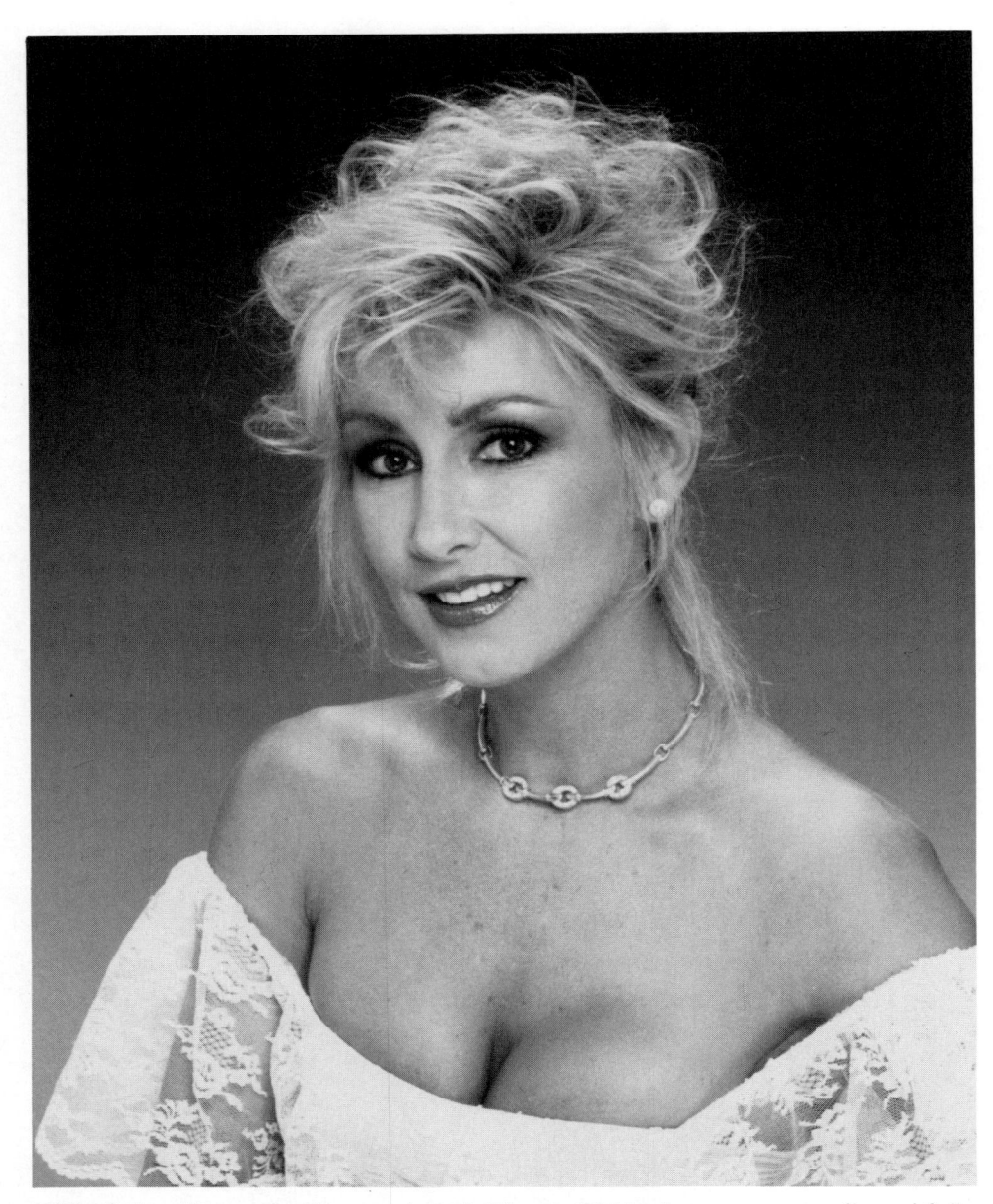

STYLE 2: A soft up-do with an almost Gibson Girl look, very, very soft and full at the crown. Waves are gathered at the crown and brought forward from a french twist. Long tendrils fall softly around the nape and frame the face. White lace dress by Mystica, Los Angeles.

Classic Beauties and Their Styles

TERI AUSTIN

A beautiful woman with a perfectly chiseled bone structure, Teri is a newcomer to southern California. She plays the intriguing Jill Bennett in the nighttime soap "Knot's Landing."

Teri is a brunette with tons of fine hair with a slight natural wave—a natural kick, as I like to call it. She has a very high forehead, and she should always wear bangs, which also bring out her very beautiful eyes.

Because Teri's hair has a natural bend, it is easy to add volume—I just add a little mousse to the hair before styling and blow it upside down, using my hands to scrunch as I dry.

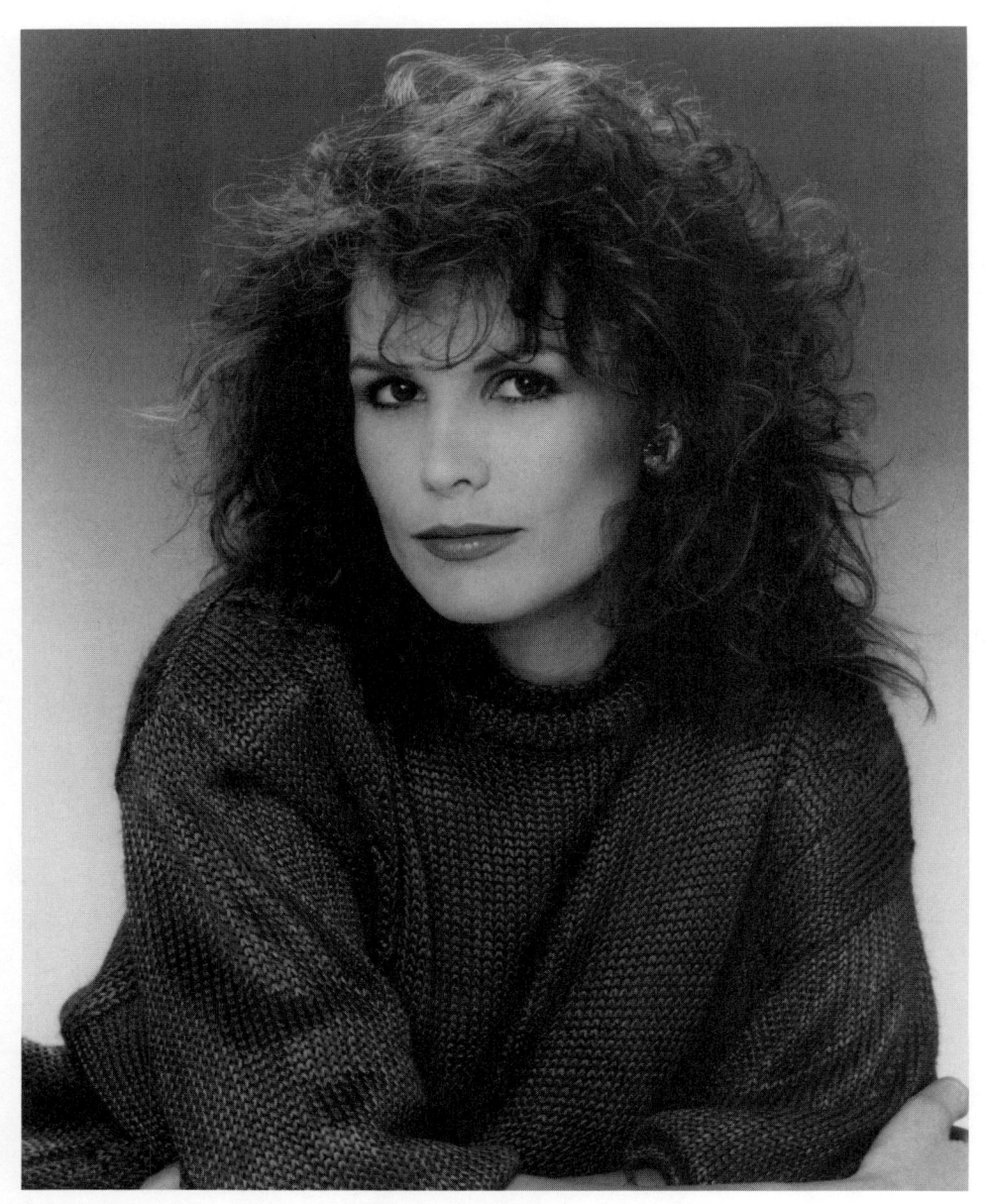

STYLE 1: Softly tousled and wavy, side-parted with side-swept, airy bangs across the forehead. Moderately high at the crown.

Classic Beauties and Their Styles

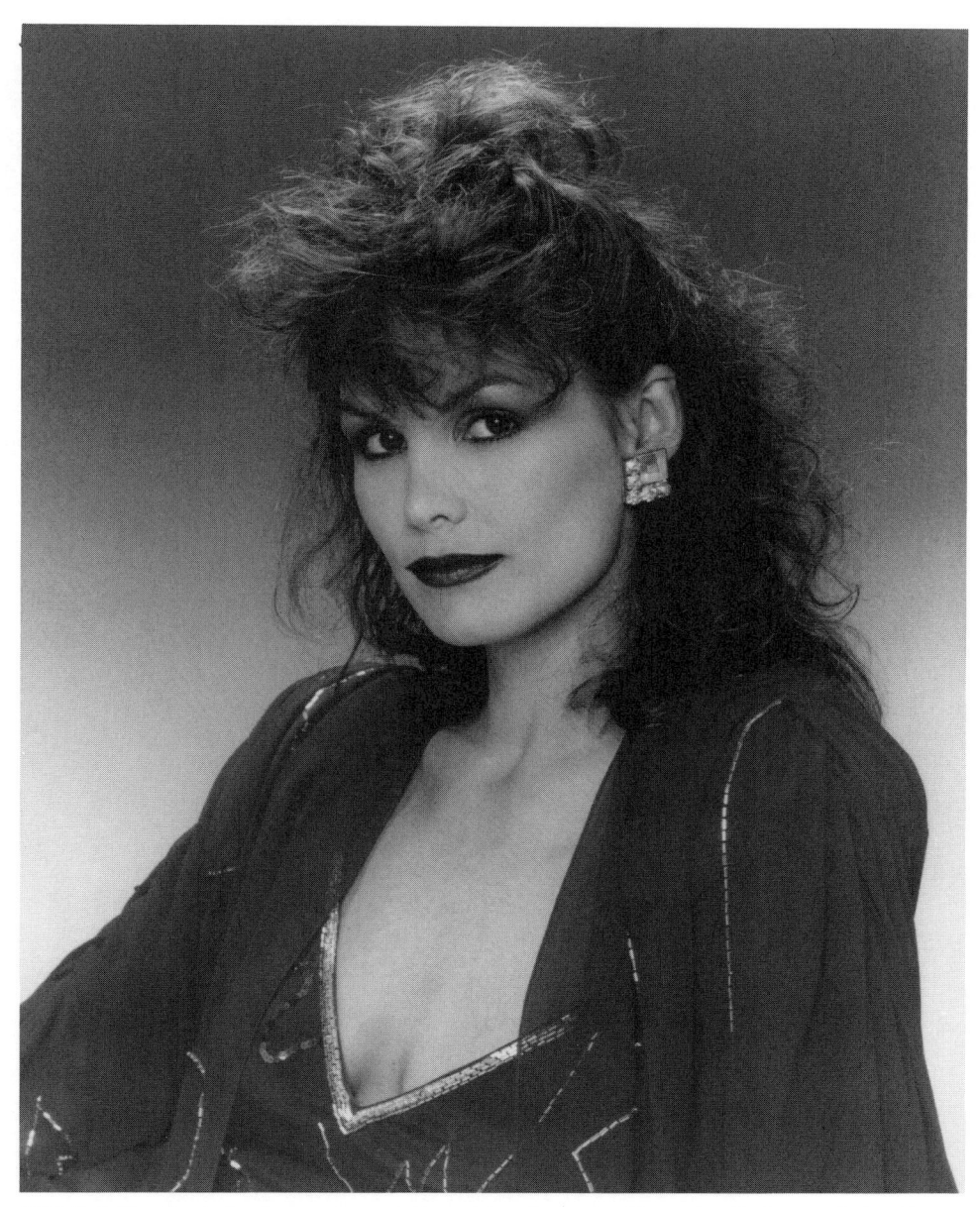

STYLE 2: The hair is drawn up at the sides for a half-up, half-down style. The crown is brought forward into an airy froth of curls ending in bangs over the forehead. Frothy waves cascade down the sides and back. Dress by Eletra Cassadei.

PATRICIA KLOUS

Pat has the classic "girl next door" look when she appears on TV as Cruise Director Judy McCoy aboard "The Love Boat." But in real life this classic blond shows off the many looks she can wear, perhaps a quality learned during her days as a Wilhemina model.

Pat has baby-fine blond hair, which is hard to manage because it is straight and almost refuses to bend. She also has a high forehead, so bangs are a great way to deemphasize this area. My formula for adding body and volume to Pat's hair is simple. I set her hair in twisted pin curls (see Chapter 6) and dry them. If you have this type of hair, you can do the same; let them air-dry if you have the time to wait. When the hair is dried, it is unpinned, shaken, and blown dry upside down for just a couple of minutes.

Avoid roller settings for this type of hair, as the results will be too matronly. Up-dos are another good solution for this type of hair. All the hair can be slicked into a french twist, a braid, or simply pinned up at the back. Concentrate volume and fullness just in the crown area.

Classic Beauties and Their Styles

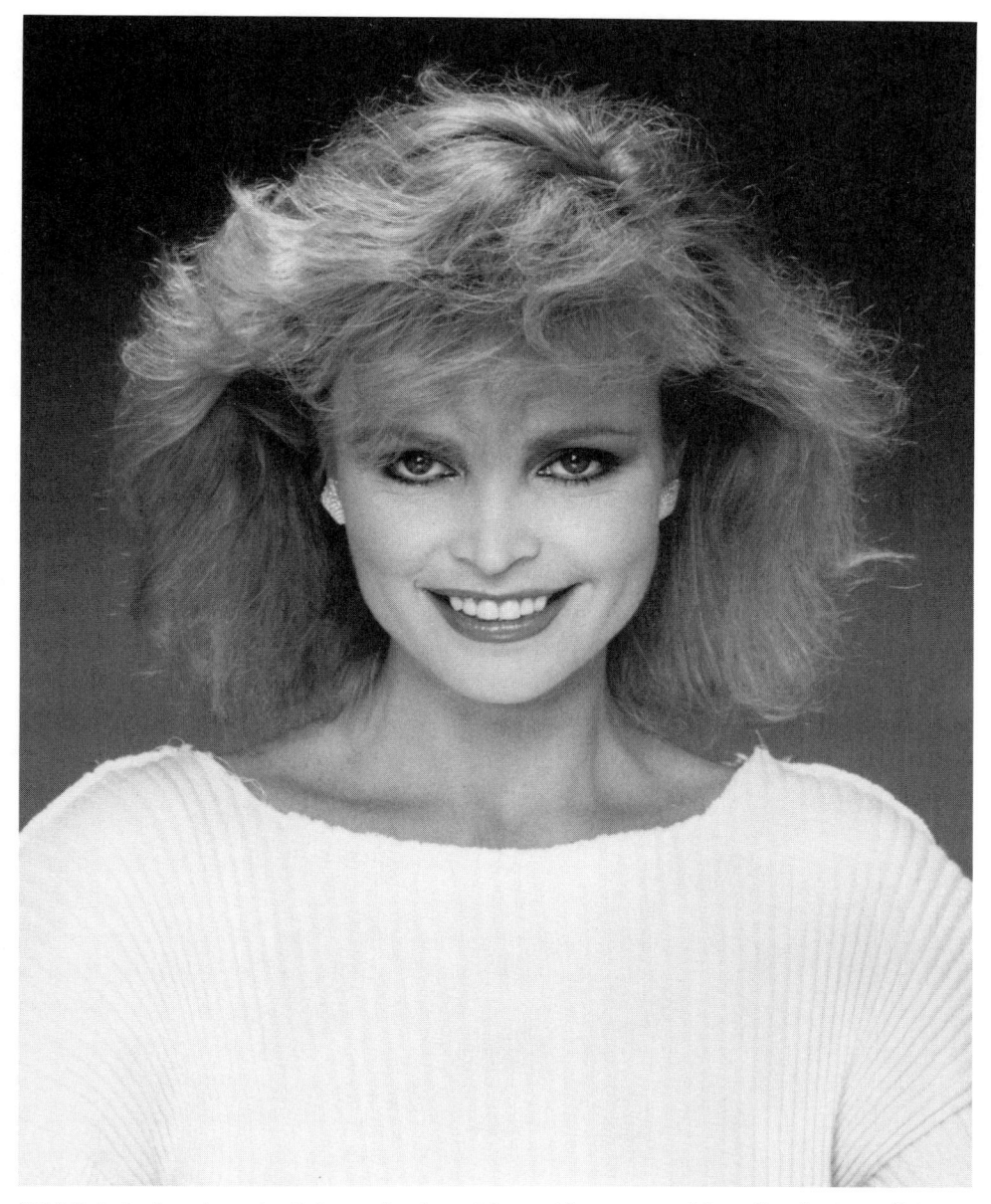

STYLE 1: A simple, windblown look achieved by scrunching the hair as it is blow-dried upside down. Diamond earrings by Nova Stylings, Inc.

TOVAR'S CLASSIC BEAUTY

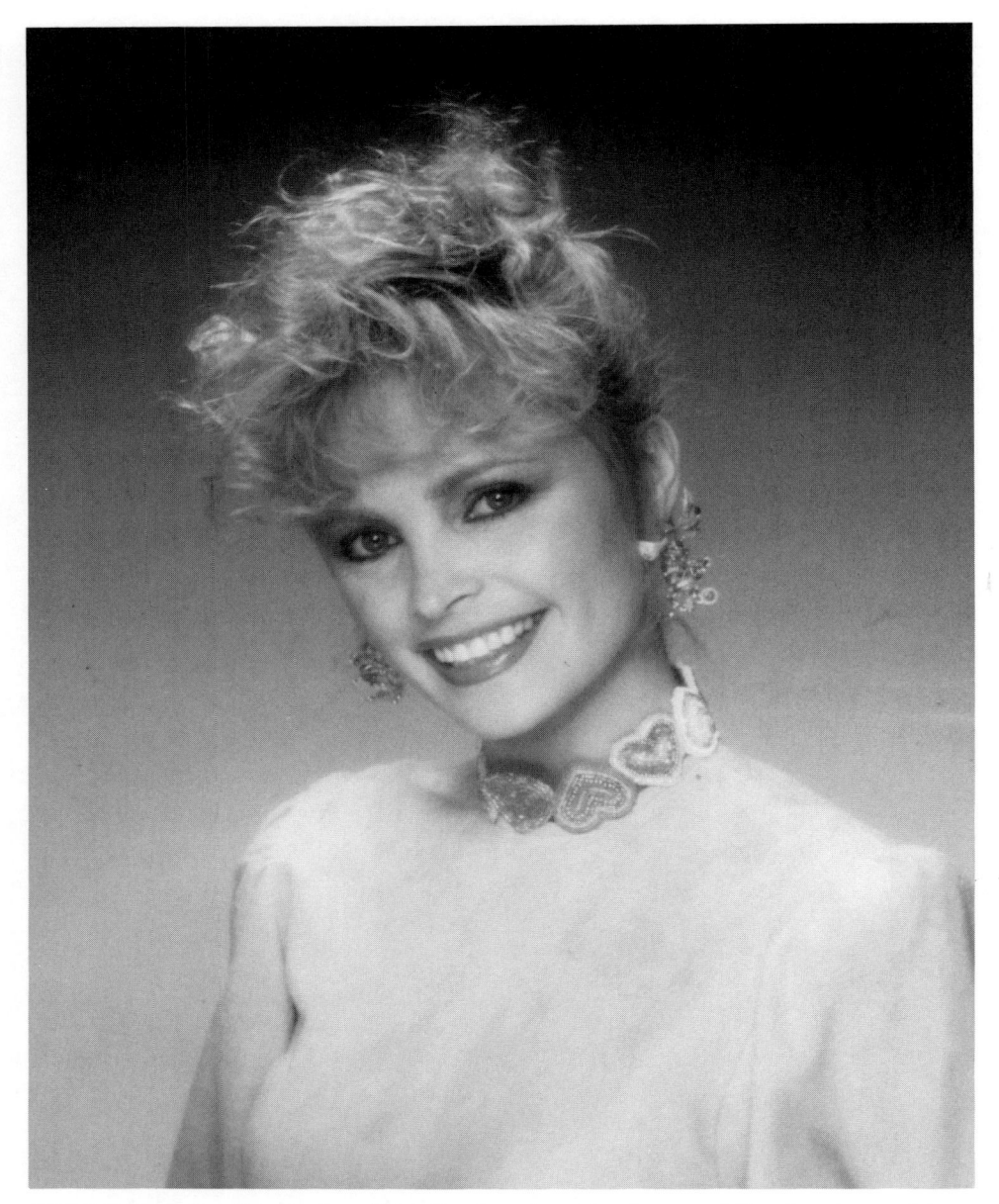

STYLE 2: The simple up-do with lots of curl and volume at the top brought forward into bangs. Pale pink suede dress by Gossamer Wings. Earrings by Bobi Leonard.

Classic Beauties and Their Styles

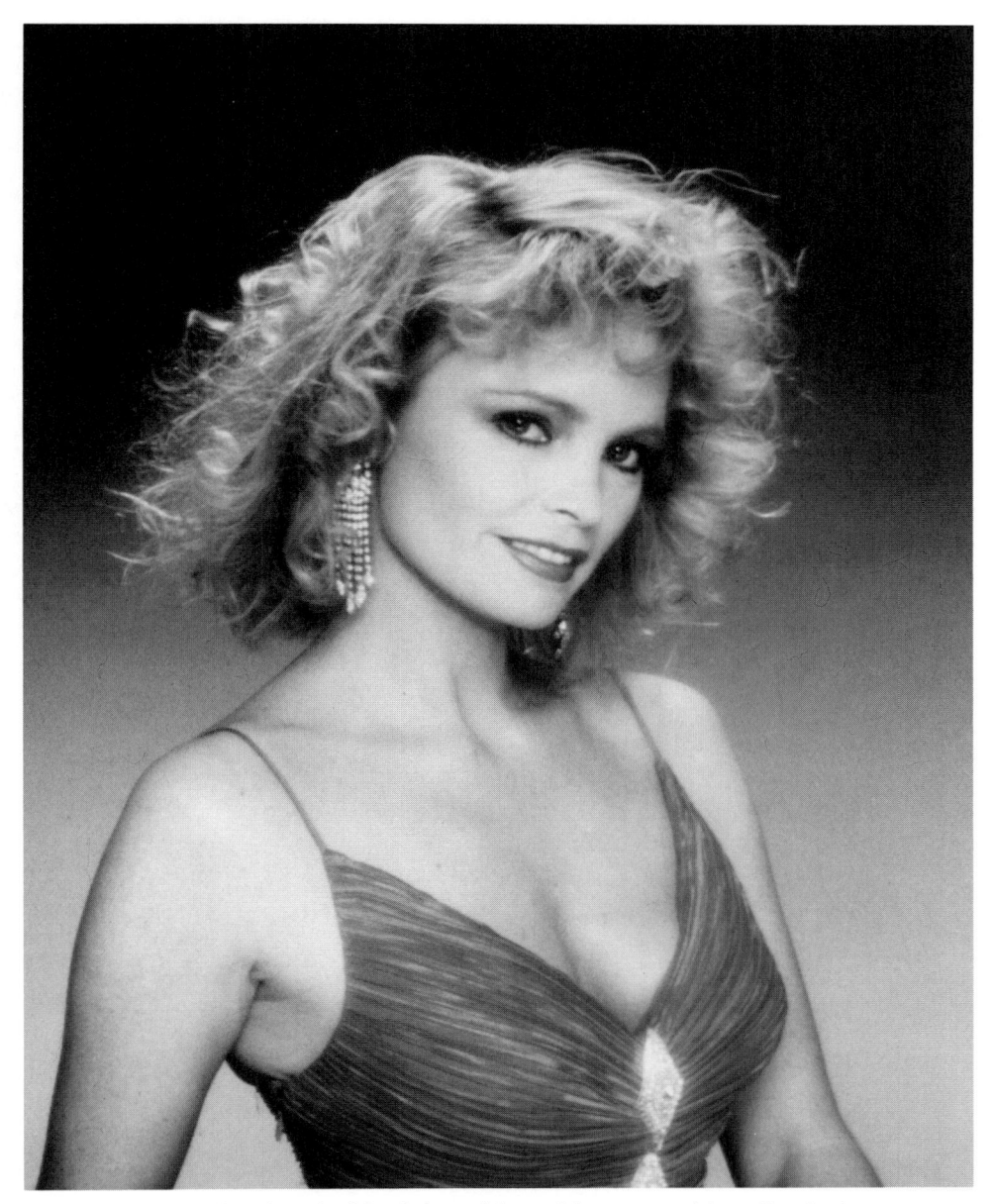

STYLE 3: The curlier, tousled look is achieved by scrunching the hair very vigorously. A curling iron is used to curl the hair around the bangs and sides in an upward and outward direction. Earrings by Bobi Leonard.

ERIN GRAY

This very beautiful lady has just finished her fourth season as the female lead in "Silver Spoons," and she is said to be the most beautiful stepmom on TV today.

A very versatile actress, Erin appeared in the film *Buck Rogers in the 25th Century* and the subsequent "Buck Rogers" TV series as the sleek, silver-clad, laser-toting Colonel Wilma Deering. But her acting scope also has been demonstrated in a variety of comedy and dramatic roles.

Erin's hair is very thick and coarse, in a lovely coffee brown shade. Because her hair is so heavy, it is very hard to work with. There is so much hair that it is difficult even to set on rollers. The best way to style Erin's hair is as naturally as possible. Her look is very classic, very simple—she is a true classic beauty.

Classic Beauties and Their Styles

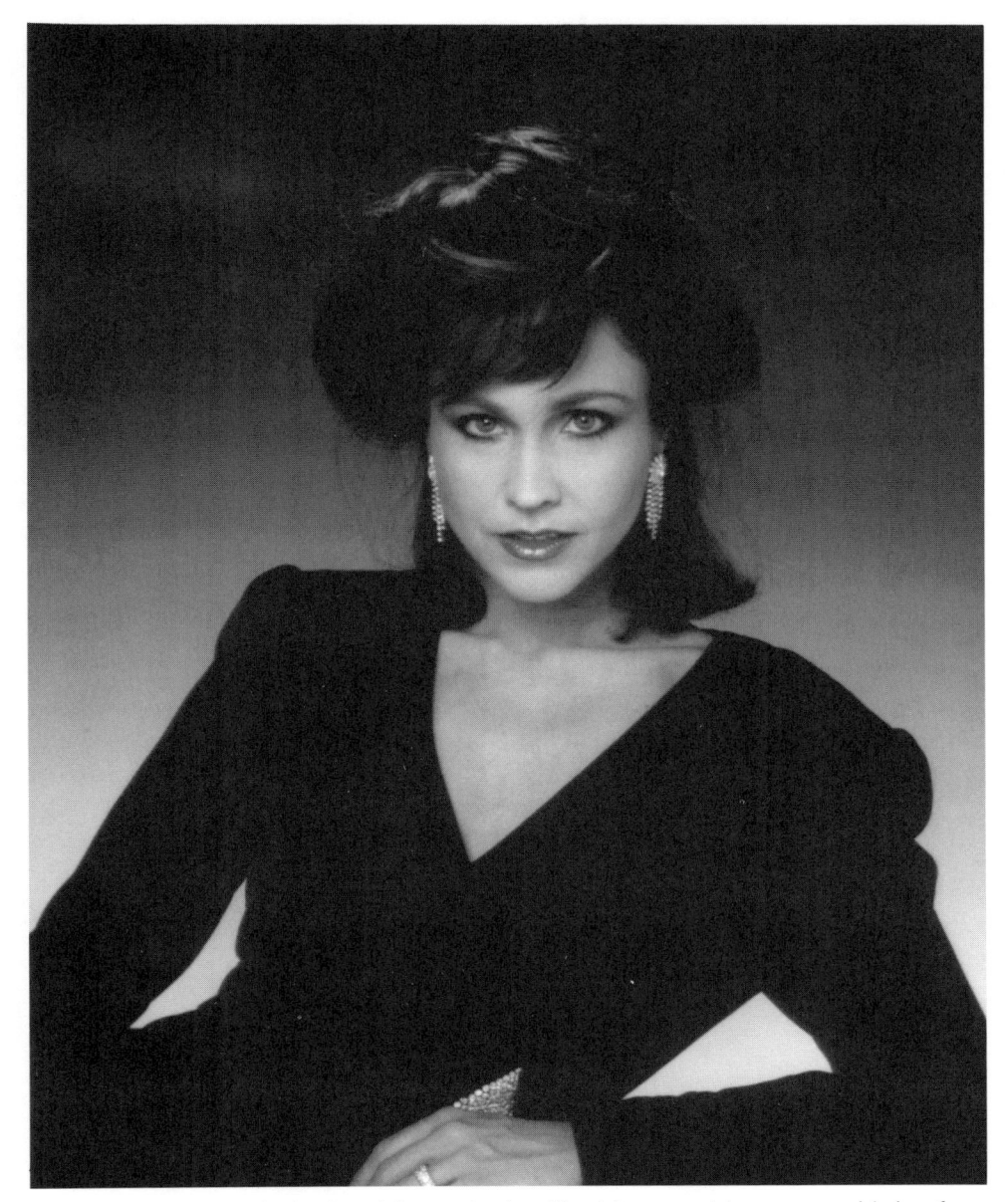

STYLE 1: Erin's classic look—side-parted, with side-swept bangs and lots of very full hair, slightly scrunched for some curve and bend.

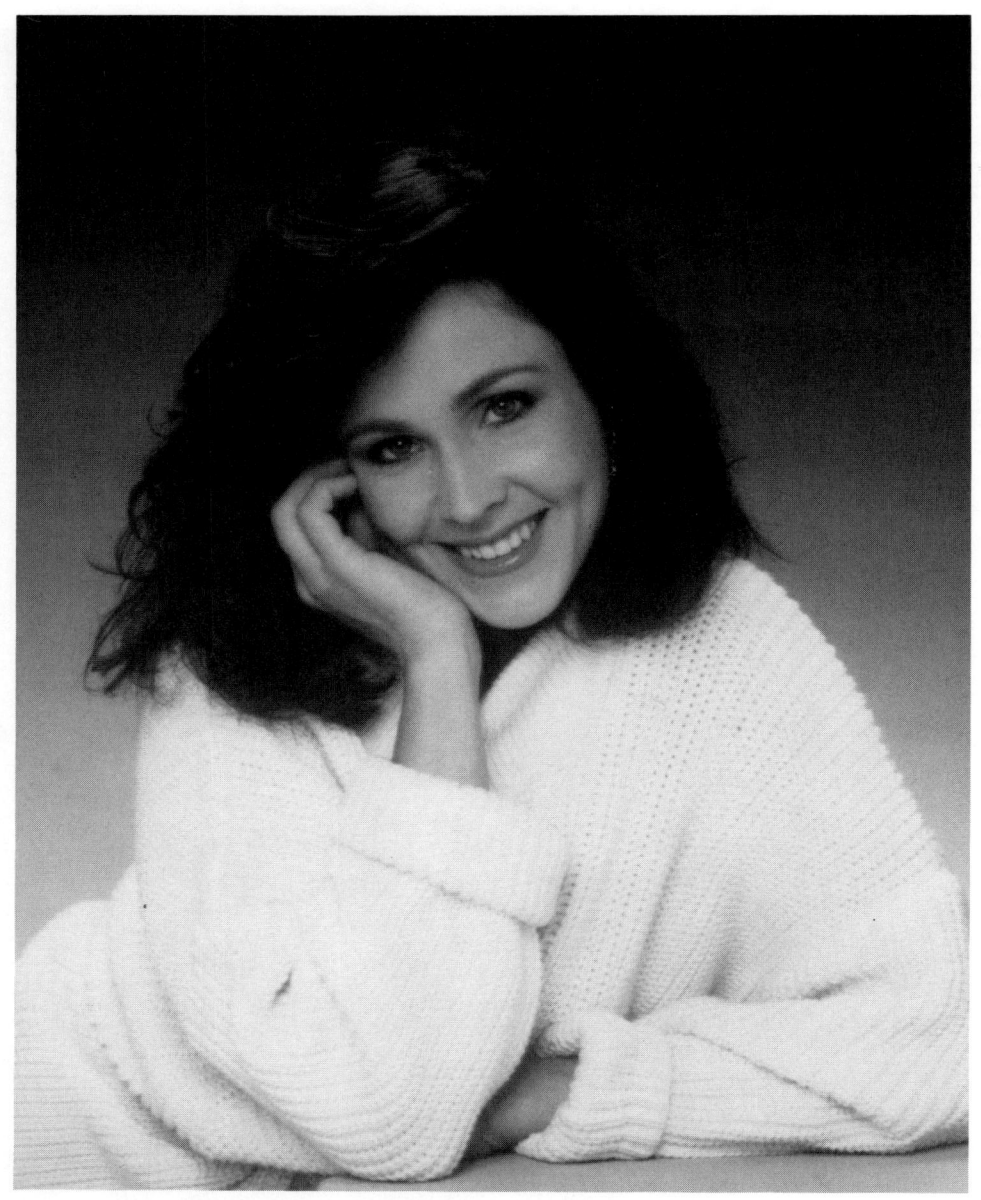

STYLE 2: A gala variation shows the crown hair gathered into a very loose, very loopy Gibson with lots of fullness. The back hair is left down, smooth and sleek.

Classic Beauties and Their Styles

ROXIE ROKER

Roxie plays Helen Willis on CBS-TV's "The Jeffersons." She combines her active acting career with community work on behalf of neglected and abused children.

Roxie's got very difficult hair to handle—fine, coarse, curly, and hard to manage. I keep it cut short for styling versatility. Roxie also wears wigs when she wants to change from her naturally curly look to a sleeker, straighter style.

TOVAR'S CLASSIC BEAUTY

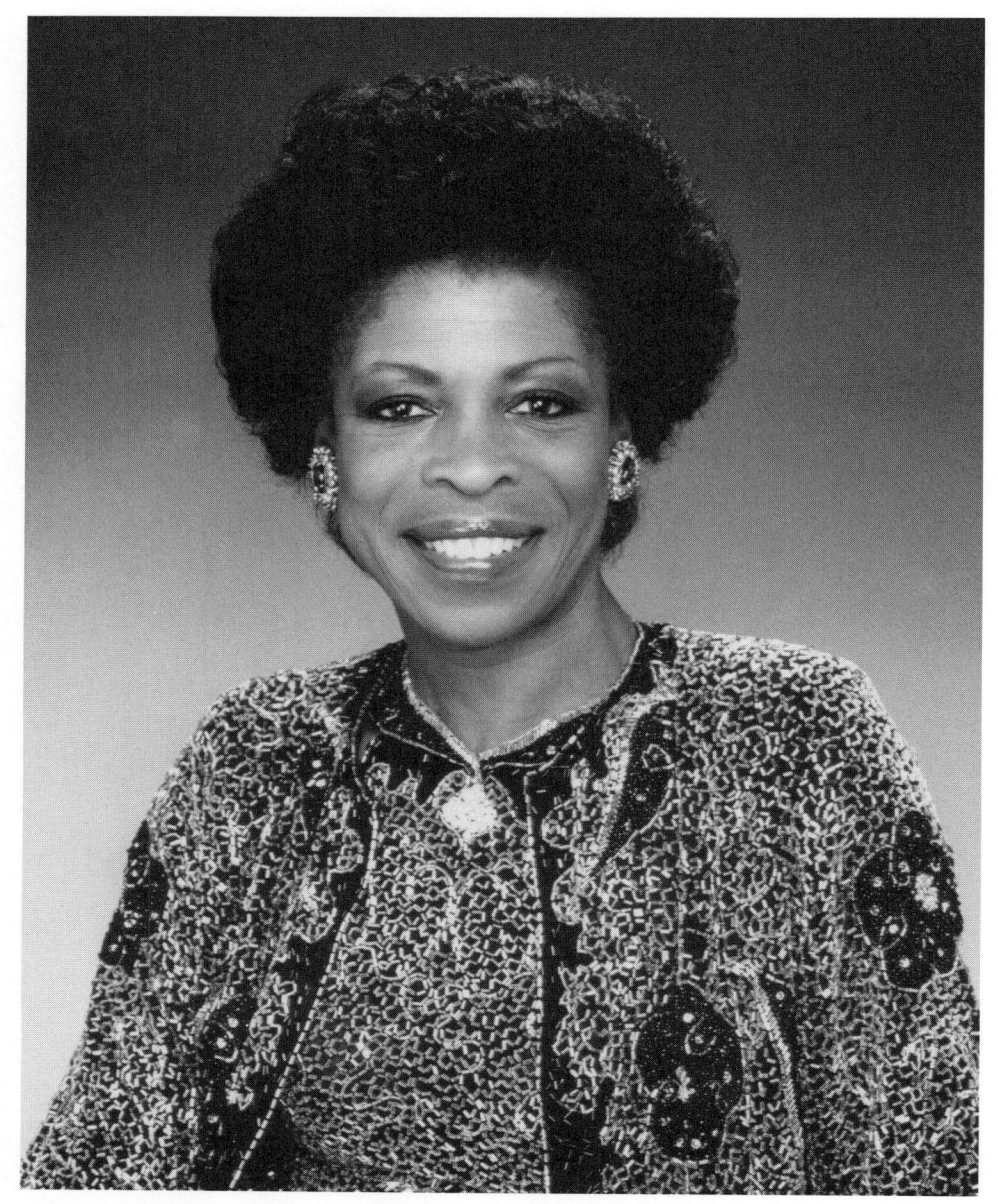

STYLE 1: Roxie's hair is styled with fullness and brushed away from the face in a very simple look, covering most of the ears. Black and silver beaded dress by Jeran Designs, Los Angeles.

Classic Beauties and Their Styles

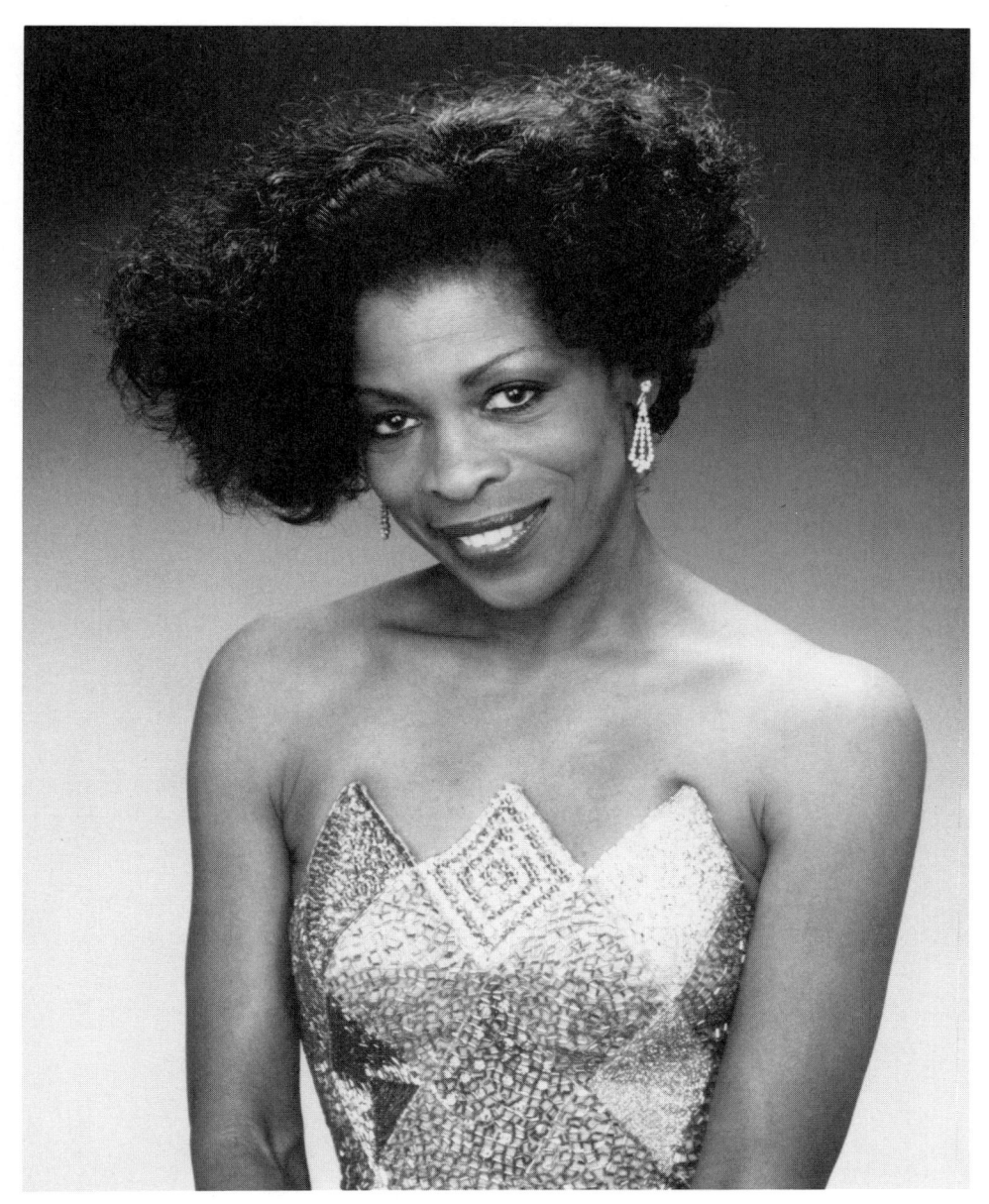

STYLE 2: A wig styled in a wedge bob, it is cut very short on top and gradually increases in volume to lots of fullness at the sides. Roxie doesn't wear bangs because she has a low forehead, but her own hair is swept over the front for a natural-looking hairline. Diamond beaded dress by Jeran Designs, Los Angeles.

ELLEN BRY

This stunning brunette is gifted with a magnificent head of hair. Her wonderful dark mane is naturally curly. The problem Ellen has is to keep her wonderful curls from frizzing in humid weather.

Ellen Bry is one of the few people who has made a successful leap from stuntwoman to actress. Her latest series role is that of nurse Shirley Daniels in the acclaimed NBC series "St. Elsewhere."

Ellen's hair is cut in moderate layers to keep it from looking too bushy. She has the type of hair that requires frequent trimmings. This mass of curls can be worn in a number of different ways—natural and wild, blown dry with a wide round brush to take out some of the curl, or slicked with some gel into a smooth up-do.

Classic Beauties and Their Styles

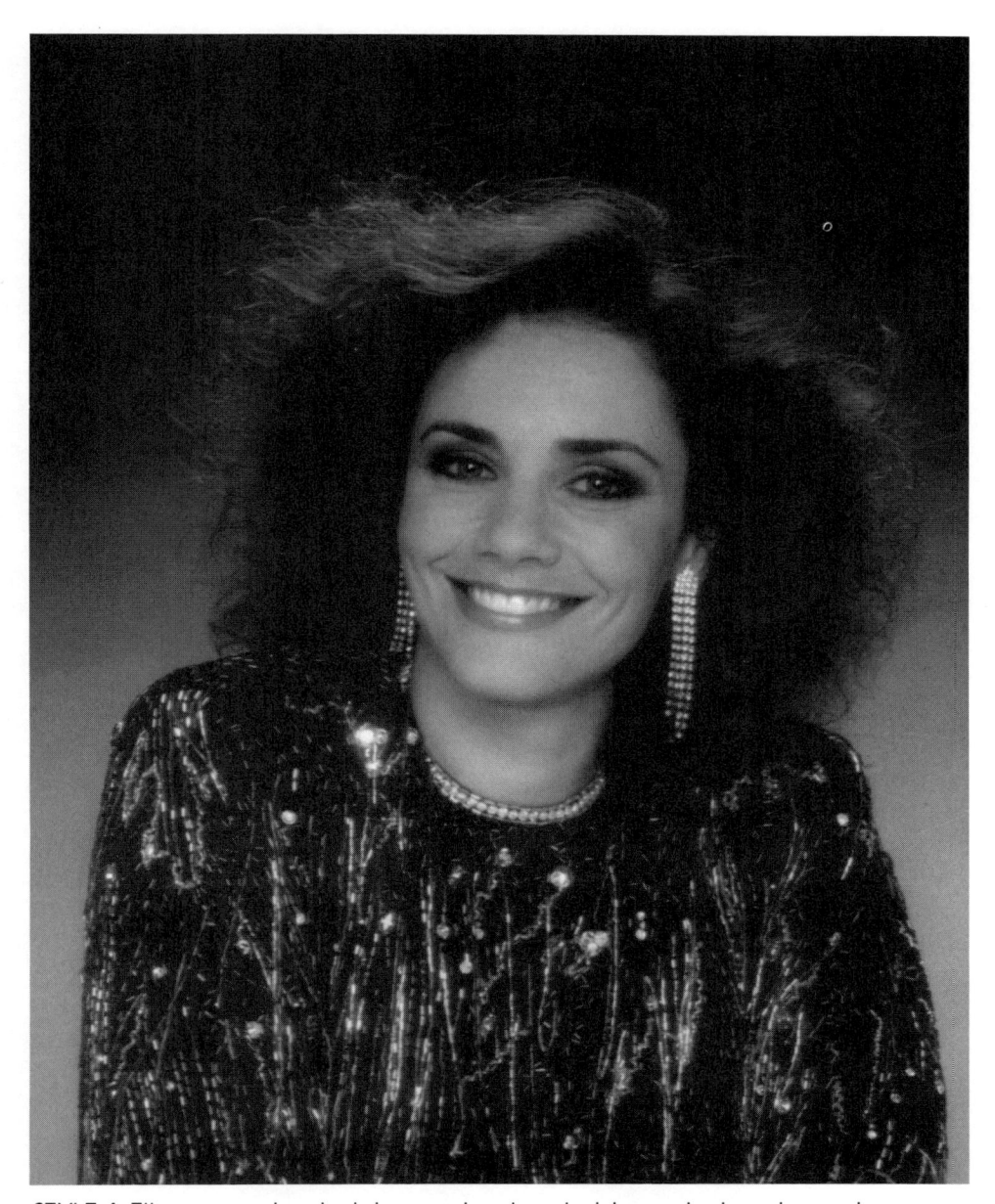

STYLE 1: Ellen wears her hair in a natural curl, side-parted and swept over the forehead. Ellen's great hair and incredible bone structure allow her not to wear bangs, although she can if she wants to for styling versatility. Beaded dress by Jeran Designs, Los Angeles.

TOVAR'S CLASSIC BEAUTY

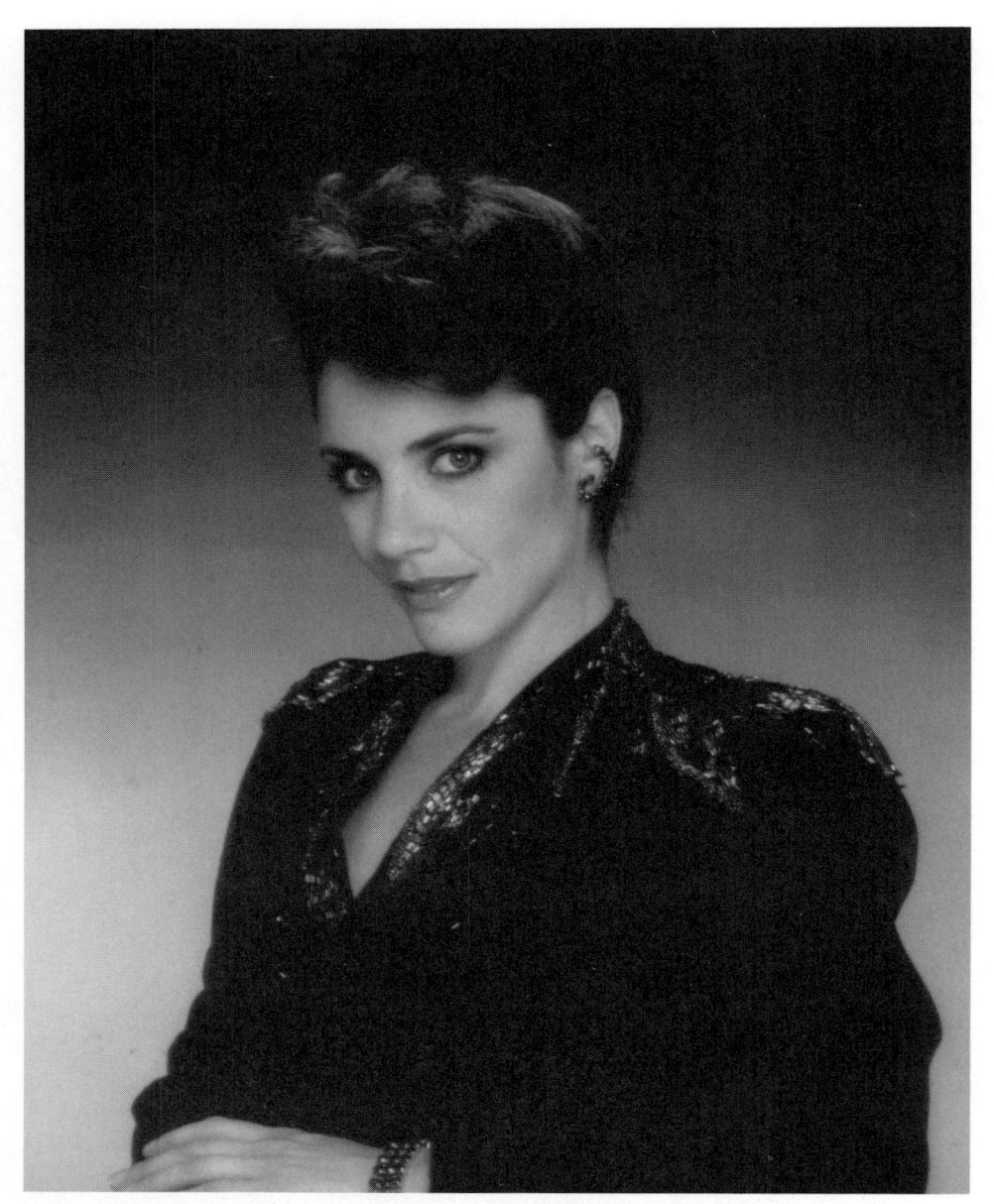

STYLE 2: With the proper methods, it is possible to get all that wild hair smooth and sleek as shown in this shining up-do. First, I use the blow dryer with the wide round brush technique to get the natural frizz out of Ellen's hair. Then, using a small amount of sculpting lotion to slick the hair, I draw it into a french twist in back and form a well-defined wave in front for softness. Velvet suit with beaded shoulders and lapels by Jeran Designs, Los Angeles.

Classic Beauties and Their Styles

DEBI RICHTER

Debi has masses of long, curly dark hair—literally tons of hair. Like many actresses, Debi wants to wear her hair long because it gives her the greatest styling versatility for the number of roles she plays. Bangs are also a favorite of hers for the same reason, but because she has a very fine bone structure, I cut very, very wispy thin bangs. Very heavy bangs would only overpower and hide her delicate face.

Debi plays Sherry, the ingenue, on a make-believe daytime soap that is the theme for the new, successful NBC series "All Is Forgiven."

When one has as much hair as Debi does, it is essential to wear it in a style that doesn't overpower and cover everything. If she wears her hair down, she can pull it up at the sides with combs, so it all doesn't fall over the face. Wearing it up is another great way to keep it controlled and neat.

TOVAR'S CLASSIC BEAUTY

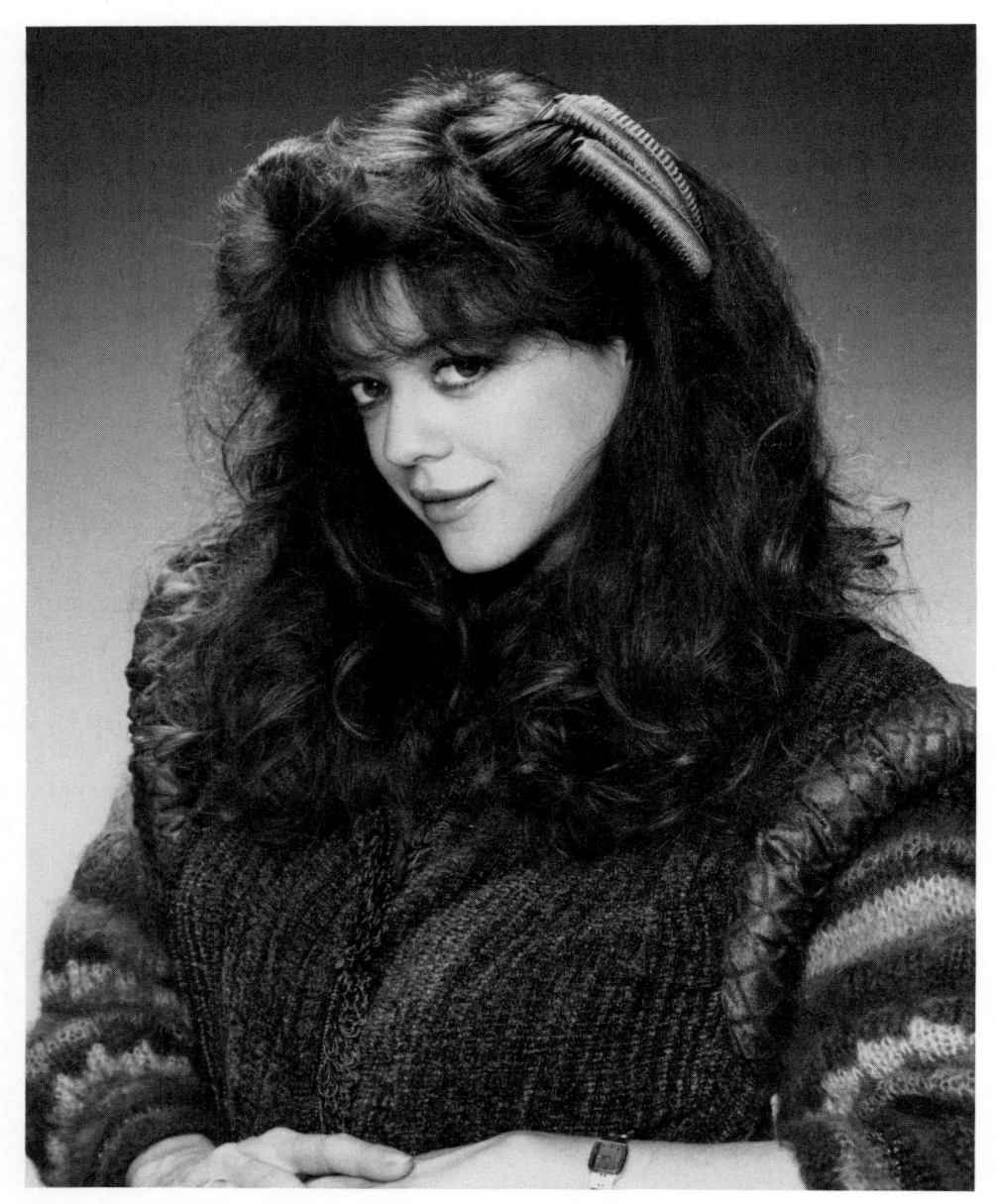

STYLE 1: Show off all that beautiful hair by wearing it down; keep it controlled by pulling up one side with festive combs. Bangs are very wispy and soft to emphasize the beautiful eyes. Sweater costume by Margi Kent, Melrose Avenue, Los Angeles. Combs by Bobi Leonard.

Classic Beauties and Their Styles

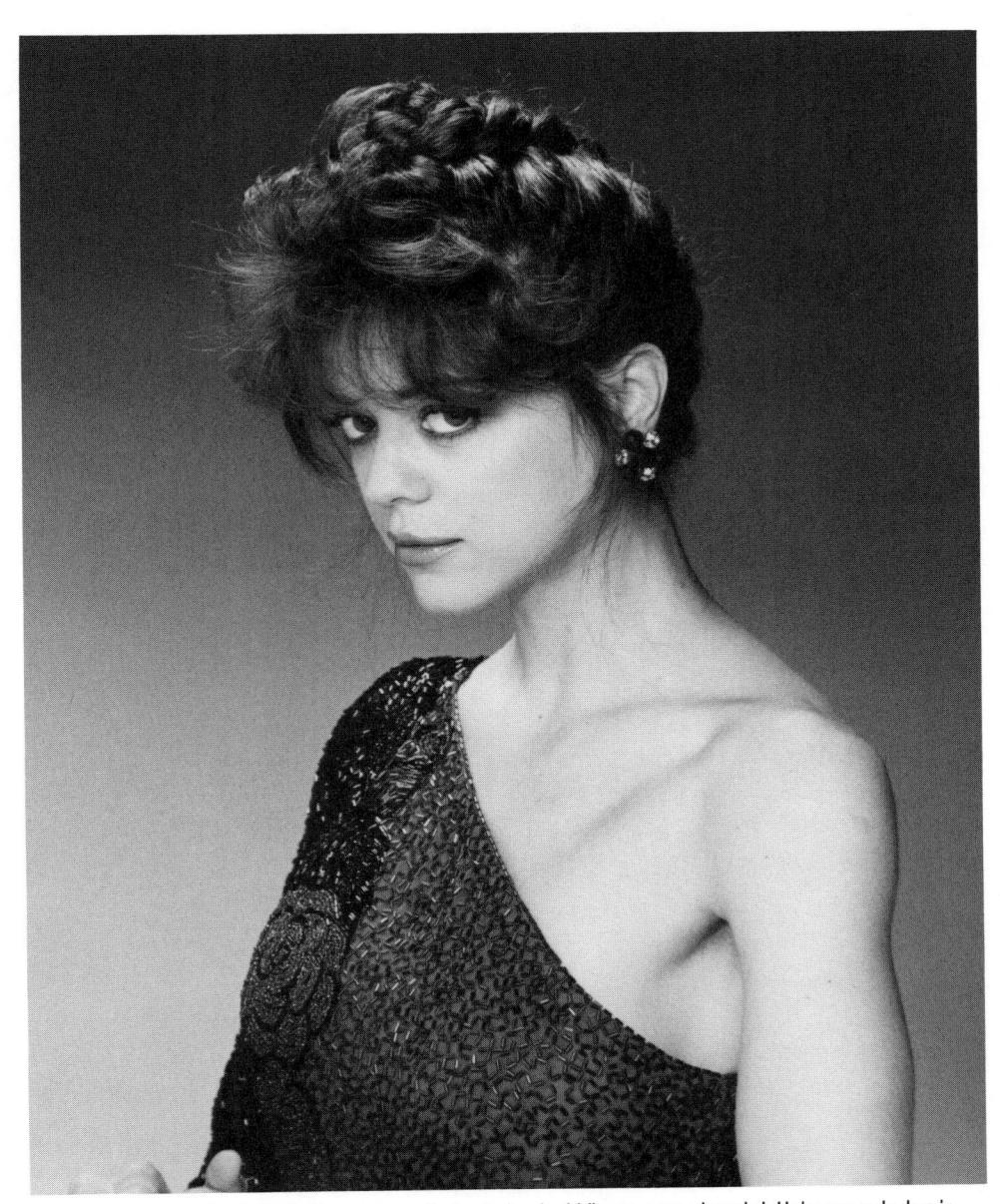

STYLE 2: I braided Debi's mass of dark hair. When you braid this much hair, be careful about where you position the braid, as it can look too bulky and awkward. I divided Debi's hair in equal parts on each side and braided the hair around from nape to front, with the most bulk placed at the crown for height. Bangs are brushed open and airy for a very soft effect. Earrings by Nova Stylings, Inc. Red and black beaded gown by Jeran Designs, Los Angeles.

CATHERINE HICKLAND

A stunning golden blond, Catherine is lucky to have masses of incredible, naturally wavy hair. Her hair is very soft and pretty, and it goes perfectly with her complexion and looks. Catherine is the typical golden-blond California girl.

Catherine plays one of the leading female parts—Julie Clegg McCandless—in the popular daytime soap "Capitol." She is a very talented actress and a very beautiful woman.

One of those ladies who just know what looks great on them, Catherine is very smart to keep her wonderful hair long. My latest addition to her look has been to cut very chunky, heavy bangs that are worn only one, two, or three strands over the forehead. This is the type of bangs you don't bring all forward, or the look would be extremely heavy and overpowering. This is another way that I use hair as an accessory.

Classic Beauties and Their Styles

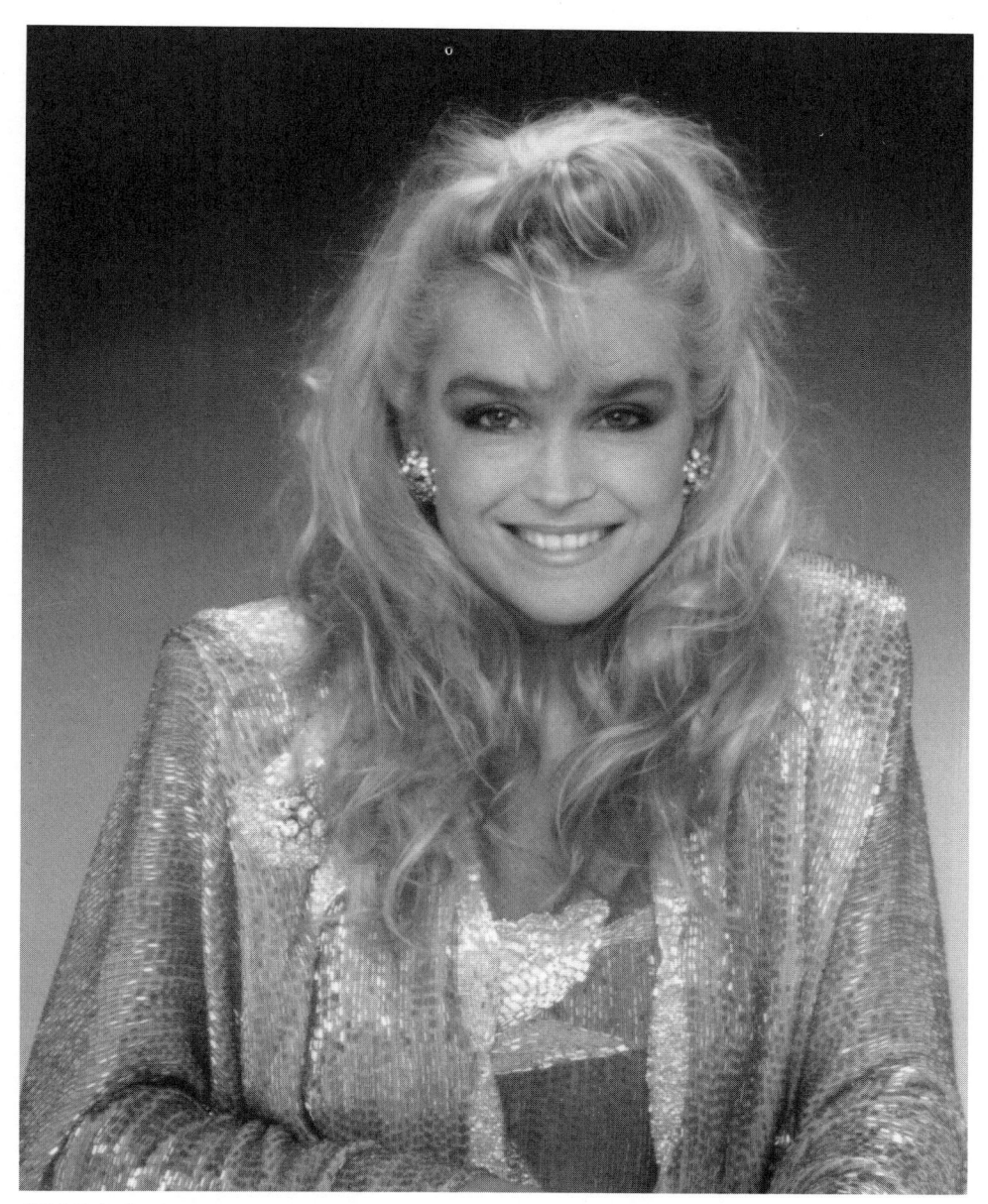

STYLE 1: Catherine wears her luxurious hair half up and half down. The crown is gathered into a loose knot right over the forehead; the rest is down, to take advantage of the wonderful natural wave. A playful piece or two of chunky bangs fall over the forehead. To achieve this style, the hair was set on hot rollers, then loosened with a bit of mousse and blow dryer to avoid a "doey" look. Golden beaded jacket and dress by Jeran Designs, Los Angeles.

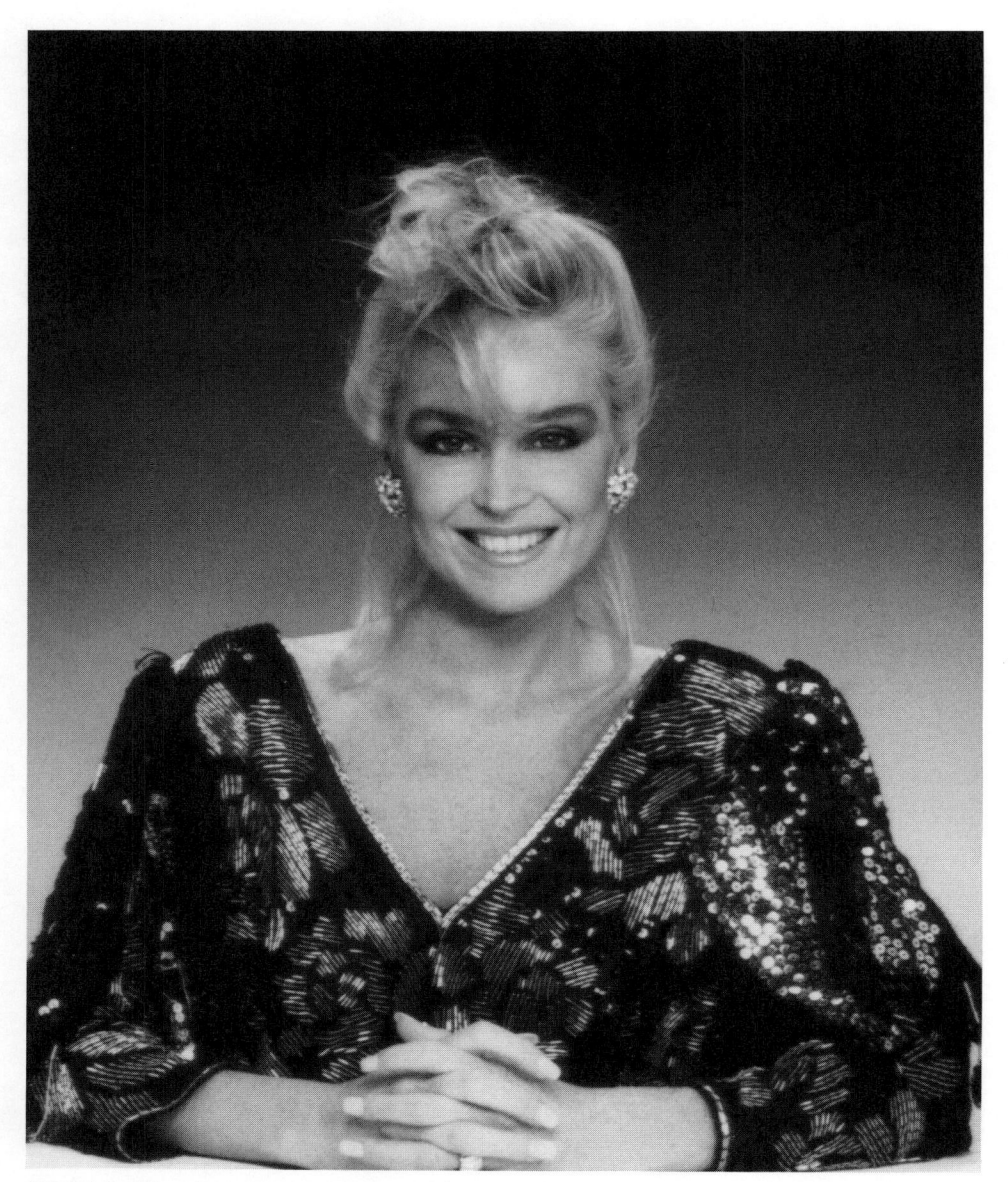

STYLE 2: This elegant up-do is achieved by pulling all the hair up into a chignon pinned off center at the top of the head. Notice that the hair is softly gathered around the hairline and not pulled tight and severe. Straight, piecey bangs over the forehead add a whimsical touch. Long tendrils are left down the neck to balance Catherine's long neck. Black beaded top by Margi Kent, Melrose Avenue, Los Angeles. Jewelry provided by Jeran Designs.

Classic Beauties and Their Styles

MERETE VAN KAMP

Merete is very, very exotic and beautiful; she has an almost shocking kind of beauty. She is one of those beauties who can break all the rules. She wears her hair dead-straight with very full bumper bangs—the kind of look that requires a great beauty to carry it off.

Merete's hair is baby fine, and it is layered around the face to frame her great features. This is the type of hair that needs some layering, or the ends begin to look skimpy.

A former international model, Merete reached acting fame when she was cast in the title role for the TV movie *Princess Daisy*. Recently, she played Grace on "Dallas."

TOVAR'S CLASSIC BEAUTY

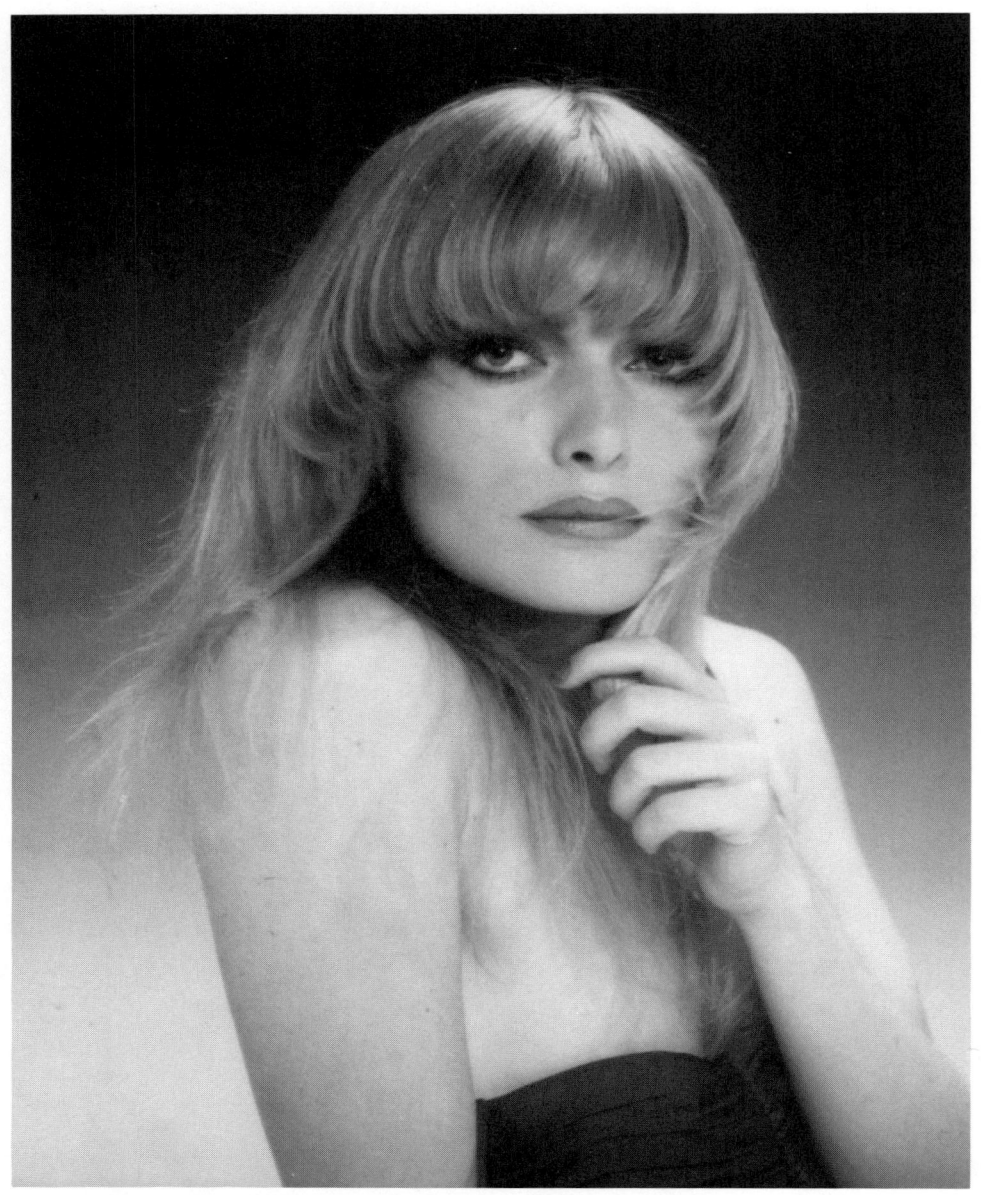

STYLE 1: Merete's favorite way to wear her hair—dead-straight, framing her face, with full bumper bangs. Dress by Jill Richard.

Classic Beauties and Their Styles

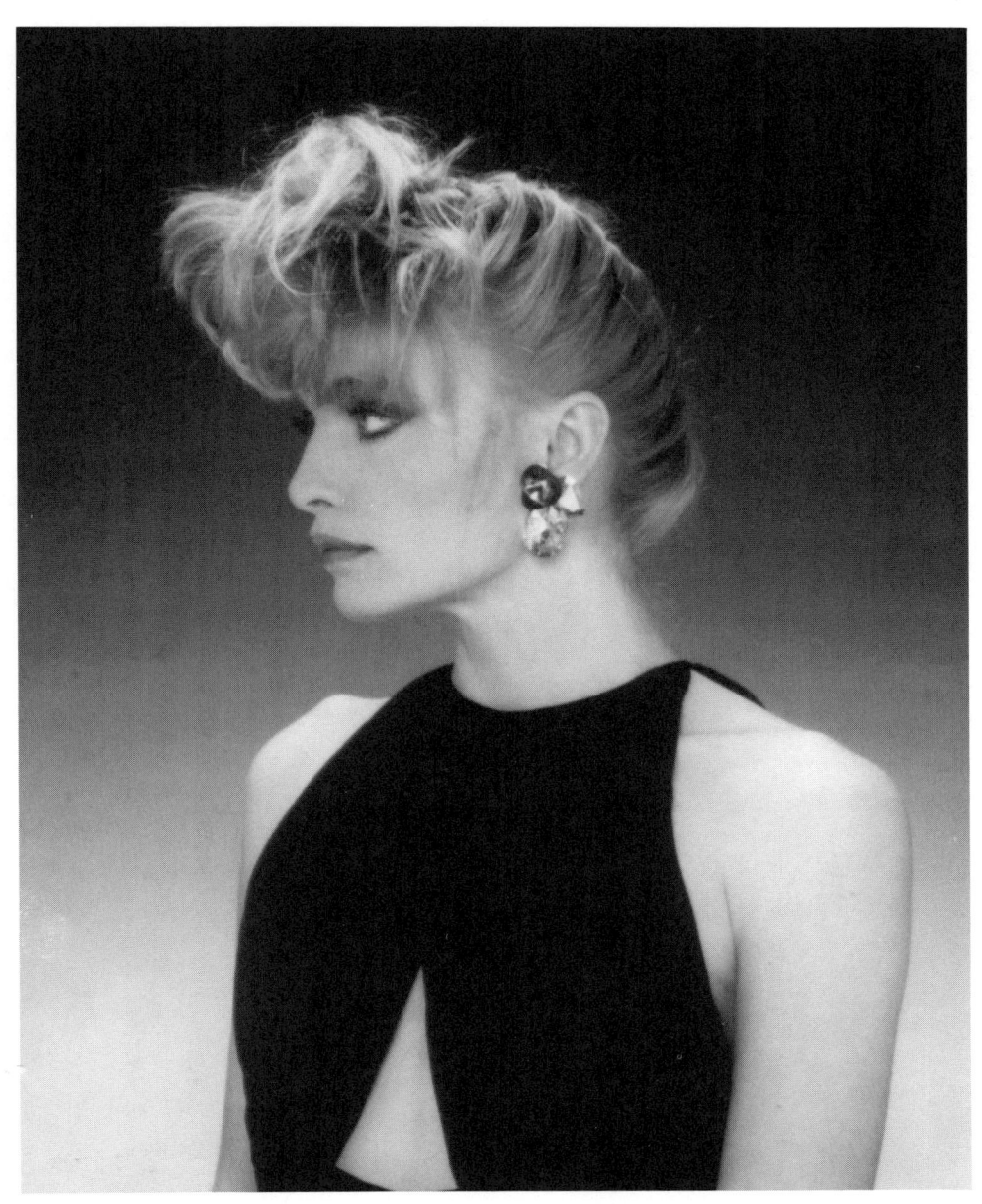

STYLE 2: Depending on how she wears her hair, Merete can look very classic and regal. Here she wears her hair up in a french braid. The bangs are curled into a frothy effect in front. Dress by Jill Richards. Earrings by Bobi Leonard.

TOVAR'S CLASSIC BEAUTY

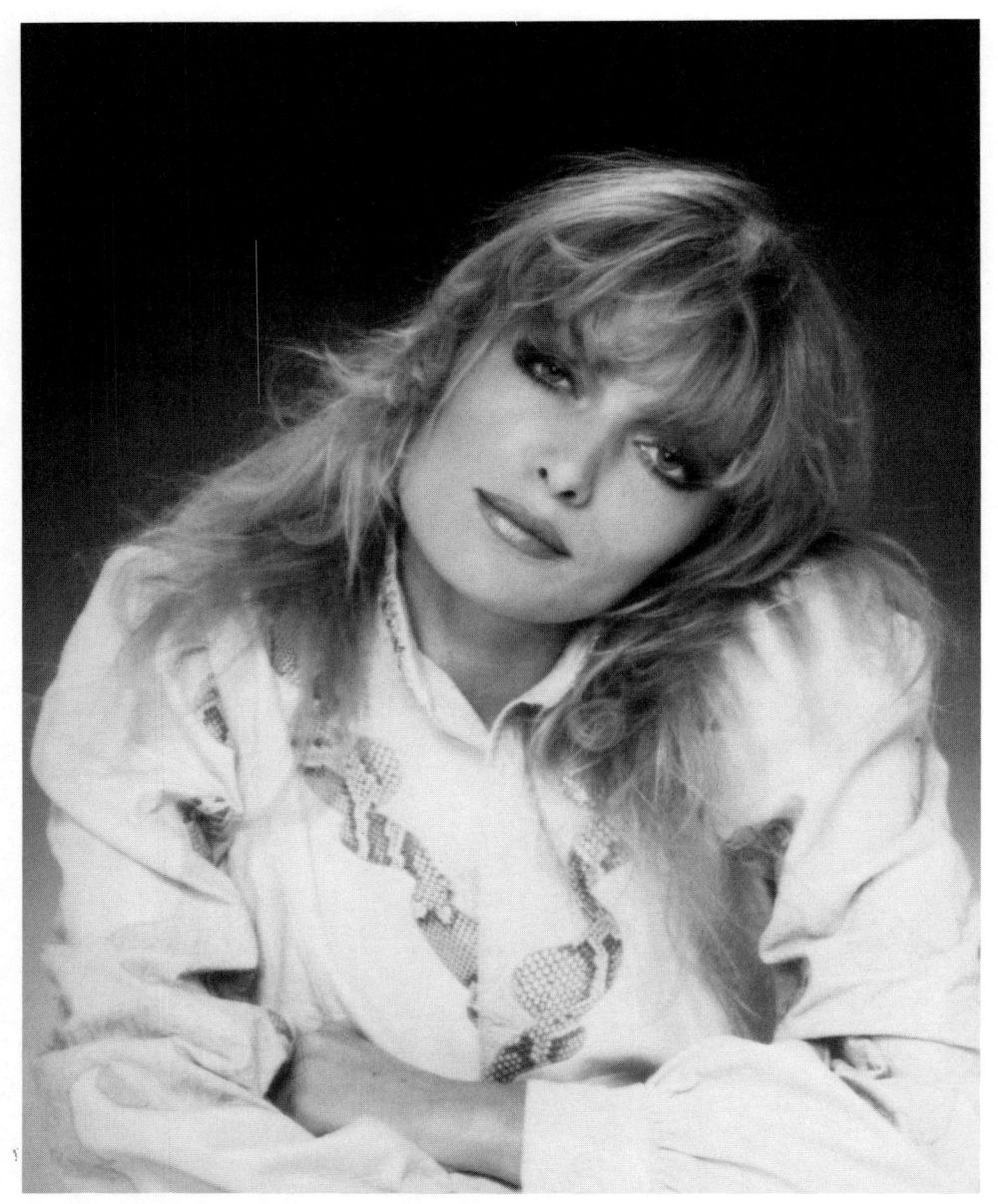

STYLE 3: A fuller, slightly wilder look is achieved by adding mousse to the hair and scrunching it at the same time the blow dryer is used. The bangs are slightly opened for an airy look. Suede jacket with snakeskin appliqués by Gossamer Wings.

Classic Beauties and Their Styles

NIA PEEPLES

Nia is an exotic beauty whose ethnic mix—Indian, Scotch-Irish, French, and Filipino—turns heads wherever she goes. Nia plays the role of Nicole Chapman in the critically acclaimed TV series "Fame."

Nia's hair is thick, coarse, and fairly straight, but it is the type of hair that is easy to work with and holds a set and curl well. I gave Nia very soft bangs to balance her very striking features and bring out those great, smoldering, dark eyes. But I cut the bangs long enough to make it possible to sweep them off to the side or back for styling versatility. I also suggested a body perm to add volume to this wonderful head of hair.

TOVAR'S CLASSIC BEAUTY

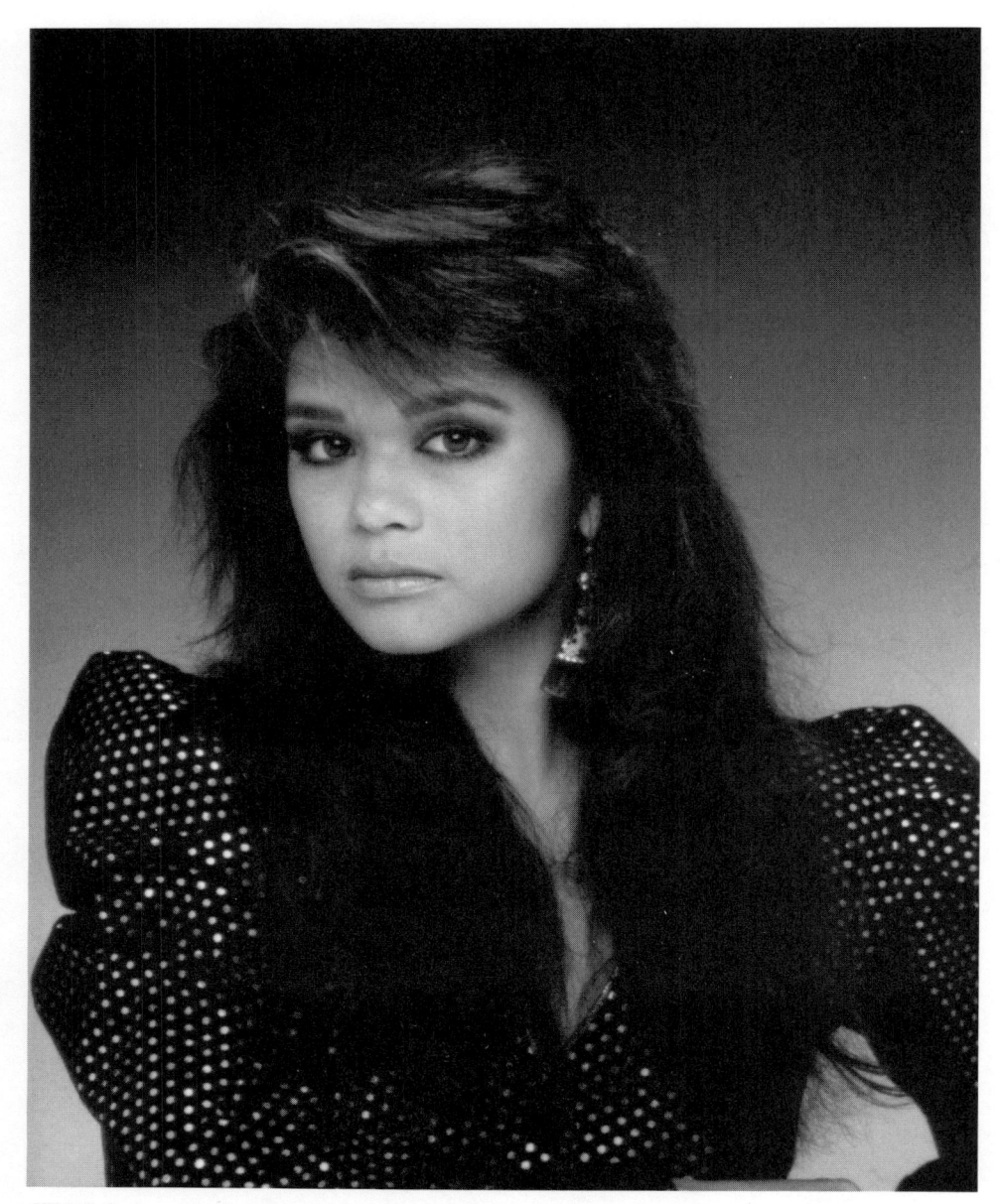

STYLE 1: A very simple, attractive, and easy-to-achieve style. Nia's hair is side-parted and scrunched with a little mousse and a blow dryer for volume. Black suede dress stenciled with gold dots by Gossamer Wings. Earrings courtesy of Ellene Warren.

Classic Beauties and Their Styles

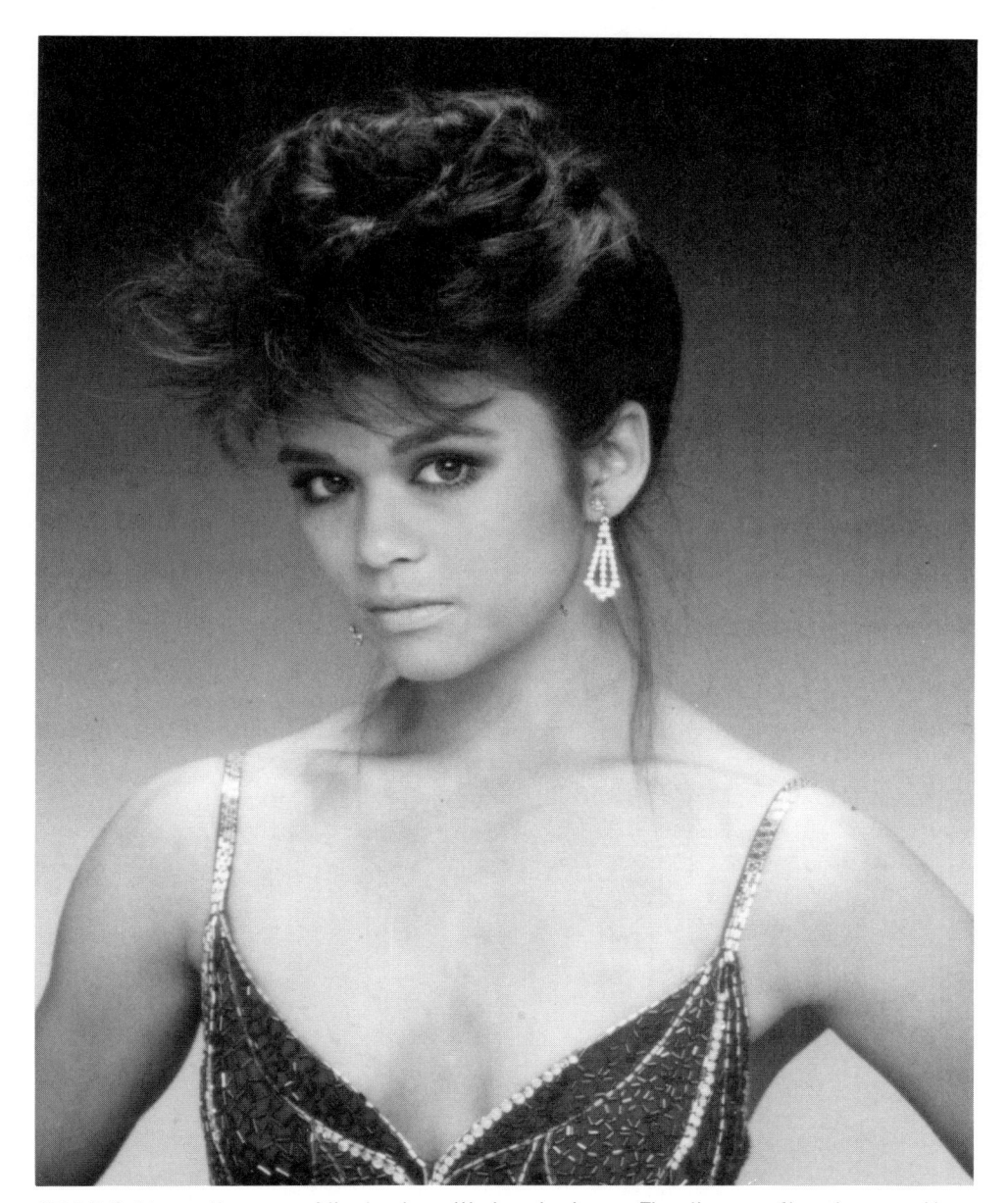

STYLE 2: I love the way Nia looks with her hair up. The lines soften her pretty face, and the controlled amount of hair is just perfect for her petite frame. Nia's hair is drawn into a twist in back, the crown and bangs swirled into soft waves. Beaded evening gown by Jeran Designs, Los Angeles.

TOVAR'S CLASSIC BEAUTY

EMMYLOU HARRIS

She was the first of my classic beauties to be photographed for this book, and is looking her best right now.

Emmylou's hair is very straight and baby fine: the kind of hair that needs lots of help—the right cut, a body wave, mousse, as many hair helpers as possible. When I first met Emmylou, she was wearing her hair just straight and long enough to be able to sit on it. It detracted from her looks instead of enhancing them.

I cut Emmylou's hair shoulder length and layered it all over to give it lots of movement and volume. But just cutting and layering were not enough. Emmylou needed lots of extra help to achieve the kind of full, pretty hairstyle she loves and which has become part of her glamorous image. I prescribed a body wave and highlights, which must be repeated as soon as they are growing out and the hair starts to become flat again.

Classic Beauties and Their Styles

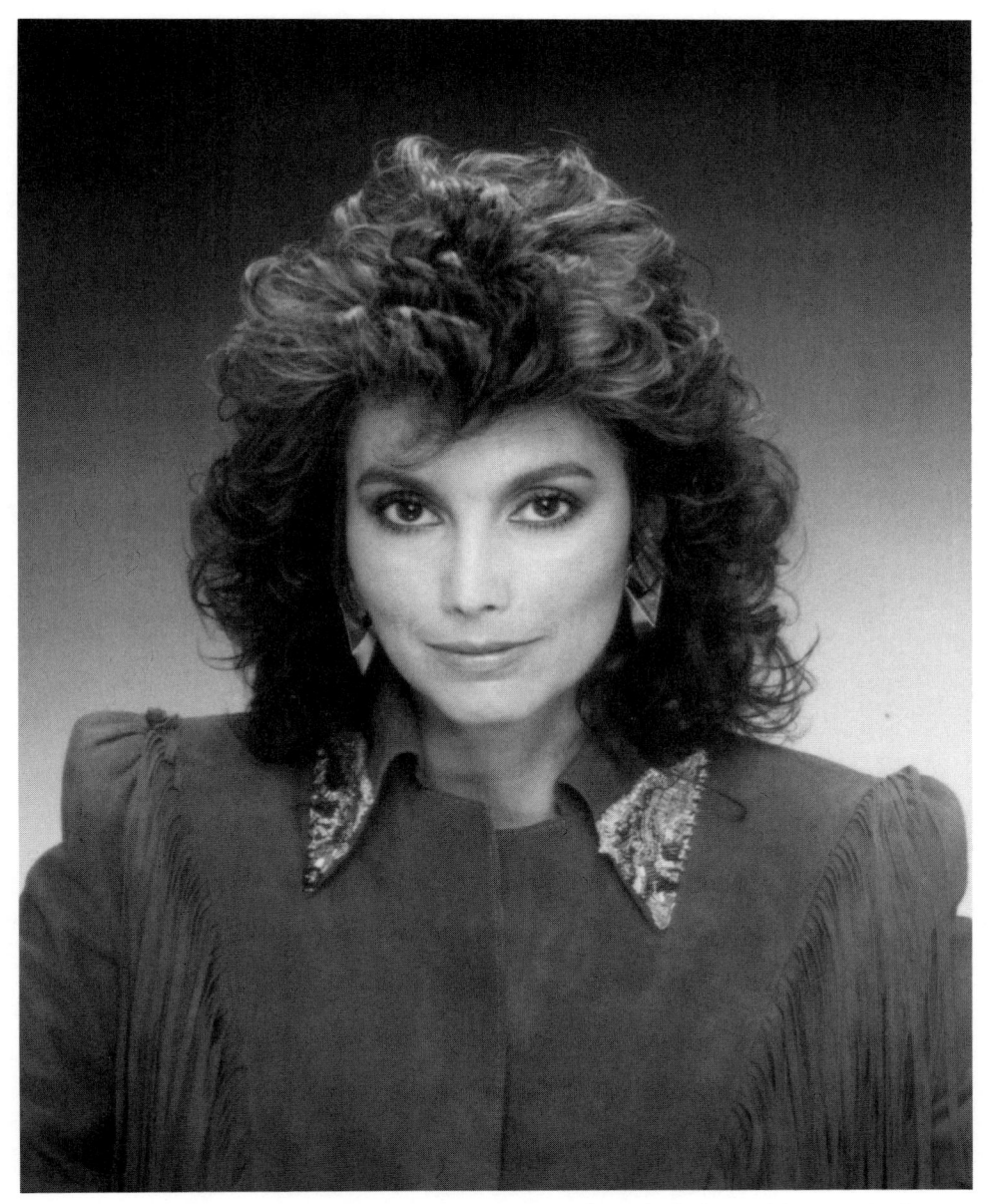

STYLE 1: Emmylou's "signature" look is very soft, very full, and layered all over. I set her hair on hot rollers to give it as much volume as possible, then blow it dry, fluffing the hair with a brush to make it look natural and not set. Soft, piecey bangs add softness around the face. Red suede jacket with beaded wing-tipped collar by Gossamer Wings.

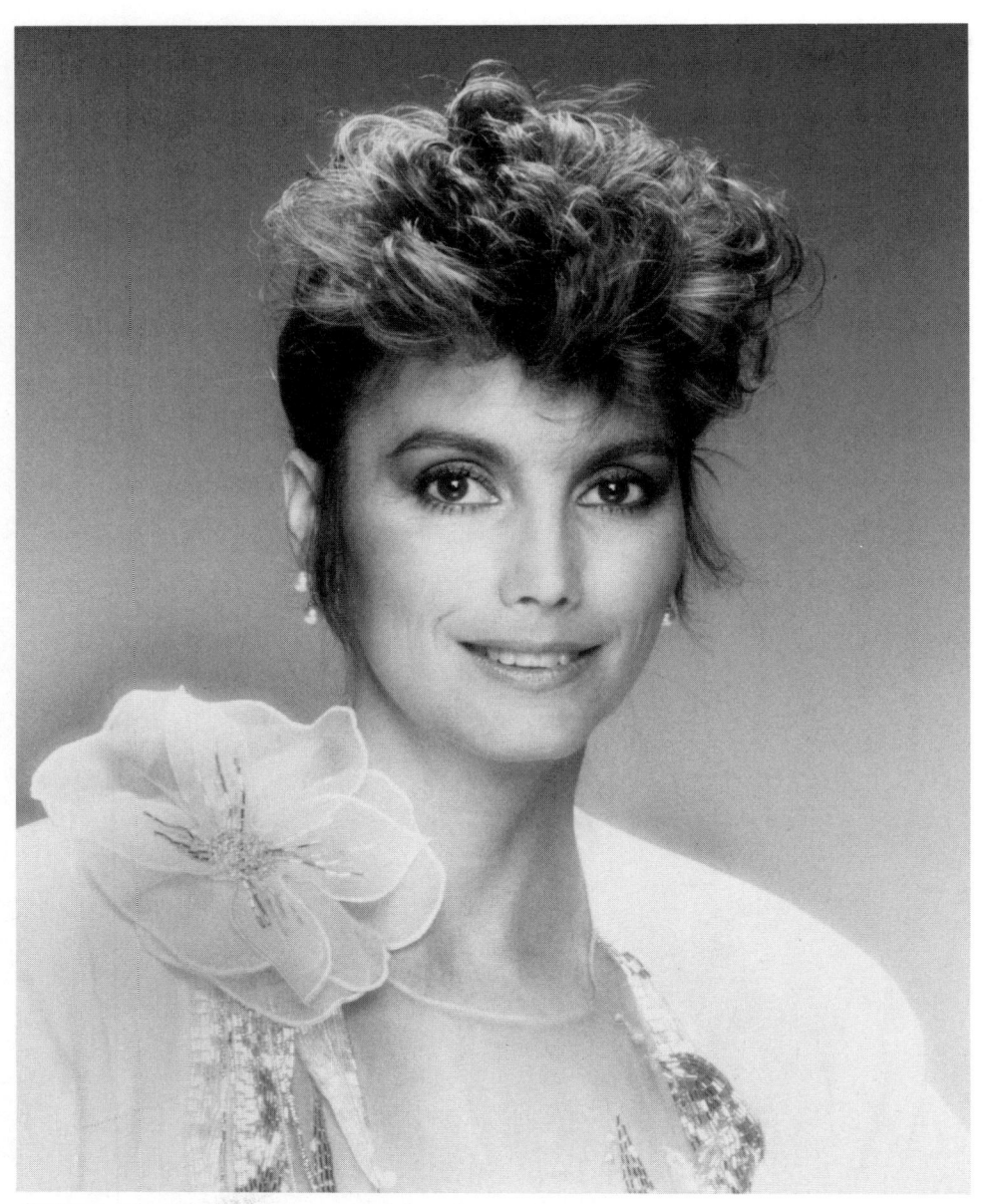

STYLE 2: The up-do with a very full, wavy, voluminous front is another of Emmylou's favorite hairstyles. This style is very soft and feminine, and it perfectly complements her romantic lady image. The back hair is folded into a french twist, the sides are slicked back, and very soft "sideburns" on each side add the finishing touches. White dress by Eletra Cassadei.

Classic Beauties and Their Styles

BROGAN LANE

She is another of my exotic beauties with a magnificent head of hair. Brogan's look is unusual and extraordinary. A top model, she soon will become Mrs. Dudley Moore.

Brogan's hair is full, naturally curly, and extremely good to work with. She has the kind of hair that can be tossed any which way and end up looking wonderfully tousled. She is a very exciting beauty who looks great in anything she wears.

TOVAR'S CLASSIC BEAUTY

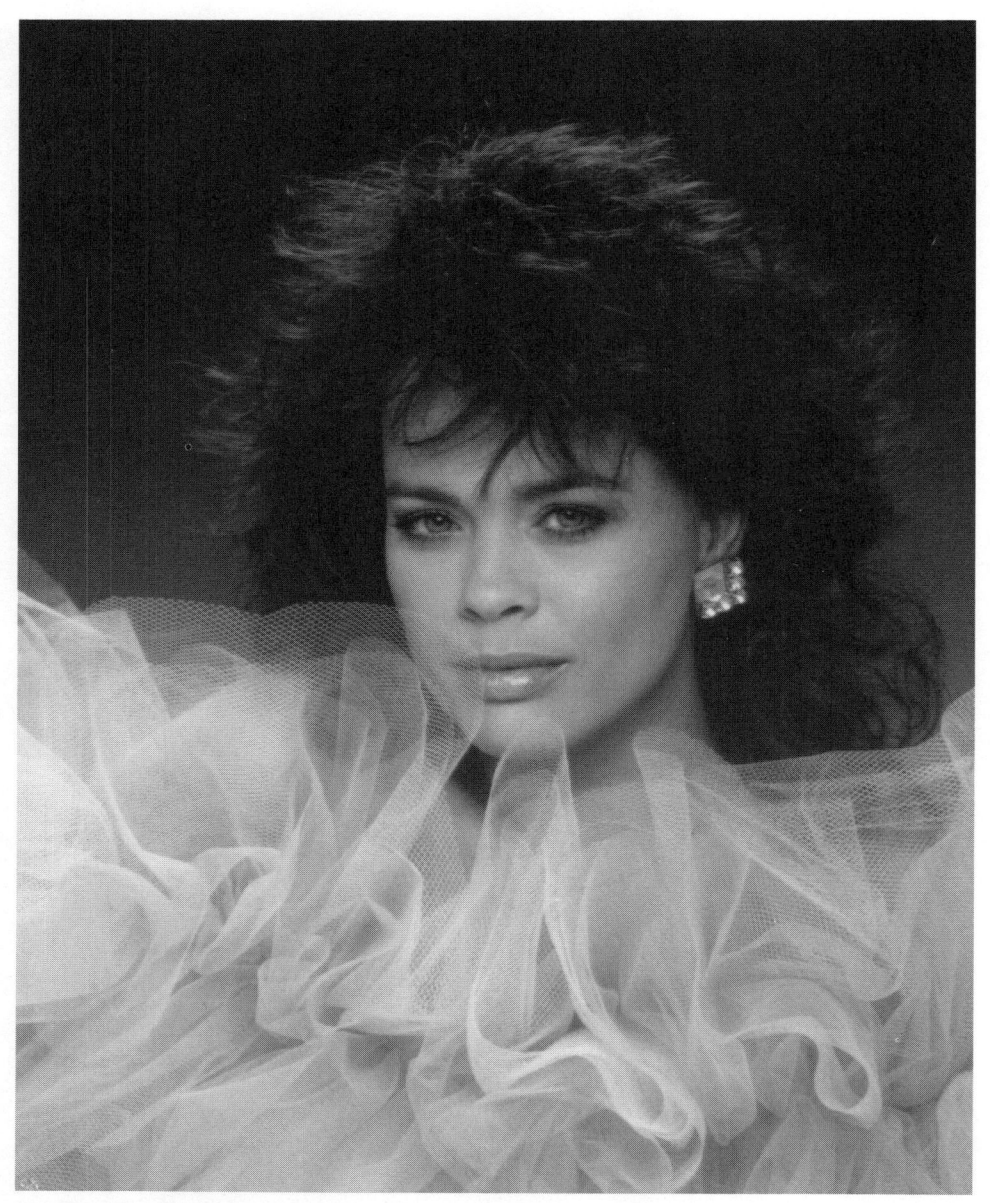

STYLE 1: The "pretty in pink" look—the hair is wildly tousled in a very exciting look. A fun look with hair that moves, bends, and kicks. It is very up and energetic. Not too many women can wear this look, but if you are the type that can, why not look magnificent? Dress by Mystica, Los Angeles.

Classic Beauties and Their Styles

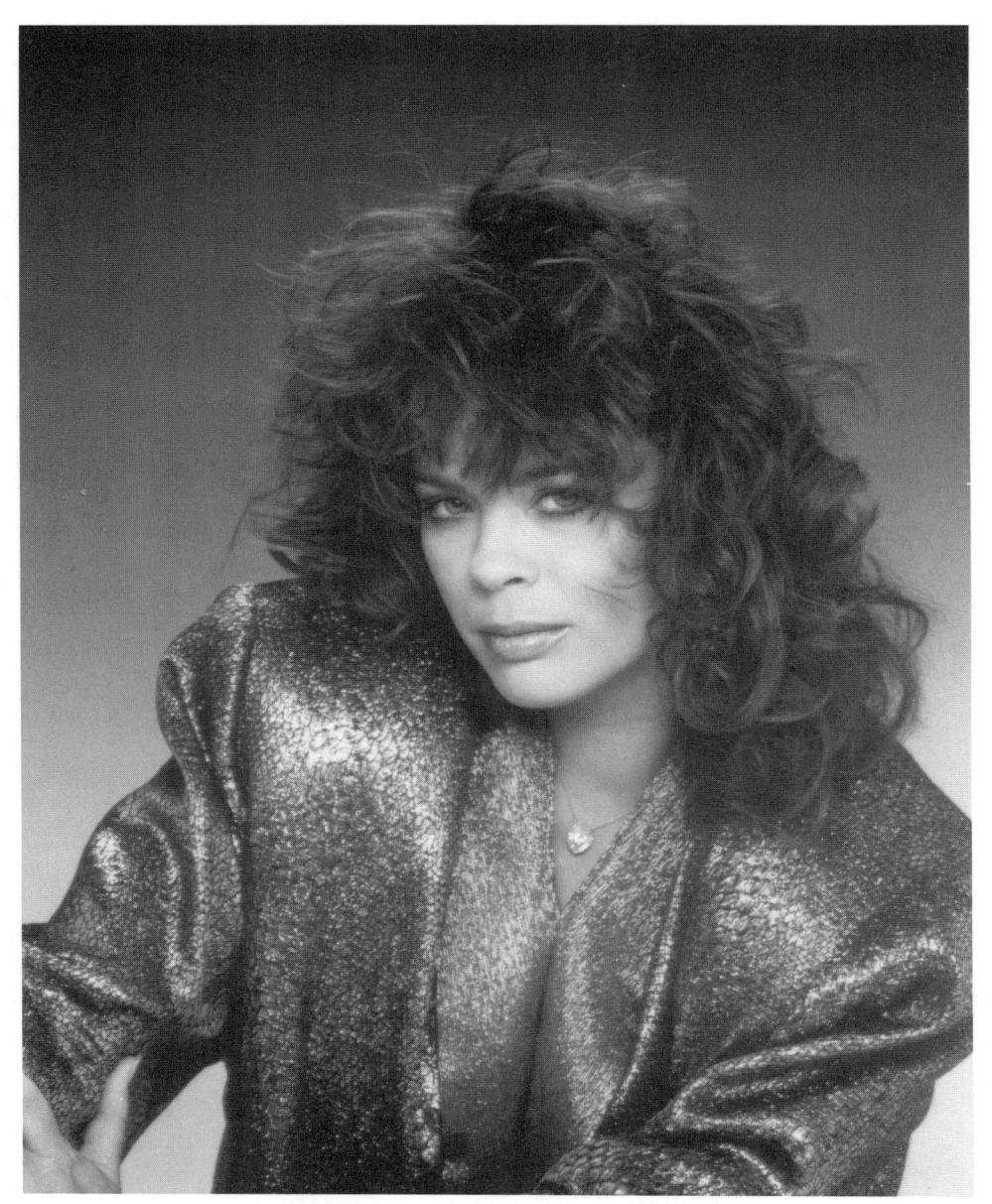

STYLE 2: A different look, still full of excitement and movement, but very light, very airy, with wispy bangs and the hair scrunched and tousled all over for lots of movement. Blue brocade jacket by Ellene Warren, Melrose Avenue, Los Angeles.

HEATHER LOCKLEAR

Blond and blue-eyed Heather is the all-American beauty and one of the celebrity cover girls in greatest demand today. Her face graces the covers of numerous national and international magazines. Heather is also the only TV actress who has the distinction of starring in two series at the same time—as the sizzling Sammy Jo Carrington in "Dynasty" and as good-girl policewoman Stacey Sheridan in "T. J. Hooker."

This very pretty girl has lots of healthy, medium-coarse blond hair, and she knows how to wear her hair very well. The length of her hair is perfect. It is very versatile since it can be worn up or down, although Heather prefers to wear her hair down and simple most of the time. Heather also likes to wear bangs to emphasize her pretty eyes.

Classic Beauties and Their Styles

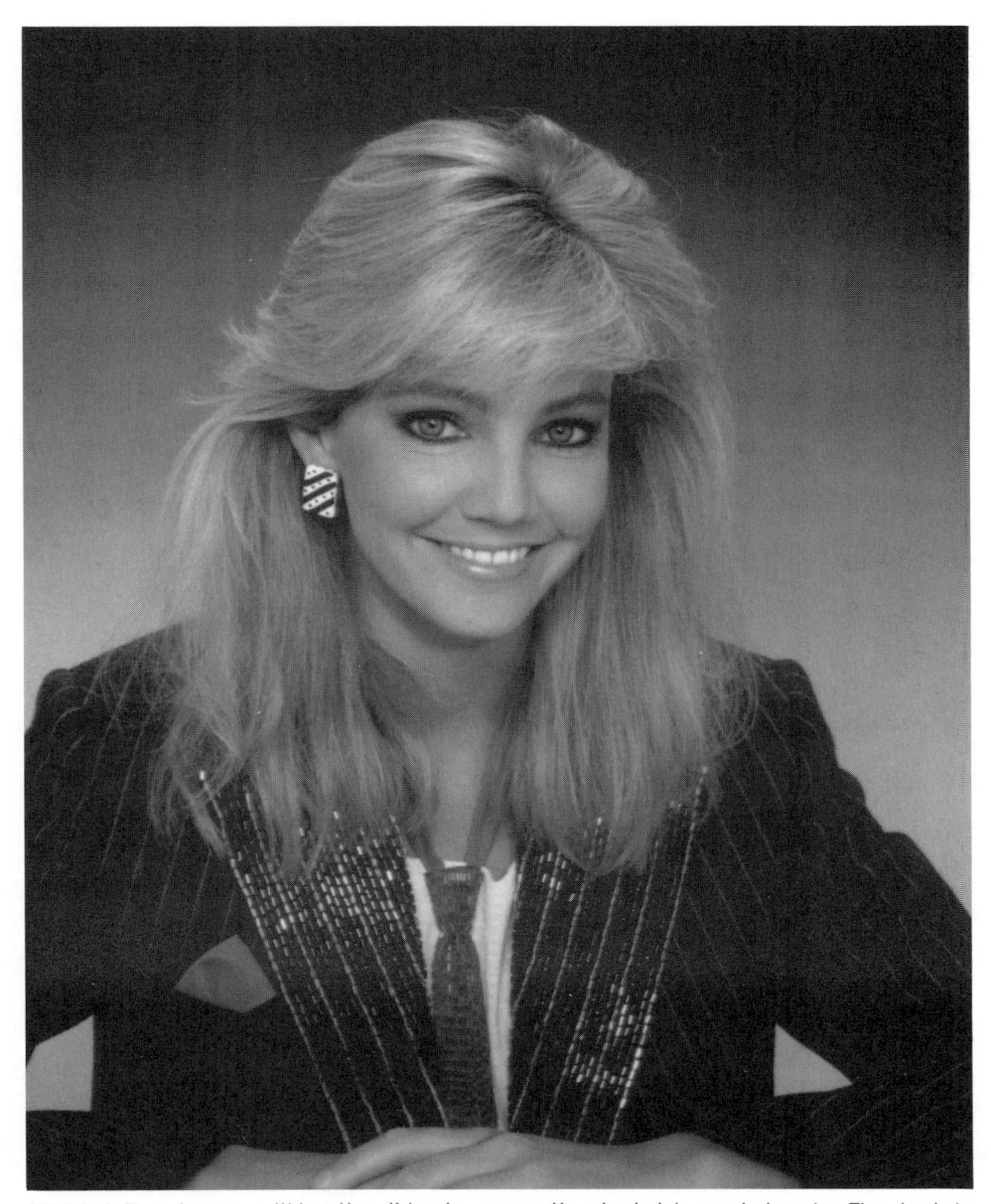

STYLE 1: The famous "Heather" look—smooth, straight, and simple. The hair is parted in a short part off the center, and full bangs are slightly side-swept for interest. Charcoal pinstripe "gangster" suit with beaded lapels and red beaded tie by Jeran Designs, Los Angeles.

TOVAR'S CLASSIC BEAUTY

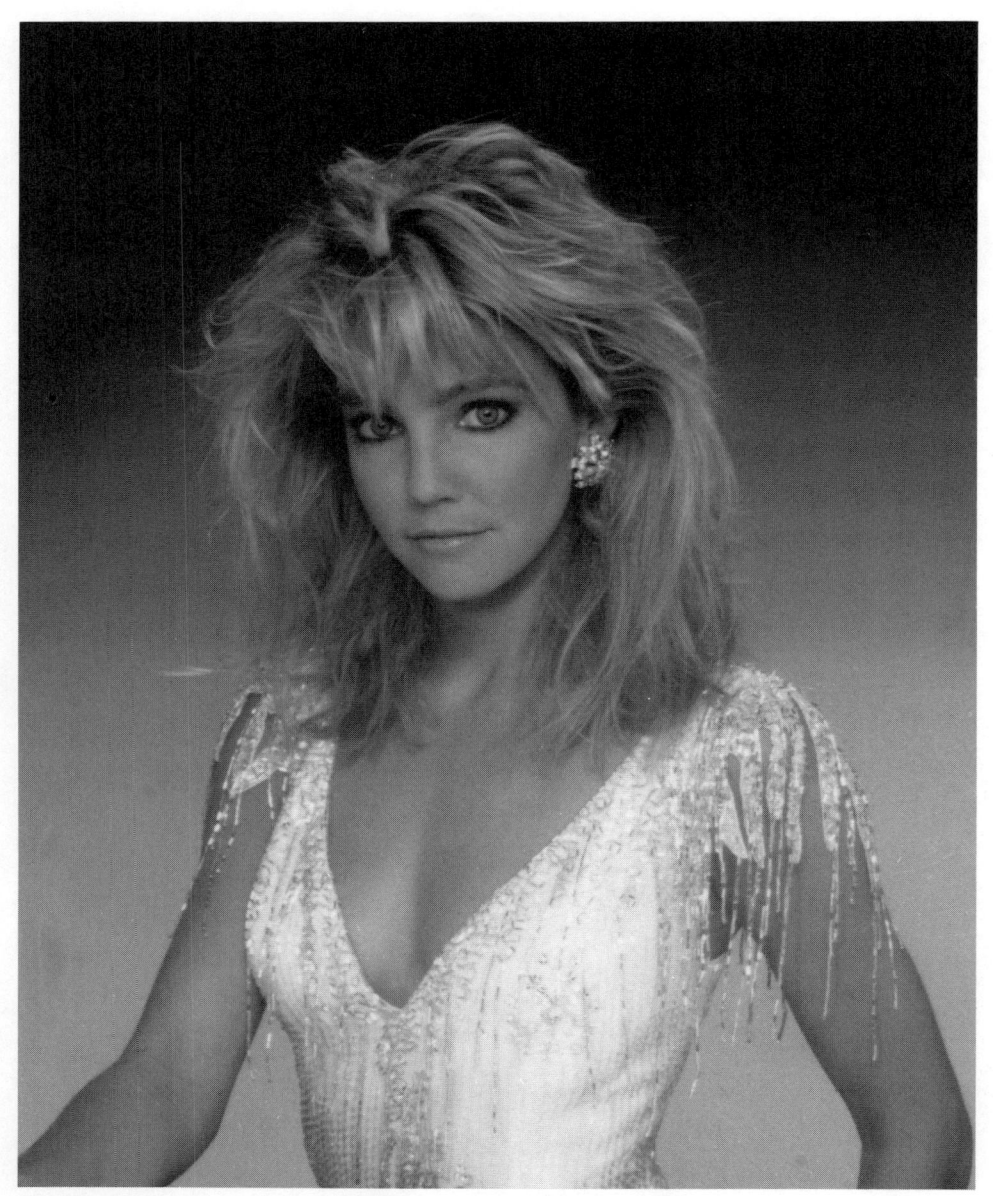

STYLE 2: My new look for Heather—I gave her hair lots of body and volume by rolling it in a twisted pin curl set (see Chapter 6). Then I blew it dry, scrunching the hair as it dried, finishing with a short upside-down blow-dry. The bangs are opened up for an airy softer look. White beaded dress by Jeran Designs, Los Angeles.

Classic Beauties and Their Styles

SEASON HUBLEY

Season is an extremely talented, multidimensional actress and a beautiful woman with very delicately chiseled features and very, very fine hair.

I keep Season's hair layered all over—shorter at the crown, with piecey bangs to balance her high forehead and long face. Season's hair lacks body, and I recommend a body perm and highlights to give her hair some added volume and fullness.

Season looks great with her hair up. The clean design lines of the up-do bring out her wonderful bone structure. When doing Season's hair up, I always give her fullness at the top to balance her facial structure.

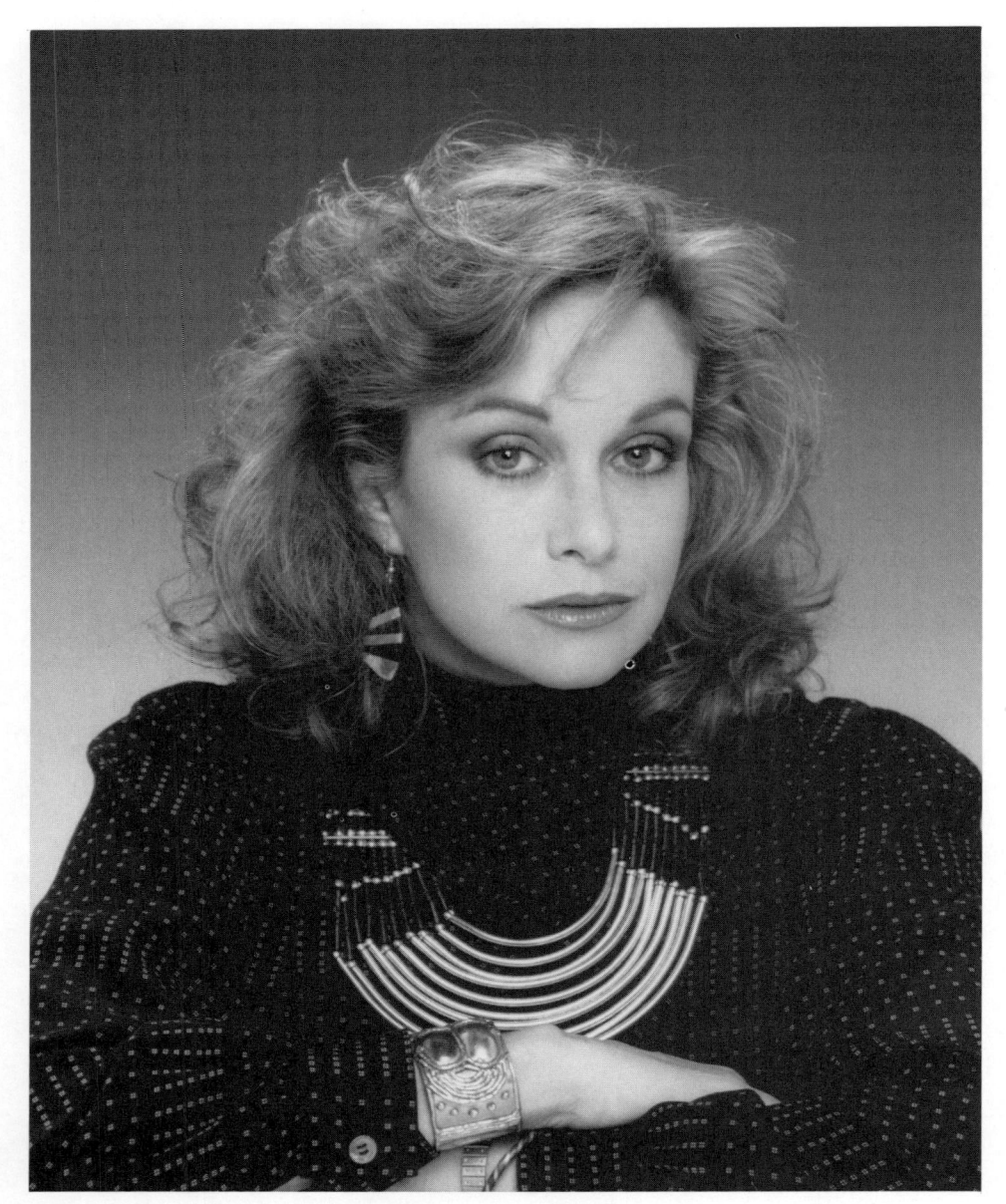

STYLE 1: Season's classic look—layered and full, with a smooth, slightly lifted crown and lots of volume at the sides to balance her long face. The wave dipping over each temple and piecey bangs work well to "hide" her wide forehead.

Classic Beauties and Their Styles

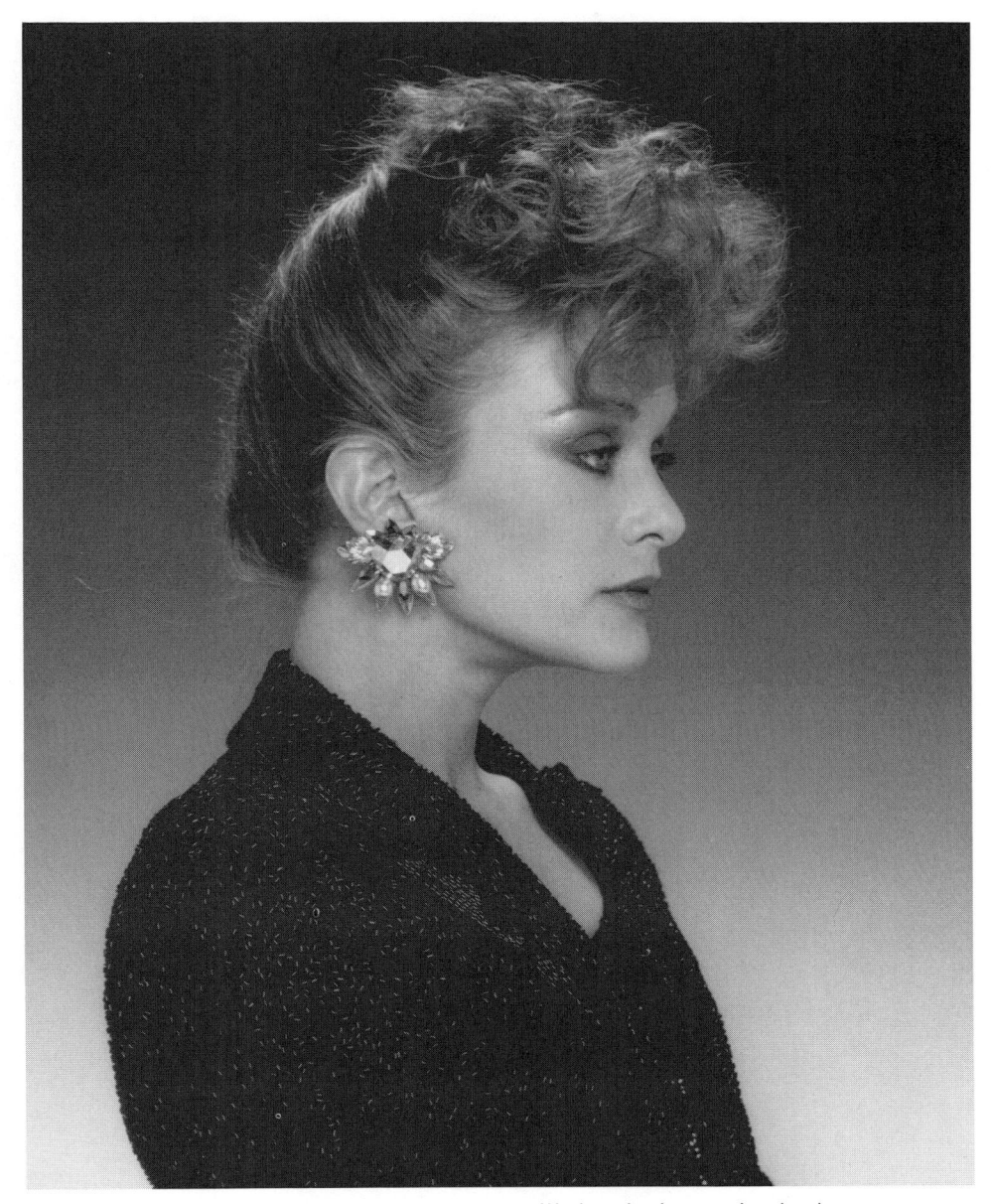

STYLE 2: I just love the way Season looks with her hair up; she looks younger and very elegant. All the hair is very slick and close to the scalp, then it literally bursts into a froth of curls over the crown, spilling forward toward the forehead. Earrings by Bobi Leonard.

CLAIRE YARLETT

Young Claire, only 21, is a flawless beauty—one of those women lucky enough to be blessed with beautiful hair and an incredible face and figure. She plays the younger Colby daughter, Bliss, in "Dynasty II: The Colbys."

   Claire has tons of natural blond, wavy, long hair with natural highlights. Her look is classic in the traditional sense. Claire's hair has incredible body, and she likes to wear it long. I cut it in long layers around the front and crown, so that it has as much movement and volume as possible. For styling versatility, I cut the type of chunky, piecey bangs that can be brought forward or blended back into the rest of the hair.

Classic Beauties and Their Styles

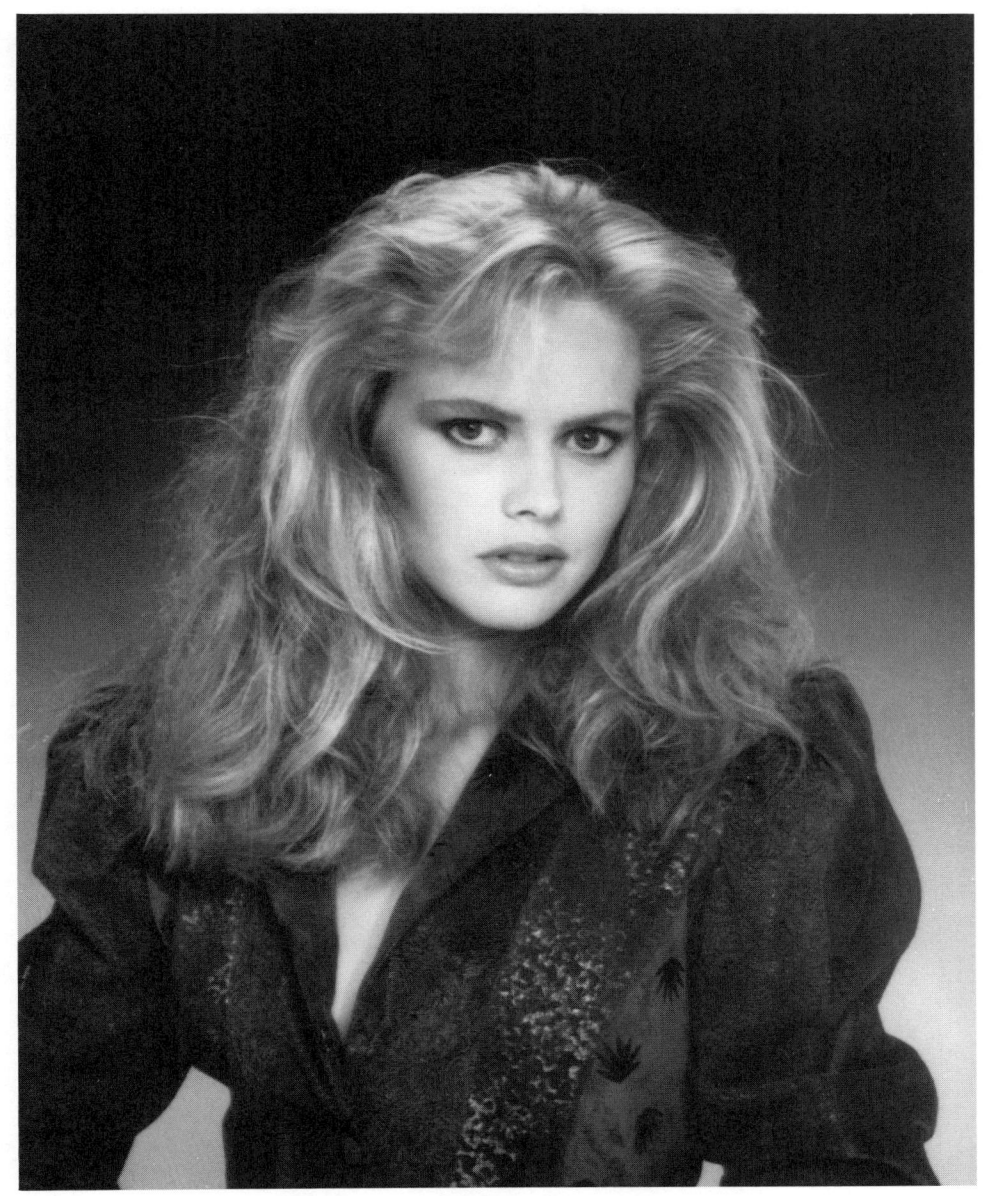

STYLE 1: A style that shows off all the wonderful qualities of Claire's natural hair. This style is so simple that I created it mostly with my fingers. I opened the sides and added a touch of spray to hold the shape and width. Suede dress by Gossamer Wings.

TOVAR'S CLASSIC BEAUTY

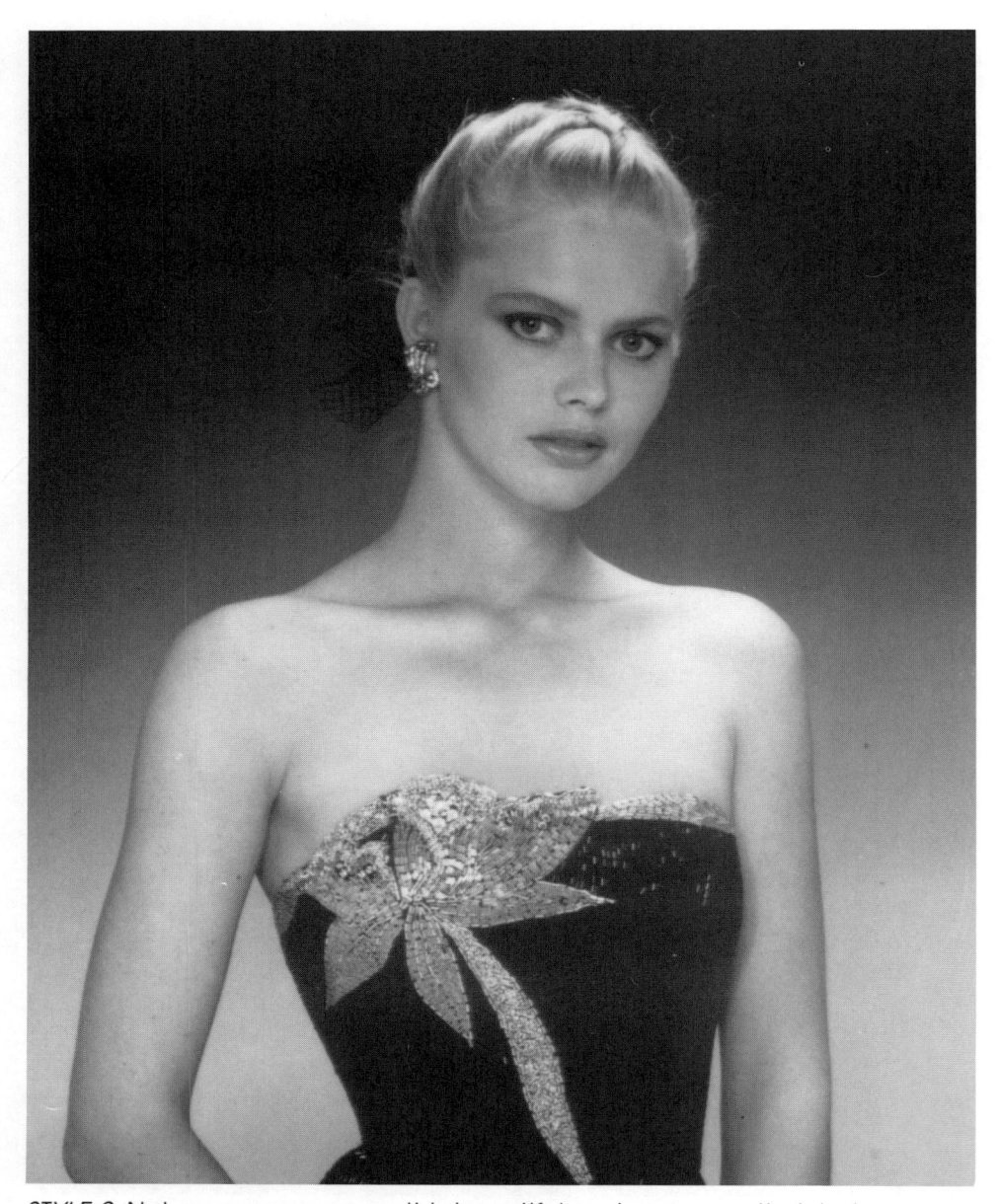

STYLE 2: Not many women are this beautiful and can wear their hair completely baring the face. I braided Claire's hair starting at the crown, arranging the braid like a chignon in back. For softness, I added an airy net hair ornament at the nape. Black and silver beaded dress by Jeran Designs, Los Angeles.

Classic Beauties and Their Styles

JAYNE KENNEDY OVERTON

The American public recently selected Jayne as the most admired black American woman. Jayne combines her acting career with sports commentary and with running her own production company.

Jayne has the type of thick, coarse hair that is easy to handle. She is one of those women who knows instinctively what looks good on her, and that is why she always wears her hair long and loose. She knows how to use that hair to bring out her marvelous bone structure.

Long hair is perfect for Jayne. She is a very tall lady and needs all that hair to balance her body proportions. I layered her hair—long hair that graduates from chin length to about four inches below the shoulders—to avoid a very bulky look and give the hair movement. Jayne collects unusual hair ornaments, and she likes to add them to her hairstyle for festive occasions. Jayne is the perfect example of a woman who knows how to use her hair as a wonderful beauty accessory.

TOVAR'S CLASSIC BEAUTY

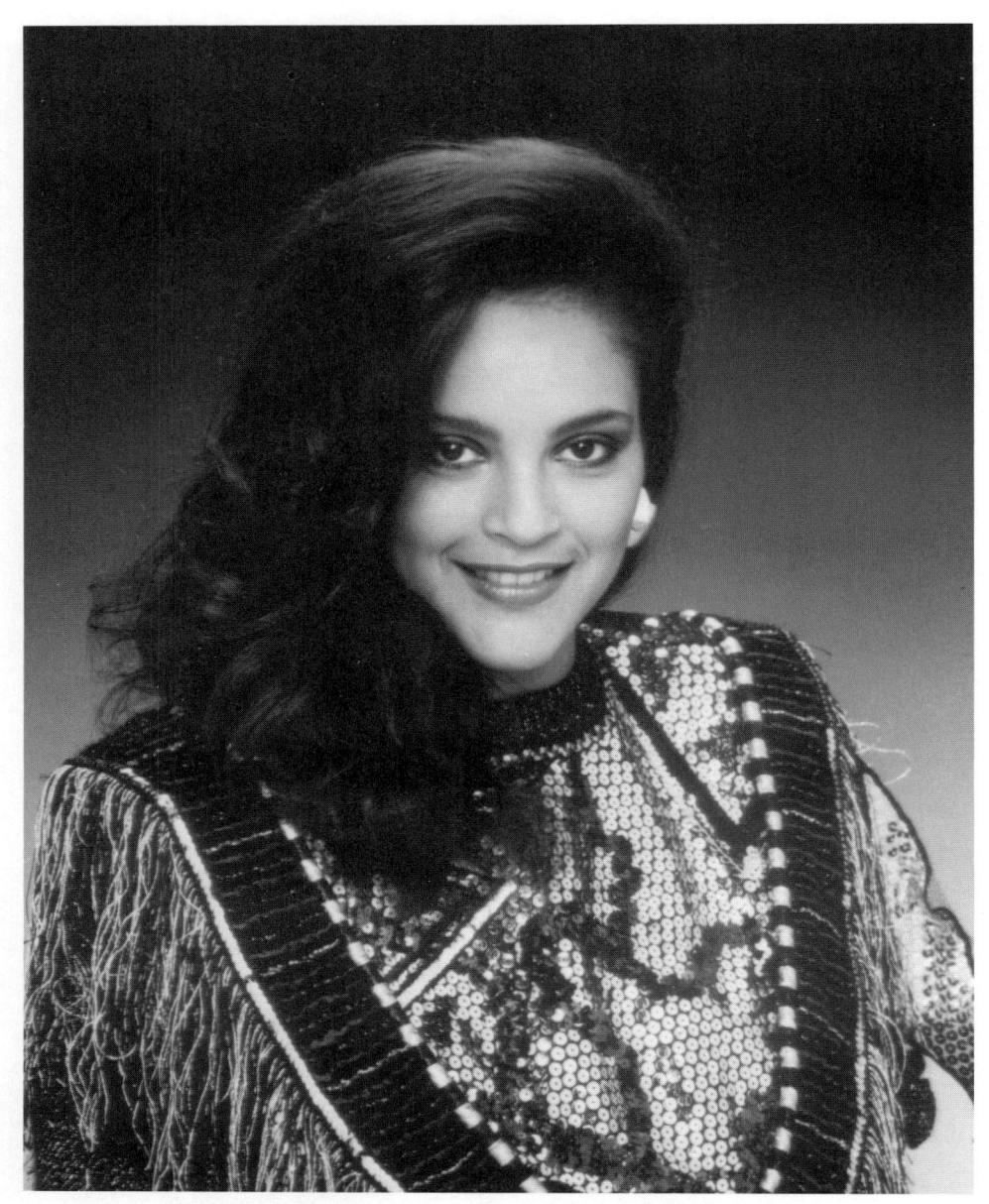

STYLE 1: Jayne wears her fabulous mane swept over one side and in a loose cascade of soft waves. A very natural, lovely, and classic look to bring out that wonderful face. Outfit by Margi Kent, Melrose Avenue, Los Angeles. Earrings by Bobi Leonard.

Classic Beauties and Their Styles

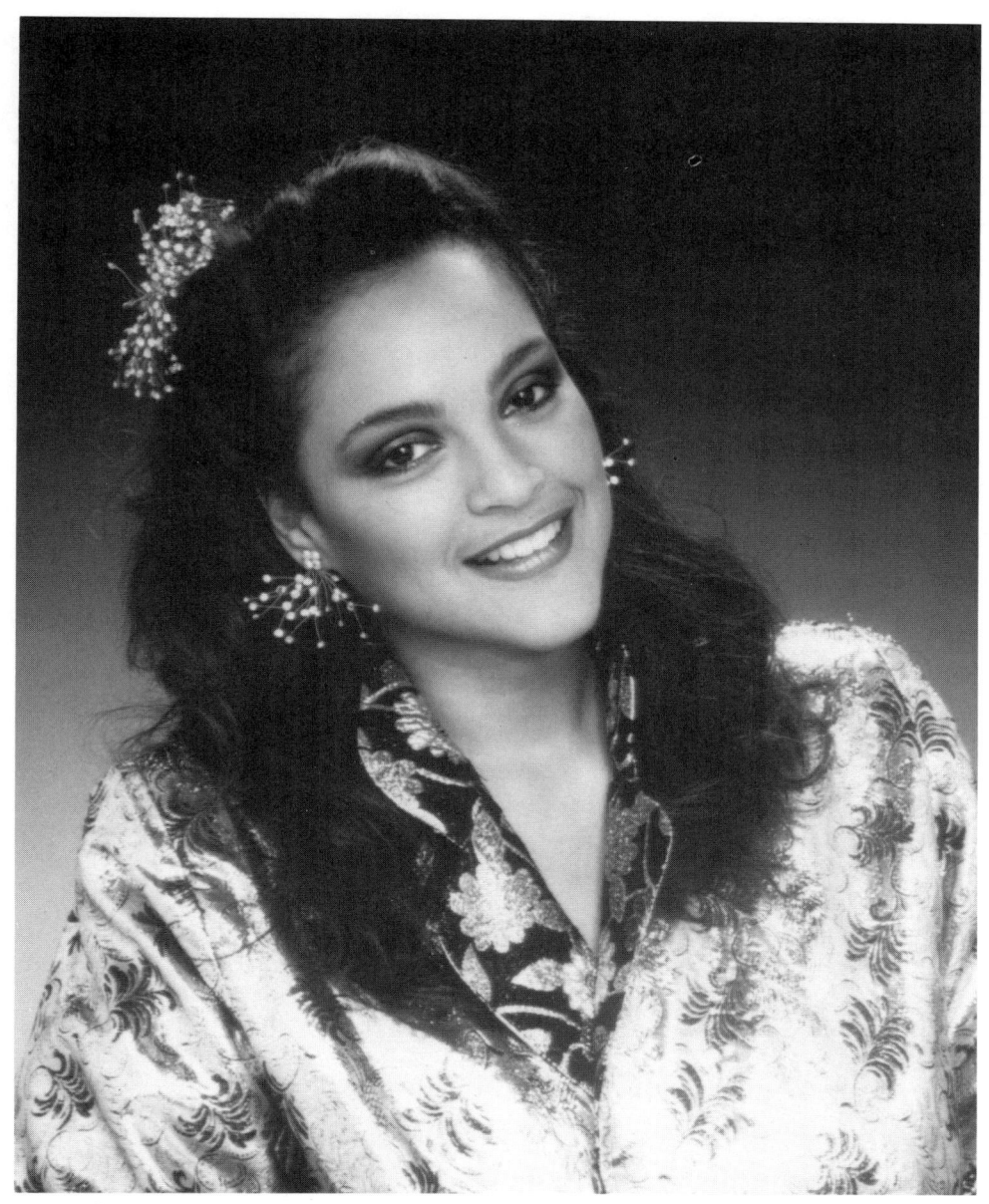

STYLE 2: Another style that underlines Jayne's preference for simplicity and elegance. I pulled the front and crown hair up and twisted it into a tiny knot off center in back. This is a great way to wear hair to show off a fabulous face. The rest of the hair is just brushed naturally in soft waves. Some delicate hair ornaments dress up the style. Black and gold lamé jacket by Margi Kent, Melrose Avenue, Los Angeles.

ABBY DALTON

Abby is one of those great-looking over-40 actresses who have achieved celebrity status in the 1980s. She is an incredibly good-looking woman with true star quality. Abby plays Julia Cumson on "Falcon Crest."

Abby shows how youthful the right hairstyle can be. I cut her hair very short, tapered in back, with lots of volume at the top. Besides taking years off, her hairstyle is also very easy to maintain. This is important for Abby, who works out at a gym about two and a half hours a day.

Like many blonds, Abby's hair is fine, but she has lots of it and it is easy to work with. When Abby wants extra fullness at the top, she can curl the crown hair with a curling iron, tease it a little bit, and add some spray for body. Abby wears her hair off the face most of the time to show off her wonderful bone structure.

Classic Beauties and Their Styles

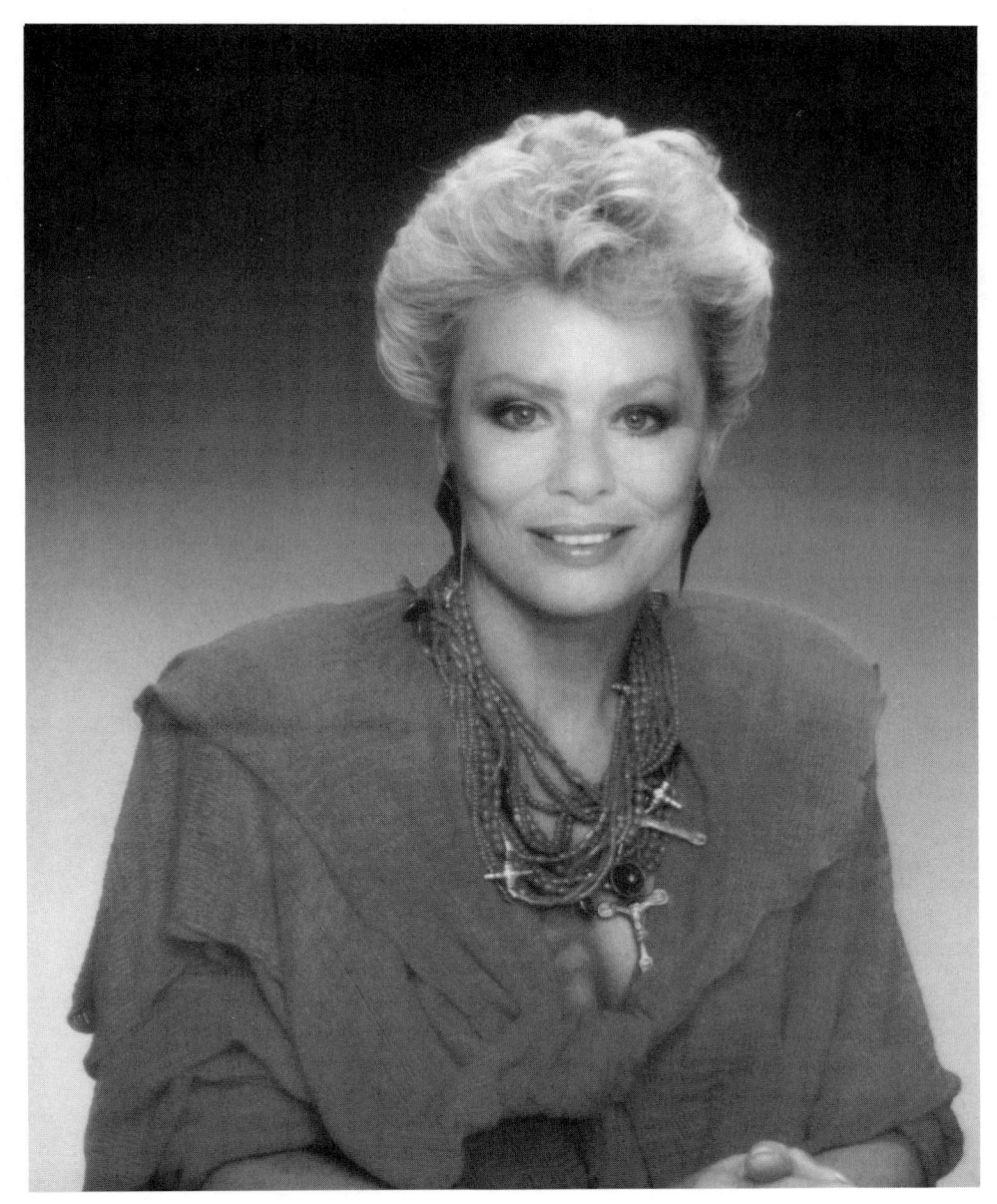

STYLE 1: Abby knows how to wear her hair to show off her great face. Here, I just curled the side and crown hair with the iron and brushed it back. One playful strand curls forward over the forehead. Outfit by Margi Kent, Melrose Avenue, Los Angeles.

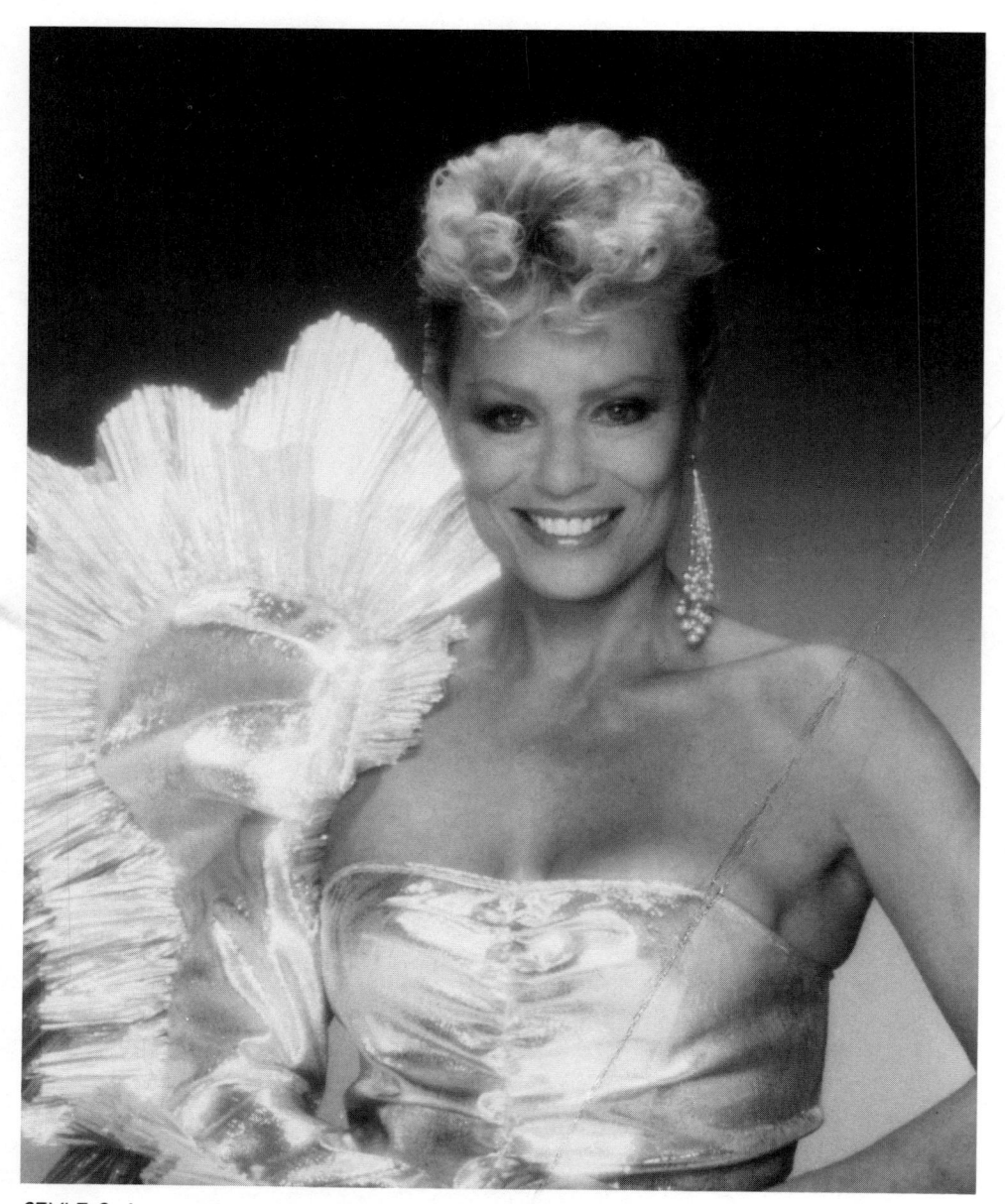

STYLE 2: A very severe, dramatic style to go with the very dramatic silver dress. I slicked the sides back with gel; curled the top in soft, loopy waves, and added a little height. The hair is brought slightly forward toward the forehead in what I call my "rockabilly" pompadour. Dress by Margi Kent, Melrose Avenue, Los Angeles.

Classic Beauties and Their Styles

MELODY ANDERSON

Her versatile looks and acting ability have won her a number of different roles. Melody has been described as a chameleon on the screen. Her most recent role was as Claudia, the "whore with a heart of gold" in the TV movie *Beverly Hills Madam.*

   Melody has masses of curly blond hair worn in a layered bob. She has the type of hair that you must be careful with layering, because if it is layered too much it can look wild. I left Melody's hair in long layers and added bangs that can be brushed back (as I did for the photographs here).

   She has a great face that lets her wear her hair severely slicked back, as in the braided up-do shown here.

TOVAR'S CLASSIC BEAUTY

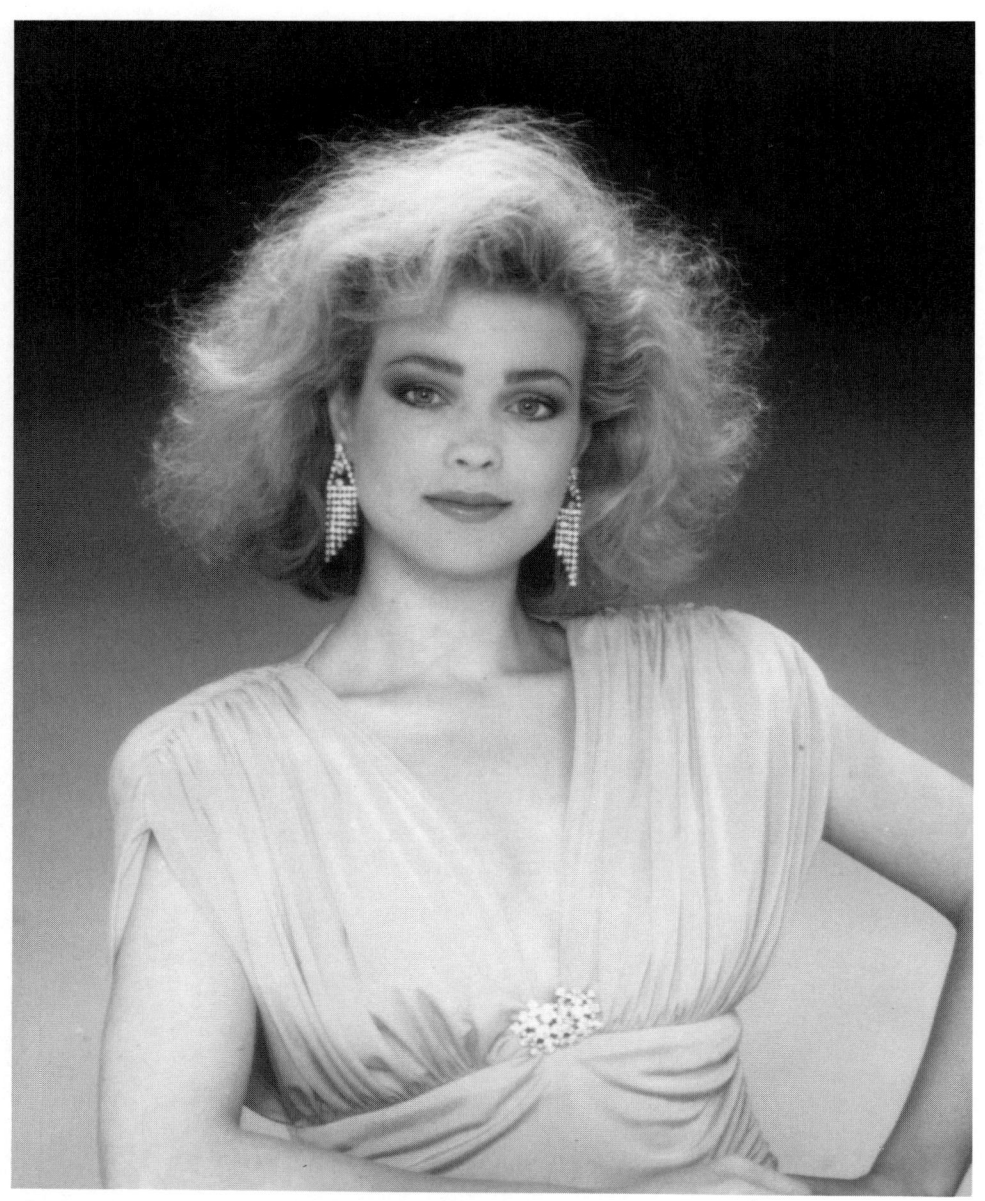

STYLE 1: Melody's coarse, curly hair is blown for lots of airy fullness and brushed back to show off her wonderful face. Dress by Eletra Cassadei. Jewelry by Jeran Designs, Los Angeles.

Classic Beauties and Their Styles

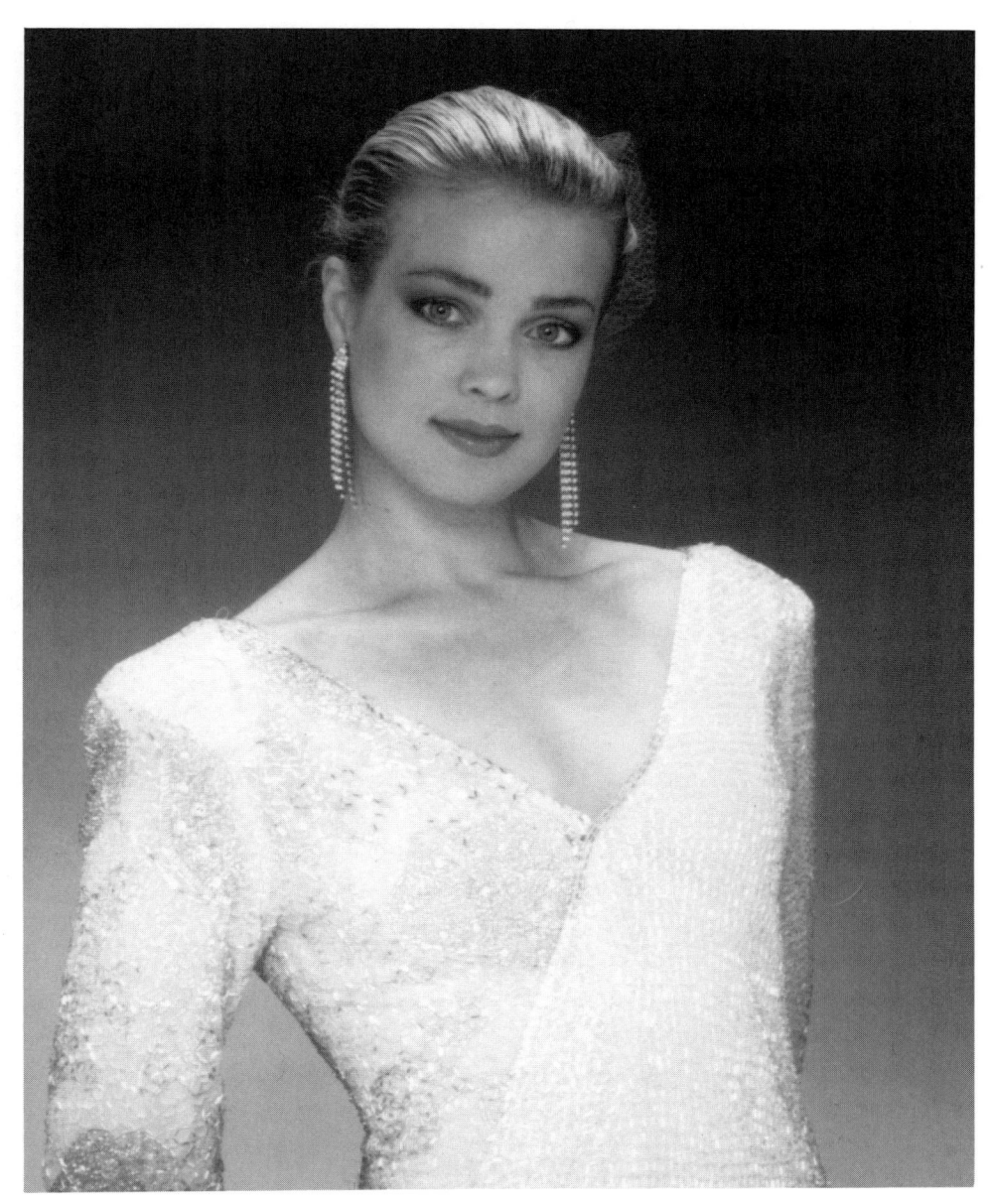

STYLE 2: A totally different look—all the hair is severely slicked back and braided from crown to nape. To break the severe lines, I added a frily net ornament at off-center back. When adding an ornament to severe styles such as this, always place it off center—from mid-back (as this one is placed) to low at the nape. Dress by Jeran Designs, Los Angeles.

DEBORAH MULLOWNEY

This self-described "Irish girl" is a native Californian with sultry, dark good looks and a full head of rich brown hair. A former model, Deborah plays Sloane Denning Clegg in the CBS daytime soap "Capitol."

I recently cut Debbie's hair in this versatile, chin-length, layered bob that gives the illusion of a one-length cut. Very fine, shimmering golden highlights were added to give some dimension to the style. Debbie's hair is full and thick, and she can wear it blown dry smooth and sleek or scrunched for a wild, very full look. Debbie's forehead is very high, and she should always wear bangs. I cut her bangs long enough to give them styling versatility, as shown in the two photographs here.

Classic Beauties and Their Styles

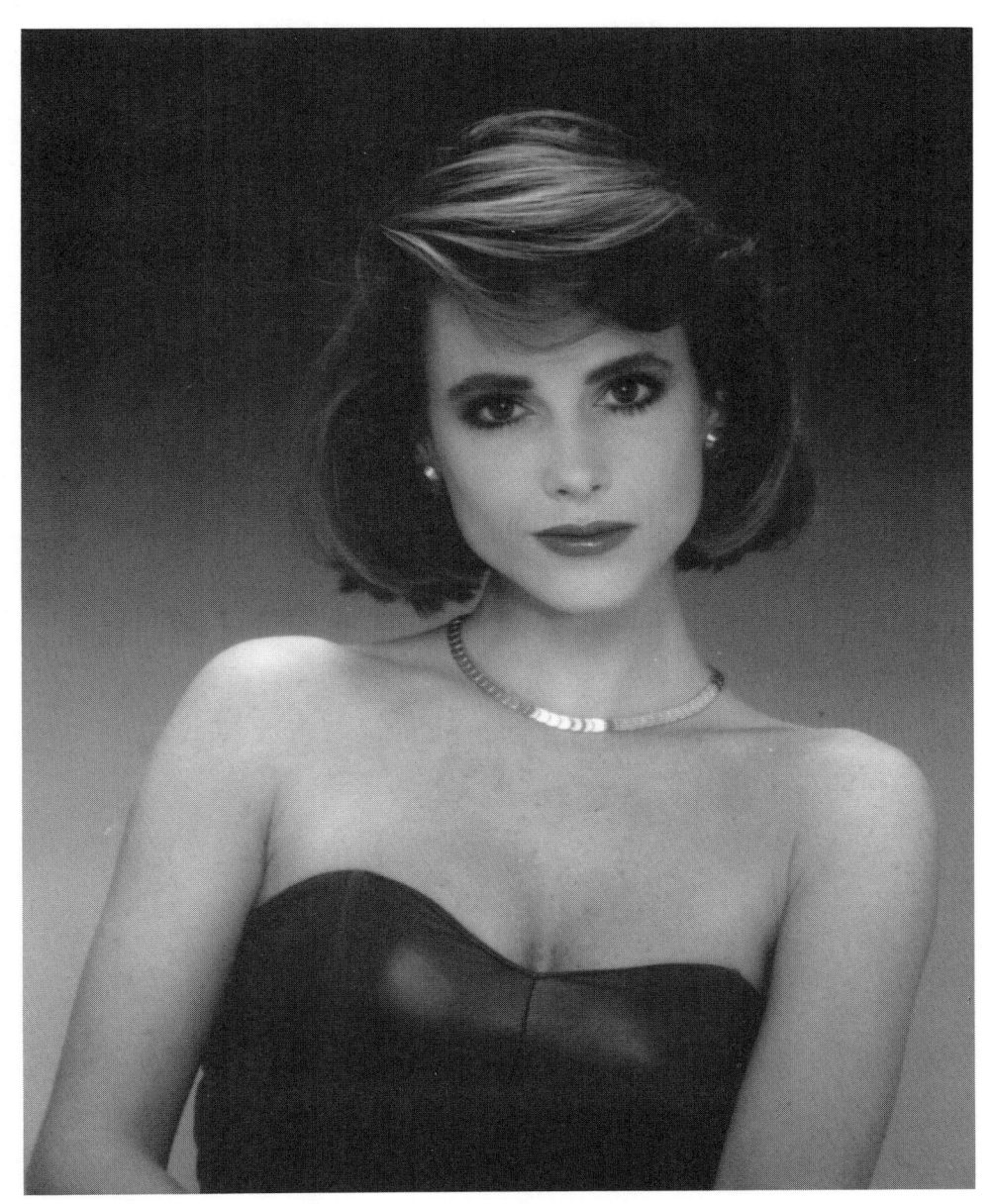

STYLE 1: Debbie's hair is blown dry in a very smooth and sleek side-swept style. Very light, airy bangs sweep across the forehead to add softness to her face. Jewelry by Nova Stylings, Inc.

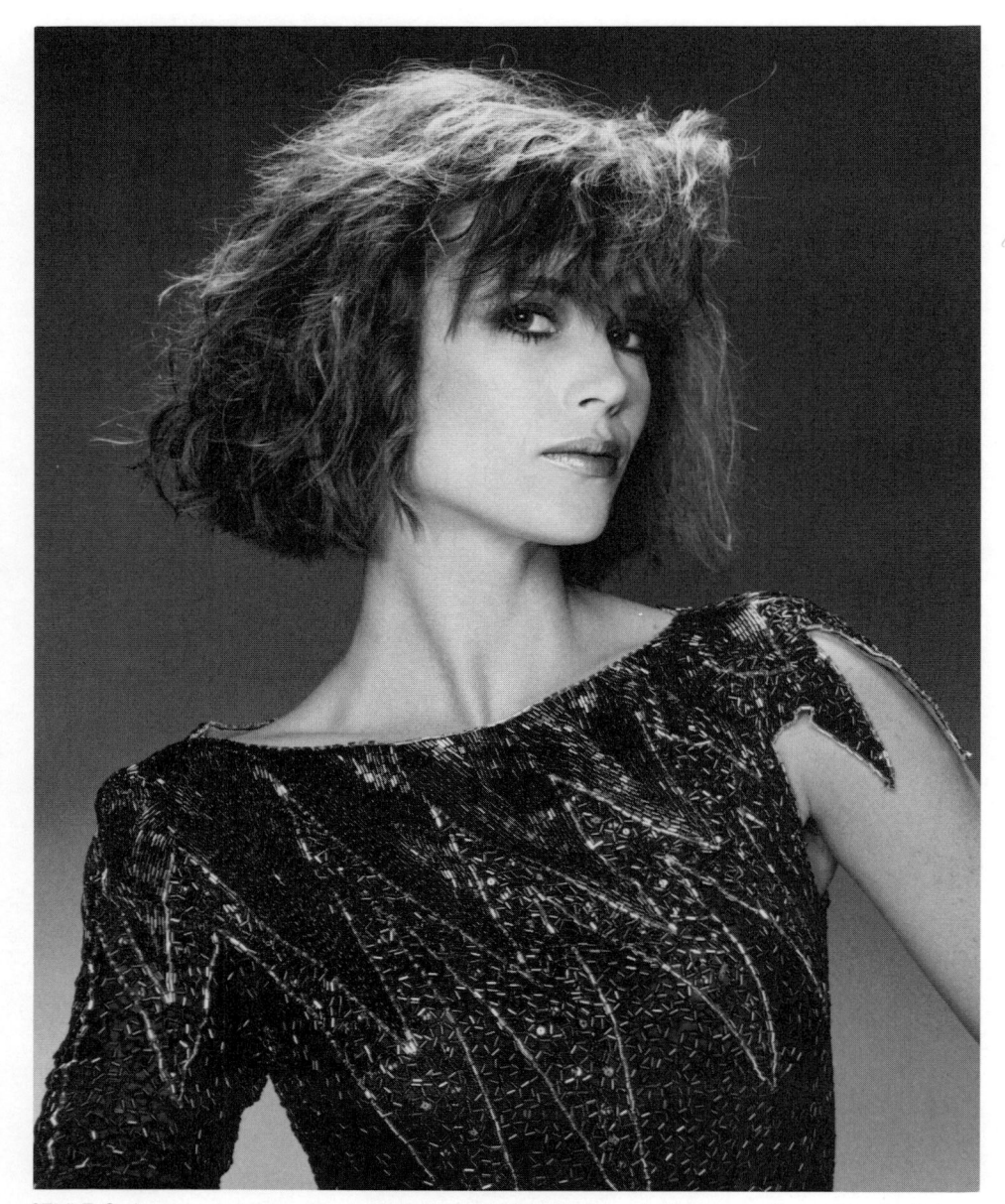

STYLE 2: A more dramatic look gives Debbie a real change. To achieve this fullness I scrunch the hair with mousse while using a blow dryer. The carefree tousled look is done with the fingers, combing the fingers through the strands of hair and adding hair spray for hold. Gown by Jeran Designs, Los Angeles.

Classic Beauties and Their Styles

ROSALIND CHAO

Pretty Rosalind has that classic "China doll" look with straight, almost blue-black hair, cut blunt with wispy bangs.

TV viewers remember her as Klinger's wife Soon Lee in "After M*A*S*H." Now Rosalind appears in a recurring role in "Falcon Crest" as Li Ying, the seismographer daughter of the Chinese butler who gets romantically involved with Lance (Lorenzo Lamas) and Cole (William R. Moses).

Rosalind has typical Oriental hair, very coarse and straight. This is the type of hair that must be blunt-cut, but I add piecey bangs that are wispy and airy, not too full.

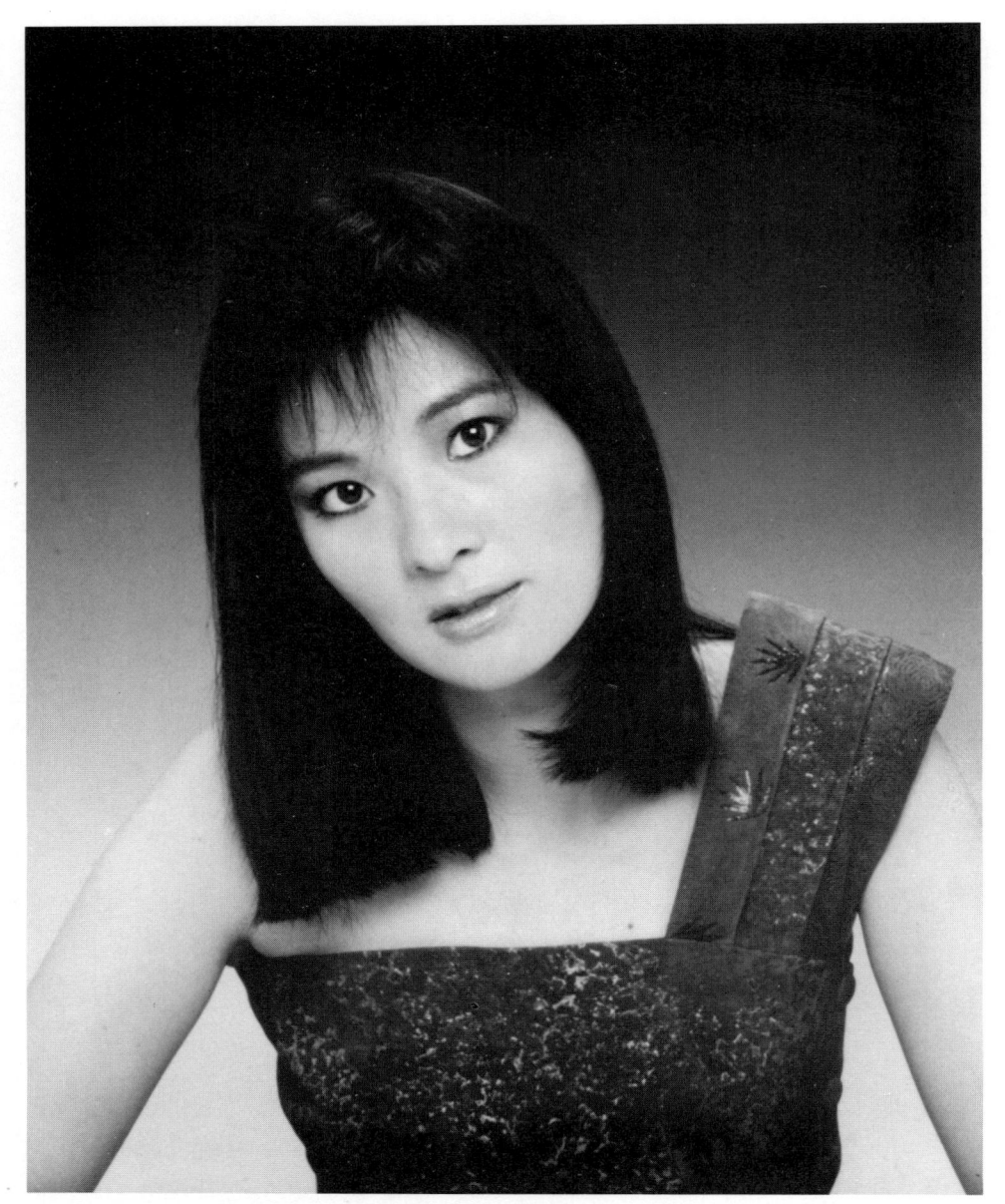

STYLE 1: Rosalind wears her hair in its natural state, the classic bob with wispy bangs. A style like this looks best with hair that is in magnificent condition, shiny and very full. One-shoulder suede top by Gossamer Wings.

Classic Beauties and Their Styles

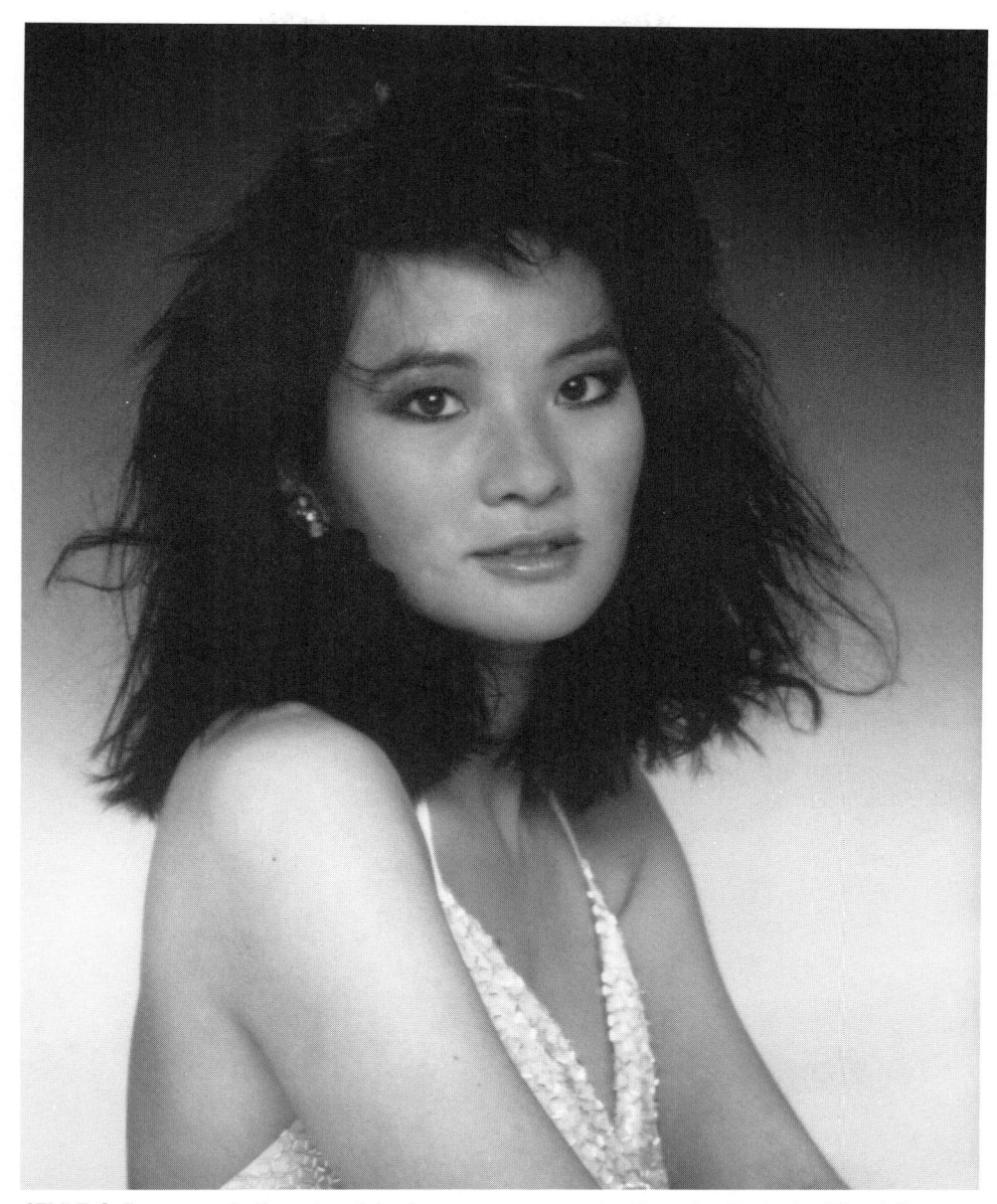

STYLE 2: For a variation, I added some mousse to Rosalind's hair, tilted the head upside down, and scrunched it vigorously to achieve this very full, wild look. Then I side-swept the piecey bangs to add some movement to the style. Beaded gown by Jeran Designs, Los Angeles.

PRISCILLA BARNES

Priscilla loves the very straight, sleek look because that is the way her natural hair is. She's learned this by trial and error: like anyone with straight hair, she once wanted curls and got a perm that was awful. According to Priscilla, she was very happy when that perm finally grew out.

A TV and feature films actress, she is best known for her role as nurse Terri Aulden in "Three Is Company." At the moment, Priscilla is studying, writing, and developing her own projects.

Priscilla is fanatical about her hair color. She has silvery golden highlights woven into her hair by Francois Noel at my salon, and when she is traveling, she has Francois flown to wherever she is, as her color must be done every two weeks. She prefers straight hair because she likes a look that frames rather than overpowers her face. Her beautiful face and wonderful bone structure look best with a subtle framing. Nothing wild for her.

Classic Beauties and Their Styles

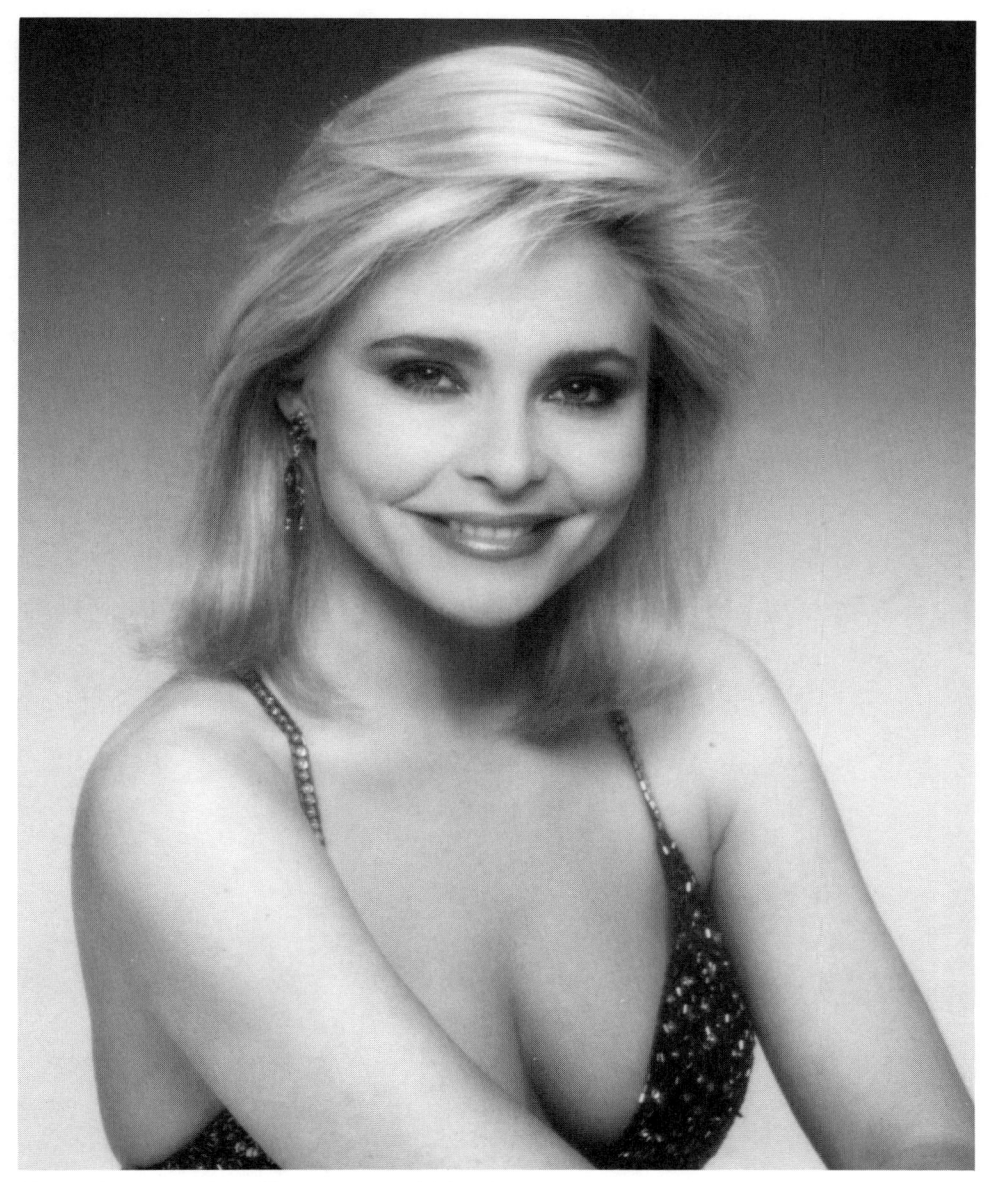

STYLE 1: I gave Priscilla a layered blunt cut to make her baby-fine, almost flyaway hair fall neatly into place. If the hair was not layered, it would lie too flat against her head. Here, the hair is lightly blown out for some softness. Dress by Jeran Designs, Los Angeles.

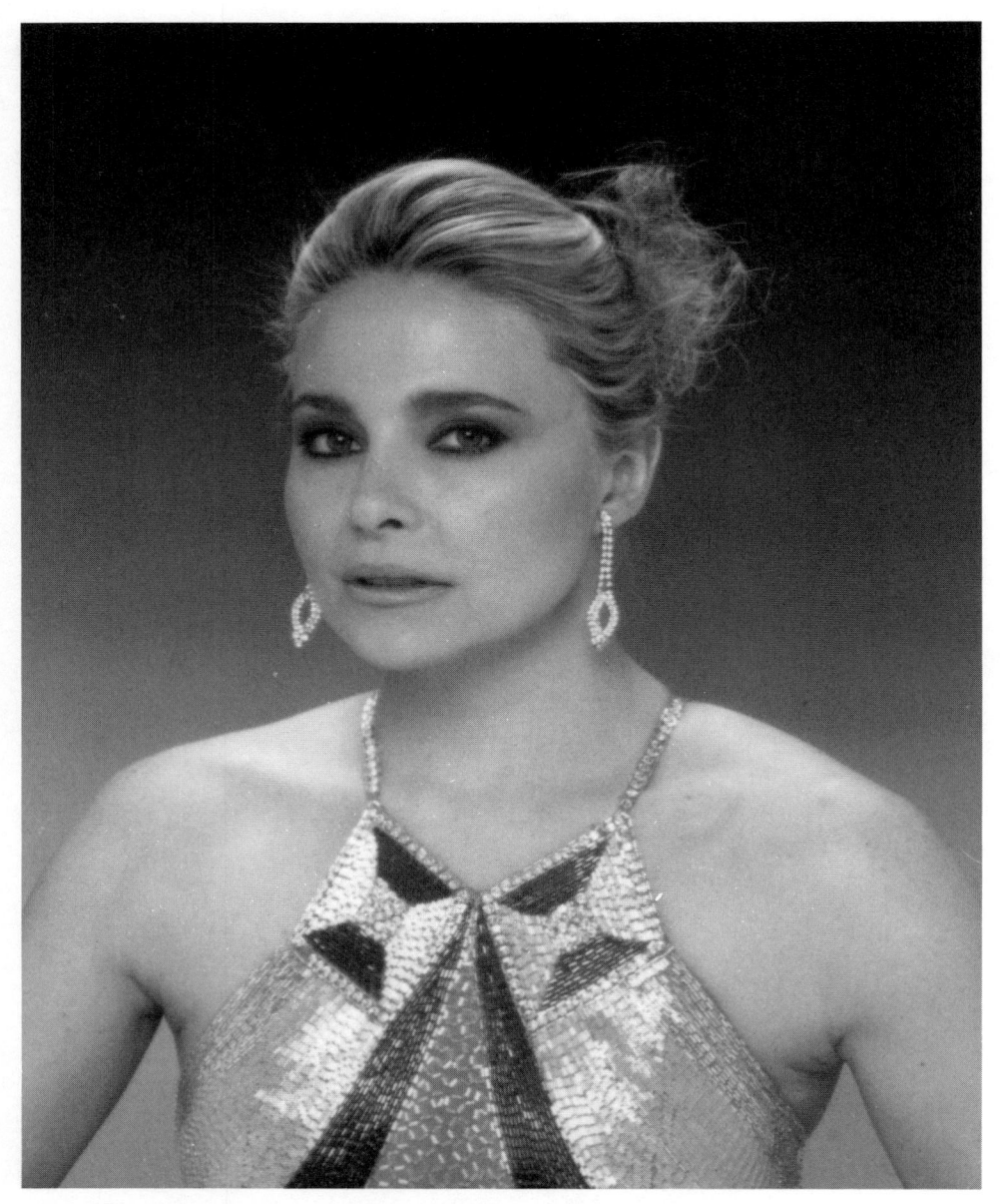

STYLE 2: Priscilla is lucky to have the kind of bone structure and features that allow her to wear this slick, severe hairstyle. Most people don't have the forehead, bone structure, or neck to wear a hairstyle like this. I added a synthetic hair ornament for color and to break the severity of the style. Beaded gown by Jeran Designs, Los Angeles.

Classic Beauties and Their Styles

BARBARA STOCK

Barbara is a striking brunette with smoldering good looks. She has that wonderful, coarse, curly hair that is very abundant, almost wild, but is kept looking right with the proper haircut and styling.

Barbara plays Susan Silverman in "Spenser: For Hire" and is actively pursuing a singing career. Her looks then must be very versatile, as she plays a high school guidance counselor in the series yet needs a different look for her glamorous singer image.

I layered Barbara's hair all over, layering it real short around the crown to keep it from looking too bushy. I suggested that she keep her hair at a collarbone length that allows her to wear it up or down.

TOVAR'S CLASSIC BEAUTY

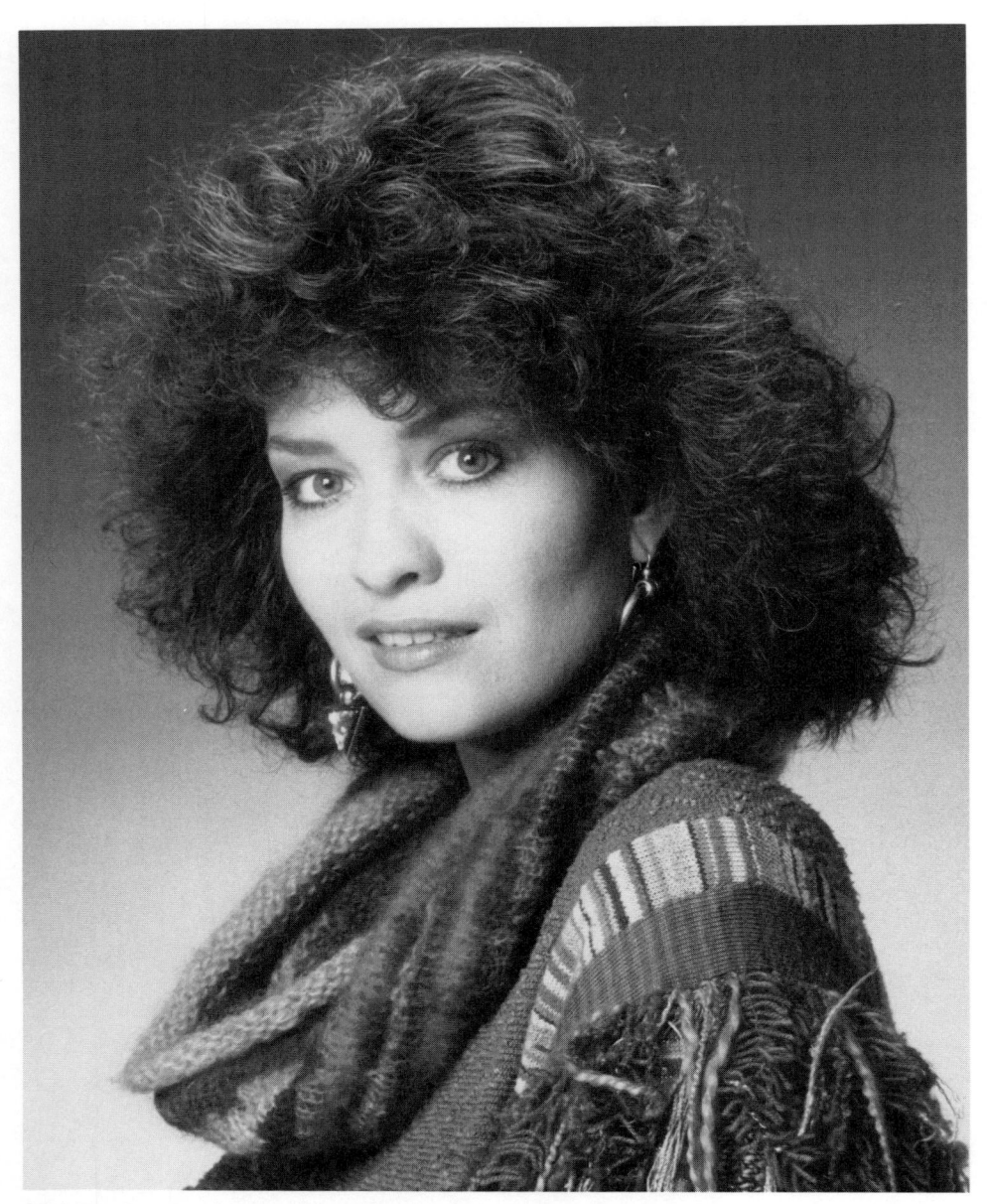

STYLE 1: Barbara wears her hair very close to its natural state. I just blew it dry to smooth out her own natural curl. Side-swept bangs balance her high forehead and long face. Costume by Margi Kent, Melrose Avenue, Los Angeles.

Classic Beauties and Their Styles

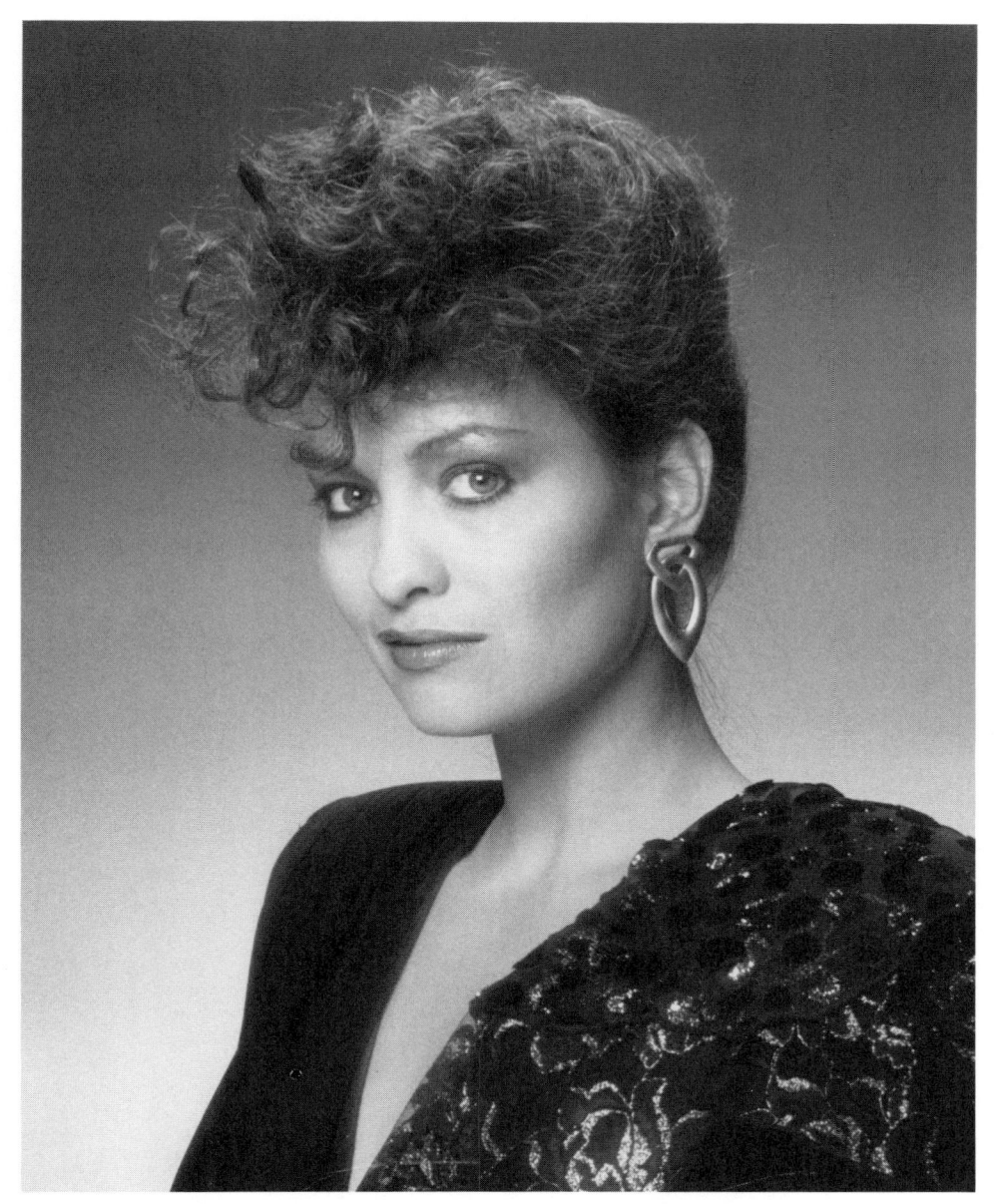

STYLE 2: The glamorous up-do adds a new dimension to Barbara's good looks. I slicked the side and back hair into a french twist, then brought the crown forward with the help of some gel in an arrangement of glossy curls. Dress by Margi Kent, Melrose Avenue, Los Angeles.

TANYA TUCKER

Tanya was my very first star, and I have changed her look many times. Although Tanya's hair used to look a lot wilder, I am trying to get my stars away from that "battered and damaged" look. Tanya's new look, which she is previewing on these pages, is a lot more controlled, still windblown but not wild—a look that has evolved with the times.

Tanya's hair is fine and hard to manage. I cut it in short layers around the crown for height and volume and longer at the sides. The longer sides are for versatility; this way Tanya can wear her hair up or down. A body perm and color highlights add still more volume to the hair.

Classic Beauties and Their Styles

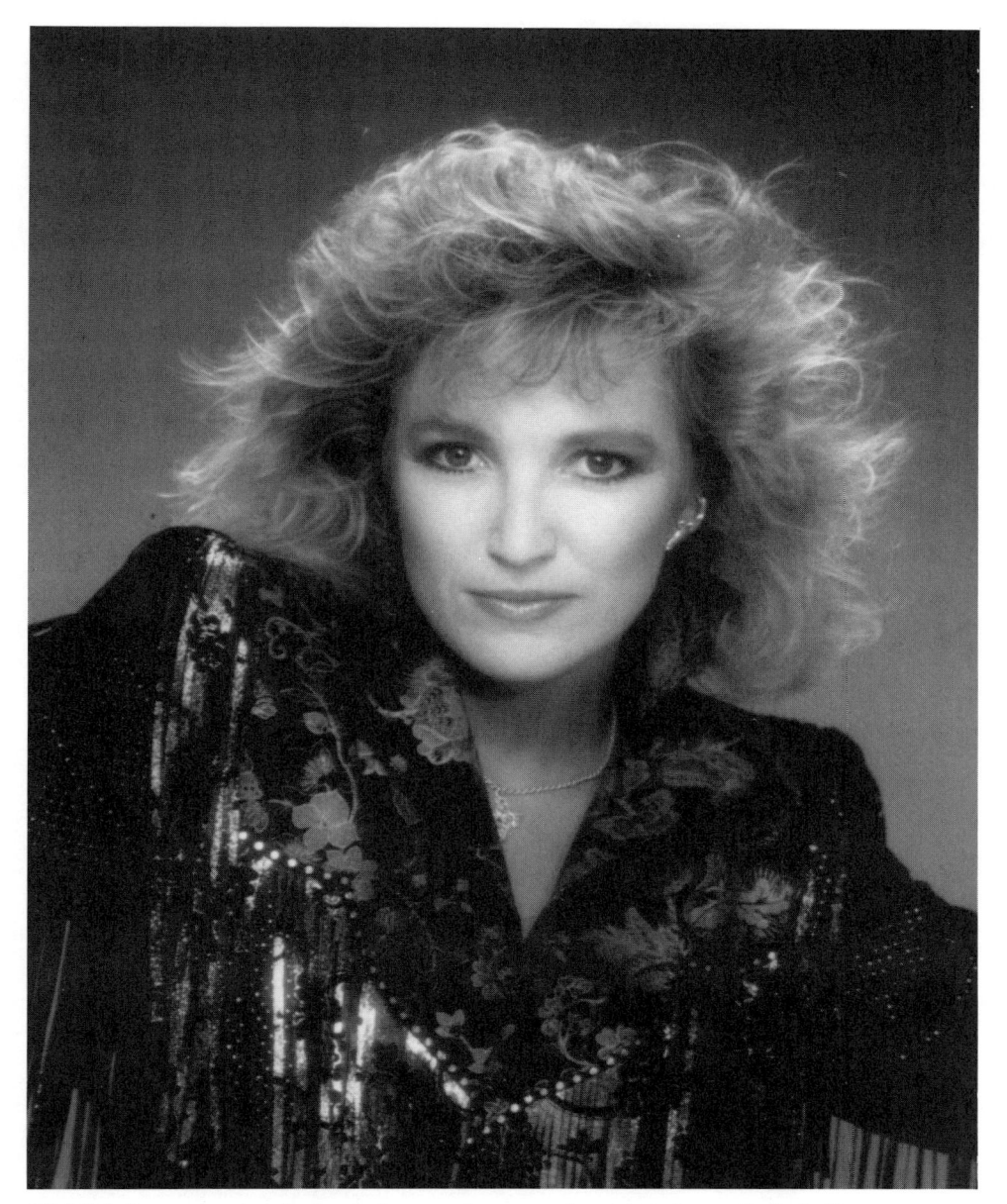

STYLE 1: Tanya's classic look: layered, scrunched, and gently full. Piecey bangs are brushed forward over the forehead to add softness to a very angular facial structure. Jacket by Gossamer Wings.

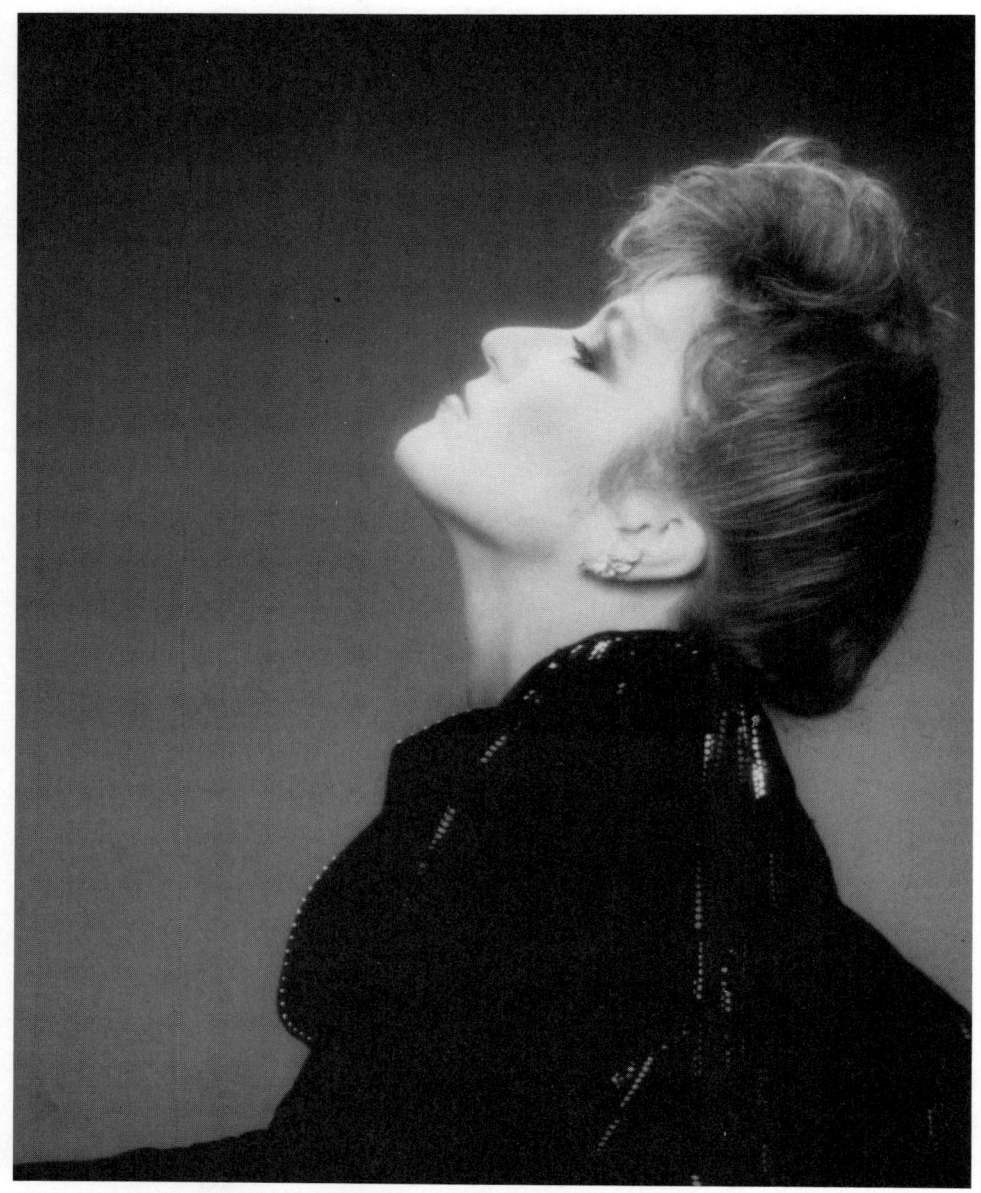

STYLE 2: The elegant, smooth, and sleek up-do. I gathered the side and back hair into a french twist. The crown is brought forward in tousled, airy waves. Bangs are open and very airy. Jacket by Gossamer Wings.

Classic Beauties and Their Styles

SYLVIA

This country-and-western singing star is one of my most famous makeovers. Sylvia used to wear her hair very long, down to her knees! And all this hair only covered up her beautiful features.

I cut Sylvia's hair into this soft, layered look that ends at the base of the neck. Quite a change from her superlong tresses, which made her look older than she was and plain.

Sylvia is really a very beautiful lady, and her contemporary hairstyle is more in keeping with her star image.

Her hairstyle is very full, swept back from the hairline with just a couple of strands left over the forehead to emphasize her pretty eyes. Fullness at the crown and sides balances Sylvia's square, angular face.

TOVAR'S CLASSIC BEAUTY

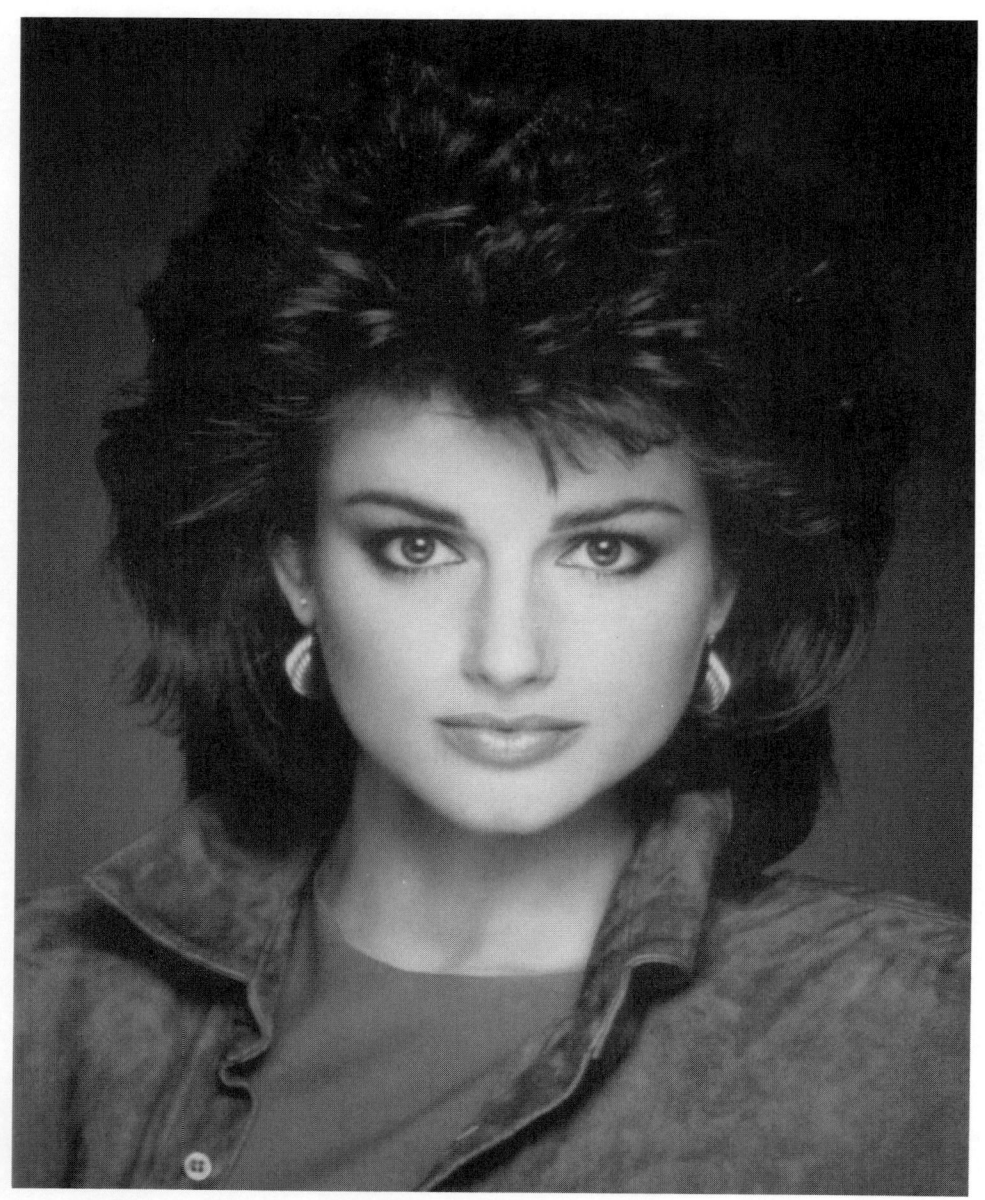

Sylvia's new trademark look calls for shoulder-length hair that is cut in layers to add volume to the crown and sides.

Classic Beauties and Their Styles

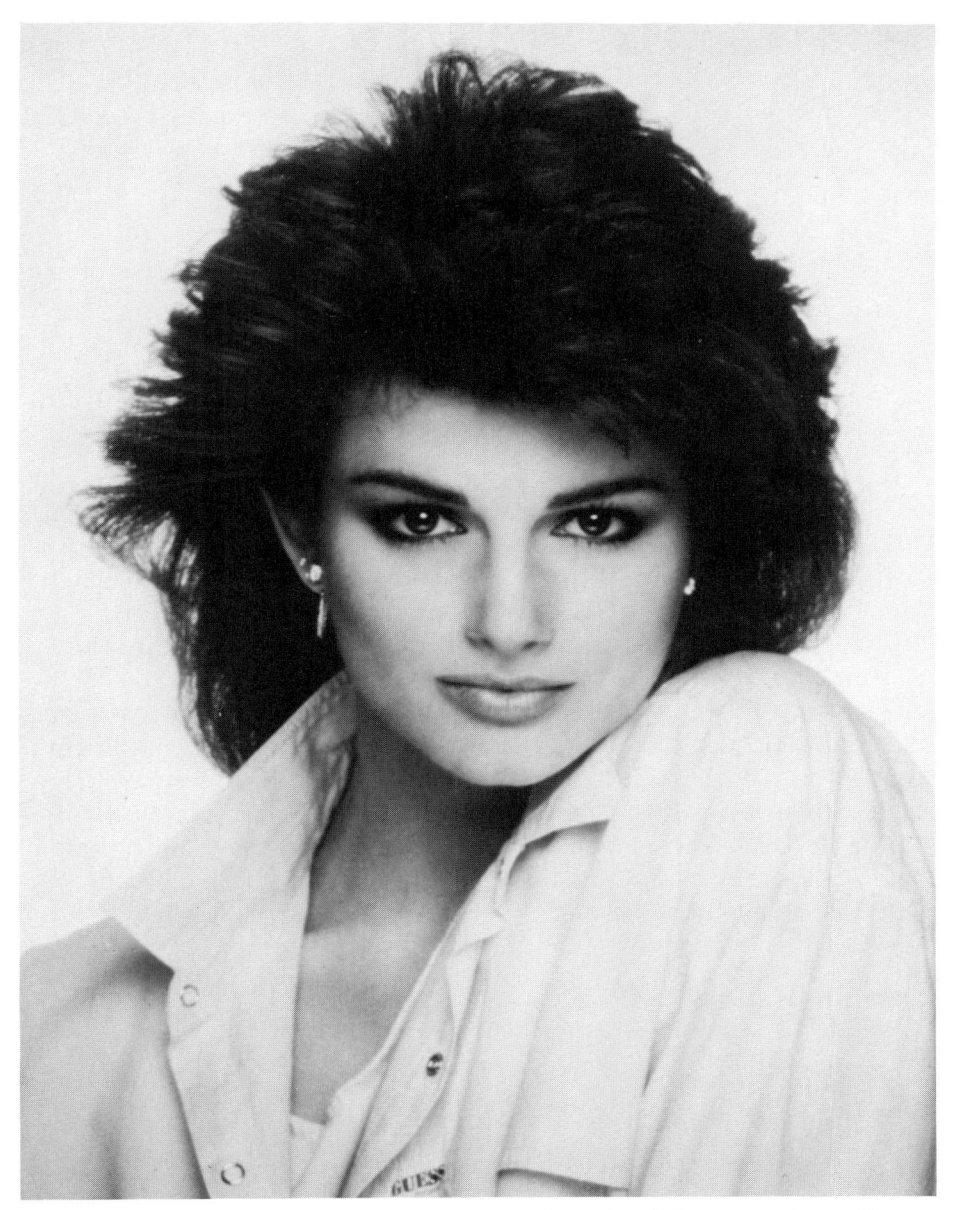

Sylvia's hair is blown dry and swept back for extra fullness and a soft, natural look.

TINA TURNER

She is a very strong lady who can carry off very, very severe looks. I was the first hairdresser ever to do Tina's hair. She had always done her own hair and makeup.

Now Tina is known for her outrageous hairdos. I designed her magnificent silver-blond wig for the video "We Don't Need Another Hero" from the film *Mad Max Beyond Thunderdome*.

Tina's latest hairstyle is a $3,000 silver platinum wig. Her own hair was shaved around the ears in a semicircular pattern. The wig is cut in steps—very short, almost sticking up at the top, graduating longer as it goes down toward the shoulders, ending at hip length.

Tina is unique—she is wild and outrageous but at the same time a classic. What other woman could wear this look? Tina is a champ, and she wears her hair like one!

Classic Beauties and Their Styles

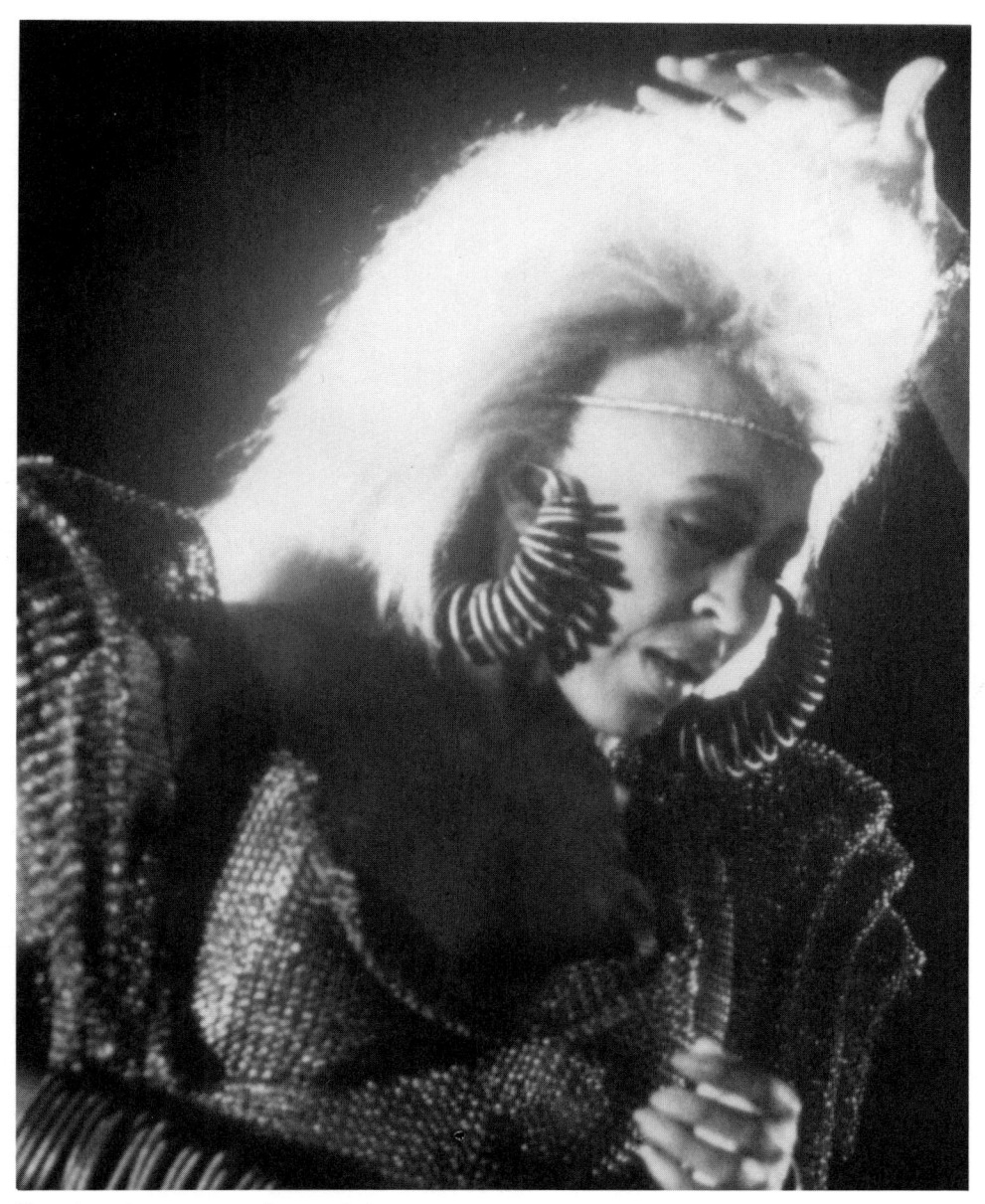

Tina has her own unique style.

DOLLY PARTON

She is one of the most beautiful, delicate women I have ever met. She is known for her cascade of soft blond curls, and she wears wigs because her own hair is too thin to be worn in her trademark hairstyle.

Dolly is wearing more different looks now than ever before, and her styles are getting less bouffant, simpler, and prettier. Dolly usually wears her own hair blended in the front for a natural-looking hairline.

Another classic beauty with a truly unique and very personal style, Dolly can wear the kind of look that shouts out STAR!

Classic Beauties and Their Styles

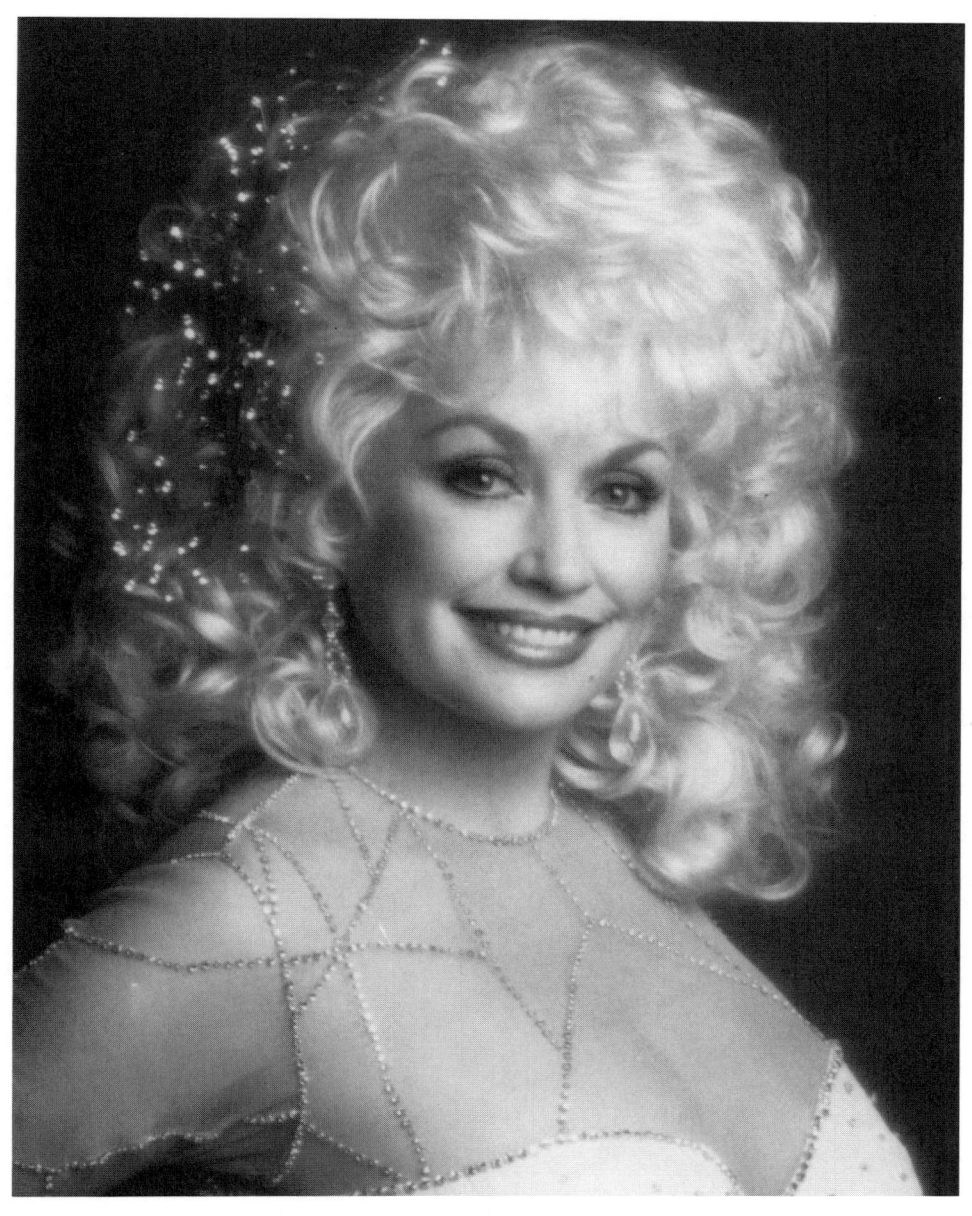

Dolly loves wearing different looks, and wigs give her this flexibility.

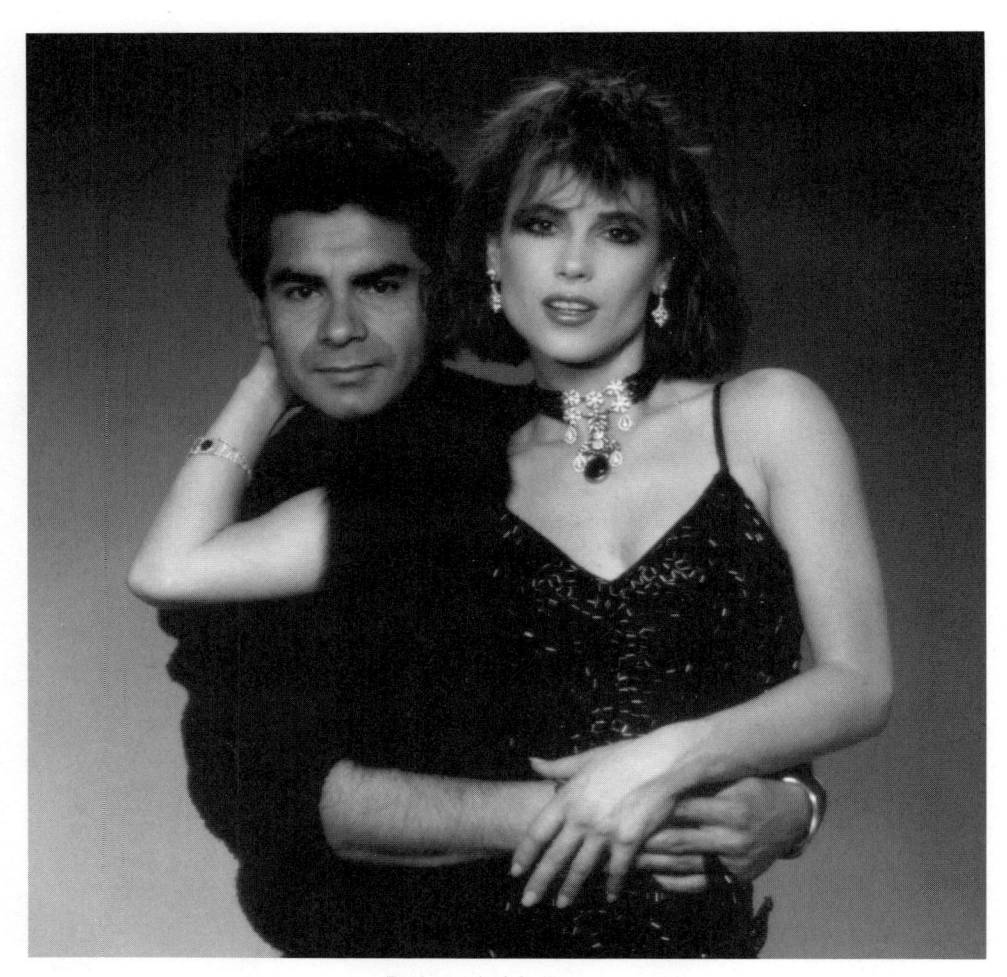

Deborah Mullowney

9
THE TOTAL LOOK

Now that you know what to do with your hair and face to make them look their best, let's go one step further to create the total look that will make you stand out, even in a crowd.

As I have said before, every woman has the potential to look great. Any woman can look 100 percent better if she learns how to achieve the total look. The total look is what makes all my star clients stand out—that special something sets them apart and makes them individual.

Although I am a hairstylist, most of the women who are my clients ask my advice when it comes to achieving the total look. Having a great hairstyle is only the beginning; the rest of the "ingredients" must combine to produce the best overall result. Makeup, skin, clothes, style, and everything else that must coordinate with the woman's looks, lifestyle, and personality must be taken into consideration.

The basic rule to follow when trying to accomplish all this is to accentuate the positive and minimize the negative. This method of achieving the total look is based on an ancient trick called *optical illusion*. Just as wearing your hair in a certain way can work wonders for your face, wearing the right makeup and clothes can give you the total image that is uniquely and beautifully yours. The success of the total look depends on how well you mix all these magic ingredients to create that *pièce de résistance*—the new you!

The first thing I tell a client when she comes to me for advice is to take every inch of her body into consideration. I tell her to do just as I do; take a good look at her whole body—her eyes, her mouth, her forehead, her neck, her weight, her height, and her lifestyle. I can do a spectacular head of hair, but if the client doesn't have the body to carry it, or if it doesn't fit into her lifestyle, the effect is wasted. She has to have the body proportions and lifestyle to carry off the look. Never wear a look just because it is trendy; wear it because it suits you well and ties into your total look.

Barbara Carrera is the perfect example of the total look—her hair, her face, and the way she dresses are in perfect balance. Barbara is the type of woman that will never look good in a short and curly hairstyle, wearing bermuda shorts and sneakers. She has a classic look, and she ties it all together with hairstyle, makeup, and dress. Barbara's look is also dramatic; she likes stylish fashions—magnificent collars, sleeve details, sweeping silhouettes, capes, and solid colors. Everything she wears projects that regal, dramatic look. Barbara is tall and carries herself with a regal attitude; her total look ties in everything perfectly for her.

Heather Locklear is just the opposite of Barbara—her look is very pretty, fresh, all-American. She is a beautiful girl, young and carefree. There is nothing dramatic or theatrical about Heather. She likes simple looks from hair to fashions. Though Heather is casual, she also can be elegantly so, as she looks in the black pinstriped gangster suit with the beaded lapels. Heather is petite and slender, and her look is scaled down to her delicate proportions.

Abby Dalton is a wonderful example of how great a mature woman can look. Abby looks magnificent from head to toe—from her sleek short hairstyle to the very distinctive, elegant clothes she wears. And Abby proves that mature doesn't have to mean dowdy—look at her in the soft, slinky red dress or the very dramatic silver gown!

I do believe that older women should wear shorter hair. Hair cut short can lift the face; long hair can tend to drag everything down. And the older you get, the shorter your hair can be, but be sure to leave some softness around the neckline to create a look that is not too extreme.

These three women and all the other stars photographed for this book have combined a number of fashion and beauty rules to create their total look. So when you see your favorite star looking stunning, you can be sure that it just didn't happen. Her style and her look are based on a number of proven tricks that her fashion and beauty advisors have given her. These tricks are as much a part of her image as the color of her hair and the shape of her body.

The Total Look

FIGURE TYPE

The first step in learning how to apply these tricks is determining your figure type. To do this, follow the same basic principles you used to determine your hair type. Like any type of self-analysis, honesty is the most direct and successful approach. That honesty will make it possible for you to stand in front of a mirror and see your reflection as it really is.

To find out your figure type, stand in front of a full-length mirror (a three-way mirror is even better because it will allow you to see yourself in profile and from behind). Wear as few clothes as possible—a leotard, a swimsuit, or your bra and panties—to bare as much as possible and come up with a true appraisal.

First determine whether you are thin, average, or plump. Then identify your height as petite, average, or tall. Study your figure carefully: Do you have a delicate bone structure? Are you large-boned and angular? Are you softly rounded and all curves? Do you have a pretty neck? a large bosom? large hips? Are you small-waisted?

Once you determine your particular proportions, faults, and attributes, make note of them. Then use some of the following fashion tricks, which will help you create the optical illusion that flatters you most.

Petite

Petite women are short and have a small, delicate bone structure. Petite types range from the boyishly thin to the voluptuous. The basic fashion rule for you if you are petite is to wear everything scaled down to your size. The thinner you are, the smaller the proportions; the more voluptuous types can get away with slightly larger proportions.

If you are of average weight, you can wear almost any fashion style as long as it is scaled down to your size. Avoid anything too dainty, too childish, or too small. The effect you want to achieve is elegant and fashionable, not that of a woman of indeterminate age.

Those of you who are thin are lucky because you can wear a number of fashion looks and pay a fraction of the usual cost for them. Today's preteen, junior, and big boys' fashions are as sophisticated as the adult versions, and with your proportions you can buy clothes in these departments.

If you are plump, you can accentuate your voluptuousness, but look for clothes that fit impeccably and are perfectly proportioned. Avoid anything too tenty or boxy.

The key factor for successful petite dressing is fit. Most small women have fitting problems in the shoulders, neckline, sleeve, and skirt length. Investing in alterations is essential. Petite women should avoid anything oversize—from clothes to fashion details like collar, pockets, trims, and prints to accessories.

Average

The average woman is of medium height and ranges from the perfectly proportioned to the thinner or heavier groups. Women in this group have the most fashion freedom. Follow the guidelines that apply to the weight category you fall within.

If you are of average height and weight, you are the closest of all women to having a perfect figure. Whatever your fashion style, you will look great in almost anything, and your fashion selection will have more to do with what you like than with what you can or can't wear.

If you are of average height but are thin, you have one of the most elegant and graceful figure types. When selecting clothes, keep in mind that you will look best in all the classic styles with impeccable lines.

If you are plump, you can look very voluptuous if you are not too overweight, or you can look like a much taller person if you have a large frame. If this is your figure type, be sure to select fashions that emphasize your positive points. You will look best in all types of classic fashions—pleated, bias, or gathered skirts, blazer jackets, and trousers. Best accessories are neat and simple. Avoid extreme or costumey looks, unless you are very exotic-looking.

Tall

Tall women fall into three categories: you're the model type, if you are thin; stately, if your weight is average; and statuesque, if you are on the plump side. If this is the group you belong to, you are lucky. Yours is the type of build that can hide a million faults. Of the three basic types, tall women have the greatest fashion freedom.

The model type is a fashion designer's dream. You can wear practically anything and everything. You look great in the newest fashion styles as well as in the classics; selection depends on your personal style.

The Total Look

The stately type is tall and graceful, and wears clothes very well. Take full advantage of your size and wear all those great fashion silhouettes that make the most of your height and shape. Showstopping accessories were also just made for you.

The statuesque type also can look great, if she is not too overweight. Do everything to emphasize your height, from walking tall to wearing clothes that call attention to it.

If you're tall, you will look great in dramatic and sweeping silhouettes like capes, swing skirts, and flared clothes. You also can wear longer skirt lengths, large plaids, bold stripes, and all kinds of oversized looks that would overpower your shorter sisters. Stay away from anything small, dainty, and frilly, and from very high heels that can make you look awkward.

HEAD TO TOE FIGURE FLATTERY

Now that you know the general guidelines, let's learn about emphasizing or hiding specific areas to complete this crash course in dressing to flatter your figure. While the following tips are not extensive enough to give you all the dos and don'ts about fashion, they will provide you with some basic guidelines for pulling together a total look.

Short Neck

Do wear . . .

open collars; V-necks, scoop or U-necklines; long necklaces and pendants; and small earrings.

Don't wear . . .

turtlenecks, cowls, or other high collars; blouses with ties or bows at the neck; chokers, multistrand necklaces, and dangling earrings.

Long Neck

Do wear . . .

turtlenecks, cowls, ruffles, lace collars; button-down shirts with ties; dramatic choker necklaces; ropes of pearls; and scarves knotted around the neck.

Don't wear...

small round collars, Peter Pan collars, square or scoop necklines, long necklaces, and pendants.

Broad Shoulders

Do wear...

halter necklines; raglan, dolman, or dropped shoulder sleeves; strapless tops; full skirts to balance the width at the top; full silhouettes on top.

Don't wear...

padded shoulders or any styles that emphasize the area; square necklines or collars; broad, horizontal stripes across the top; and big on top, narrow at the bottom silhouettes.

Narrow Shoulders

Do wear...

shoulder pads, puffed sleeves, set-in sleeves; necklines with horizontal lines to create the illusion of width at the top; light on top, dark at the bottom combinations.

Don't wear...

body-hugging tops, oversize blouses that droop at the shoulders; jackets and coats with too much fullness at the top.

Large Bust

Do wear...

loose-fitting cardigan jackets; Chanel jackets; classic shirts; V-necks, cowl necks, and open collars; and most important, the best fitting bra you can find.

The Total Look

Don't wear...

tight-fitting sweaters, tube tops, clingy knits; blouses with lots of ruffles, gathers, and tucks in front; horizontal stripes and large prints; and very tight belts.

Small Bust

Do wear...

jackets with padded shoulders, wrap fronts, ruffles in front; blousy tops and layered looks; horizontal stripes; and light colors.

Don't wear...

anything tight-fitting, such as sweaters, camisoles, or leotard tops; very full skirts with skinny tops; vertical lines; very loose-fitting dresses.

Small Waist

Do wear...

anything that emphasizes your waist; good-looking belts and other accessories at the waist.

Don't wear...

blouson tops, tunics, or bulky sweaters that hide the waist; shapeless or straight dresses, boxy jackets, and layered looks.

Thick Waist

Do wear...

blouson tops, overblouses, tunics, and other silhouettes that cover the waist; also dropped-waist dresses and skirts; elastic waists.

Don't wear...

tight dresses, nipped-in waistlines, tops tucked into skirt or pants; skirts or pants with too much gathering at the waist; elaborate belts.

Small Hips

Do wear...

dresses with a gathered waistline, full skirt, or patch pockets at hip; unpressed pleats; circle, dirndl or tiered skirts; loose-fitting trousers, baggy pants, or culottes; peplum skirts or oversized, belted tops.

Don't wear...

tight-fitting clothes; stretch fabrics that hug the body like a second skin; hip-hugger pants.

Large Hips

Do wear...

A-line skirts, wrap skirts, and flared skirts; tunics, long jackets, and vests that cover the hips; jewelry, scarves, and accessories to bring the eyes away from the hip area.

Don't wear...

large prints, bold plaids, horizontal stripes, heavy fabrics like wide-wale corduroy or loopy wools; clingy fabrics and stretch clothes; divided skirts and shorts.

The Total Look

This book is based on my philosophies of beauty and style, my belief that each and every woman has the makings of a classic beauty in her.

As you can see, the models in my book cover a wide range of styles. Their total look is comprised of the right hairstyle, makeup, and dress, all of which fit a particular lifestyle. By taking the time to carefully assess your beauty assets, you, too, can make the most of them by applying the tips and techniques I have shared with you. Work with your chosen hairstylist and use this book to help you look the best you have ever looked in your life!

INDEX

Aldridge, Sheila, 115–19
Anderson, Melody, 17, 201–3
Austin, Teri, 66, 151–53
Barnes, Priscilla, 61, 210–12
Bry, Ellen, 17, 61, 164–66
Carrera, Barbara, 4, 7–8, 23, 31, 46, 61, 143–47
Chao, Rosalind, 17, 60, 207–9
Dalton, Abby, 23, 60, 61, 198–200
Dennison, Rachel, 13, 14
Gray, Erin, 31, 37, 46, 158–60
Green, Joan, 24–25
Henson, Nastassia, 68–69
Harris, Emmylou, 11, 13, 22, 61, 180–82
Herrera, Veronica, 100–101
Heston, Marilyn, 24–25
Hickland, Catherine, 18, 170–72
Hubley, Season, 43, 46, 189–91
Jannick, Susan, 26–27
Jenner, Linda Thompson, 148–50
Klous, Patricia, 154–57

Kennedy, Jayne. *See* Overton, Jayne Kennedy
Lane, Brogan, 30, 40, 41, 49, 61, 183–85
Locklear, Heather, 8–9, 31, 49, 60, 186–88
Madame, 9–10
Mullowney, Deborah, 23, 56, 60, 125, 204–6, 226
Overton, Jayne Kennedy, 17, 31, 47, 49, 61, 142, 195–97
Pappas, Jessica Norman, 62–65, 99, 102–6
Parton, Dolly, 13, 21, 46, 224–25
Peeples, Nia, 177–79
Persson, Alana, 75–77
Persson, Gunilla, 107–14
Phillips, Chynna, 127–31
Richter, Debi, 17, 38, 61, 167–69
Roker, Roxie, 47, 48, 49, 61, 161–63
Song, Tamela, 132–35
Sterret, Shelley, 95–97

Stock, Barbara, 23, 213–15
Sylvia, 15, 20, 22, 82, 219–21
Thompson, Linda. *See* Jenner, Linda Thompson
Tucker, Tanya, 12–13, 22, 84, 216–18
Turner, Tina, 9, 46, 222–23
Uranga, Rima, 138–41
Van Kamp, Merete, 17, 23, 35, 49, 60, 122, 173–76
Van Kleist, Wanda, 86–89
Weintraub, Jane Morgan, 28–29, 84
Yarlett, Claire, 31, 61, 192–94